NEUROPLASTICITY

and its

DARK SIDES:

I0481475

Disorders of the Nervous System
Second Edition

by

Aage R. Møller, PhD (DMedSci)

The University of Texas at Dallas
Richardson, TX

Aage R. Møller Publishing, 2018

Neuroplasticity and its Dark Sides: Disorders of the Nervous System
By Aage R. Møller, Ph.D. (D. Med. Sci.)
School of Behavioral and Brain Sciences,
The University of Texas at Dallas
800 W. Campbell Road
Richardson, TX 75080
Front cover: Artwork by Zahra Akhavi.

Dr. AAGE R. MØLLER is a Distinguished Lecturer in Behavioral and Brain Sciences, and he is the Founders Professor of The University of Texas at Dallas.

Dr. Møller has a cand. med. degree, followed by a dr. med. degree (Doctor of Medical Sciences), all from the Karolinska Institut, (School of Medicine), Stockholm, Sweden. He was on the faculty of the Karolinska Institut for 12 years, on the faculty of the University of Pittsburgh School of Medicine for 19 years, first as Associate Professor of Otolaryngology, and later as Tenured Professor of Neurological Surgery. For the last 20 years, he is Professor of Cognition and Neuroscience at The University of Texas School of Behavioral and Brain Sciences, and he is the holder of the Founders Endowed Chair. He is the author of 17 professional books, author of more than 200 articles in peer-reviewed journals, more than 100 chapters in clinical and neuroscience books. He is the editor or co-editor of 9 professional books, the founder of an international journal, Hearing Research, published by Elsevier. He was the Journal's Editor-in-Chief for 27 years.

Now he teaches in the Neuroscience Program of The University of Texas at Dallas School of Behavioral and Brain Sciences. He teaches courses on "Biology of Pain," "Human Functional Neuroanatomy," "Sensory Physiology," "Neural Plasticity and Disorders of the Nervous System," "Intraoperative Neurophysiologic Monitoring, Part I and II" and "Neuroscience of Fear and Anxiety."

ISBN-13: 9781981464906
ISBN-10: 1981464905

© Aage R. Møller, Publishing, 2018

Table of Contents

Acknowledgements

I had many valuable comments and suggestions from Dr. Klaus Truemper. Jeff Cai and Savo Rujak helped with the cover.

I would not have been able to write this book without the support of the School of Behavioral and Brain Sciences at the University of Texas at Dallas.

Dallas, December 2017

Aage R. Møller, Ph.D. (D. Med. Sci).

Other recently published books by this author:

Møller, A.R. "A new Epidemic: Harm in Health Care. – How to make rational decisions about Medical and Surgical Treatment" Nova Publishers, New York, 286 pages, 2007.

Møller, A.R. "The Malleable Brain." Nova Publishers, New York, 2009

Møller, A.R. "Intraoperative Neurophysiologic Monitoring, Intraoperative Neurophysiology" 3rd Edition, Springer, New York, 403 pages, 2010, ISBN-13: 978-1441974358

Møller, A.R. "Hearing: Anatomy, physiology, and disorders of the auditory system," 3rd Edition, 415 pages. Plural Publishing, Inc. 2012. ISBN-13: 978-1-59756-427-4, ISBN-10: 1-59756-427-3.

Møller, A.R "Sensory Systems," 2nd Edition. Aage R. Møller Publishing, Dallas 2012. 417 pages, July. 2012. ISBN-13: 978-1478175872, ISBN-10: 1478175877.

Møller, A.R. "Pain: Its Anatomy, Physiology, and Treatment," Aage R. Møller Publishing, 2011, 364 pages; 2nd Ed. 2014, 403 pages, ISBN-10: 1466395109 | ISBN-13: 978-1466395107

Preface

This book "Neuroplasticity and its Dark Sides: Disorders of the Nervous System" covers the basis for neuroplasticity and it stresses some less well-known aspects of neuroplasticity. While activation of neuroplasticity is important for learning new skills, and adapting to changing demands it can also create symptoms and signs of common and widespread diseases such as chronic neuropathic pain and severe tinnitus. Spasticity and some forms of spasm are also caused by such *maladaptive* neuroplasticity. Recently it was found that activation of neuroplasticity is also a contributing factor together with stress and inflammation in several other diseases such as some forms of muscle spasm and probably also fibromyalgia and the chronic fatigue syndrome. In this book, we will use the term *plasticity disorder* to describe diseases where the symptoms and signs are caused by activation of neuroplasticity.

Understanding these dark sides of neuroplasticity is important for treatment of many common disorders. For example, reversing maladaptive neuroplasticity would be an ideal treatment of some common disorders such as chronic neuropathic pain, some forms of tinnitus and spasticity, and probably also diseases such as fibromyalgia and the chronic fatigue disease if it could be done effectively and with little adverse side effects.

The book discusses the ability to change the efficacy of synapses and change in protein synthesis are discussed in detail.

The book also discusses another less well-understood property of neuroplasticity, namely that not all brain systems are plastic. The fact that attempts to change sexual preferences have been unsuccessful indicates that the function of some neural circuits in the brain cannot be changed or are difficult to change, which means that some circuits are "hard-wired." Other examples of functions that are difficult to change are some forms of handedness. The personality of a person is difficult to change indicating that some very complex circuitry in the brain may be less plastic than normally assumed.

Long-term memory is another example of brain circuits that are difficult to change. Failed success in the treatment of the posttraumatic stress syndrome (PTSD) shows that some memory functions are difficult to change. Hard-wires neural circuits are also involved in the symptoms that are apparent in addiction.

The action of neuroplasticity can change the strength of functional connections in many parts of the brain and the spinal cord. The role of connectivity and changes in the strength of connections in the brain now emerges as important factors in many neural diseases, and it is involved in the changes in the function of the nervous system that occurs with aging.

Understanding the basis for neuroplasticity can benefit diagnosis and treatment of many disorders of the nervous system. The results of basic neuroscience studies of neuroplasticity are fundamental for the understanding the normal as well as many forms of abnormal function of the central nervous system. This book promotes the use of knowledge about neuroplasticity in diagnosis and treatment of disorders of the nervous system.

The book is a revision of a book with the same title, and it is based on an earlier book, Aage R. Møller: "Neural Plasticity and Disorders of the Nervous System" published by Cambridge University Press, 2006.

The book has four sections:

The first section, "Basics about neuroplasticity" provides an overview of the role of the expression of neuroplasticity and the physiological and anatomical basis for the expression of neuroplasticity and it discusses the role of expression of neuroplasticity in the creation of some neurological disorders.

The second section "Beneficial effects of activation of neuroplasticity" has chapters on adaptation to changing demands and recovery from injuries and postnatal development. It also discusses matters related to the immune system, in particular, the interactive immune system that is affected by prior exposure to pathogens, which change its response, thus a form of adaptation to environmental demands.

The third section, "Harmful effects of plastic changes *Plasticity Disorders* " has chapters on central neuropathic pain, tinnitus and movement disorders such as spasm and spasticity. It discusses the different symptoms and signs that are caused by the expression of neuroplasticity.

The section briefly discusses other aspects of the central nervous system where great advances have been made recently, such as those related to the immune system. The adaptive immune system is also plastic and can change its function in response to the way it has been activated. This section also has a chapter on the treatment of plasticity disorders.

The fourth section "Common disorders of the sensory and motor systems" discusses disorders of the nervous system where activation of neuroplasticity may play a role in generating the symptoms and signs.

Appendices A, B, C and D cover anatomy and physiology of nerves, the organization and function of sensory systems, the neuroscience of pain and the anatomy and physiology of motor systems.

Abbreviations

5-HT: serotonin

A1: Primary auditory cortex

ABR: Auditory brainstem responses

ALS: Amyotrophic lateral sclerosis

AMPA: -amino-3-hydroxy-5-methyl-4-isoxazolepropionic acid

AP: Action potential

BDNF: Brain derived neurotrophic factor,

BK: Bradykinin

BPPV: Benign paroxysmal positional vertigo

CAD: Glutamic acid decarboxylase

CBD: Cannabidiol

CCK: Cholecystokinin

CGRP: calcitonin gene-related peptide,

CM: Centromedian (nucleus of thalamus)

CMAP: Compound muscle action potentials

CMT-I Charot-Marie-Tooth

CN: Cranial nerve

CNS: Central nervous system

CPG: Central pattern generator

CRPS I: Complex regional pain syndrome type I

CRPS II: Complex regional pain syndrome type II

DBS: Deep brain (electrical) stimulation

DLPT: Dorsolateral pontomesencephalic tegmentum

DPV: Disabling positional vertigo

DREZ: dorsal root entry zone

DRG: Dorsal root ganglia

EMG: Electromyography

EP: Epinephrine

EPSP: Excitatory post synaptic potentials

FRA: Flexor reflex afferents

GABA: Gamma aminobutyric acid

GBS: Guillian-Barre Syndrome

Gly: glycine

GPe: Globus pallidus external part

GPi: Globus pallidus internal part

GPN: glossopharyngeal neuralgia

H+: proton

HD: Huntington's disease

HFS: Hemifacial spasm

HMSN-I Hereditary motor sensory neuropathies

HTM: High threshold mechanoreceptors

IASP: International Association for the Study of Pain.

IC: Inferior colliculus

ICC: Central nucleus of the IC

IPS: Intraparietal sulcus

LGN: Lateral geniculate nucleus

LGP: Lateral segment of pallidus

LTM: Low threshold mechanoreceptors

LTR: Local twitch response

MGB: Medial geniculate body

MGP: Medial segment of globus pallidus

MI: Primary motor cortex

MLF: Medial longitudinal fasciculus

MLR: Middle latency responses

MPTP: Methylphenyltetrahydropyridine

MS: Multiple sclerosis

MSA: Multiple system atrophy

MVD: Microvascular decompression

NA: Noradrenaline (Norepinephrine)

NE: norepinephrine

NIHL: Noise induced hearing loss

NMDA: N-methyl-D-aspartate

NST: Nucleus of the solitary tract

PAG: Periaqueductal gray

PD: Parkinson's disease

PF: Prefrontal (cortex)

PMA: Premotor (cortical) areas

PTS: Permanent threshold shift

RBD: Rapid eye movement sleep behavior disorder

REM: Rapid eye movement (sleep)

REZ: Root entry (exit) zone

RPC: Reticularis pontis caudalis

RSD: Reflex sympathetic dystrophy

RVM: Rostral ventromedial medulla

SC: Superior colliculus

SCI: Spinal cord injuries

SDR: Selective dorsal root rhizotomy

SG: Sympathetic ganglion

SI: Primary somatosensory cortex

SII: Secondary somatosensory cortex

SMA: Supplementary motor areas

SMP: Sympathetic maintained pain

SNc: Substantia nigra pars compacta

SNr: Substantia nigra pars reticulata

SOC: Superior olivary complex

SP: Substance P

SSRI: Selective serotonin re-uptake inhibitor

STN: Subthalamic nucleus

STT: Spinothalamic tract

TENS: Transdermal electric nerve stim.

TGN: Trigeminal neuralgia

THC: delta-9-tetrahydrocanabidiol

TIA: Transient ischemic attack

TMJ: Temporomandibular joint

TRT: Tinnitus retraining therapy

TTS: Temporary threshold shift

V1: Primary visual cortex (striate cortex)

V2-5: Extrastriate visual cortices

VB: Ventrobasal nuclei (of thalamus)

Vim: Ventral intermediary nucleus (of the thalamus)

VLL: Ventral nucleus of the lateral lemniscus

VLo: Ventralis lateralis pars oralis

VMpo: Ventromedial posterior oralis (nuclei of thalamus)

VOR: Vestibular ocular reflex

VPI: Ventral posterior inferior (nuclei of thalamus)

VPL: Ventral posterior lateral (nuclei of thalamus)

VPM: Ventral medial (thalamic) nucleus

WBS: Williams-Beuren Syndrome

WDR: Wide dynamic range (neurons)

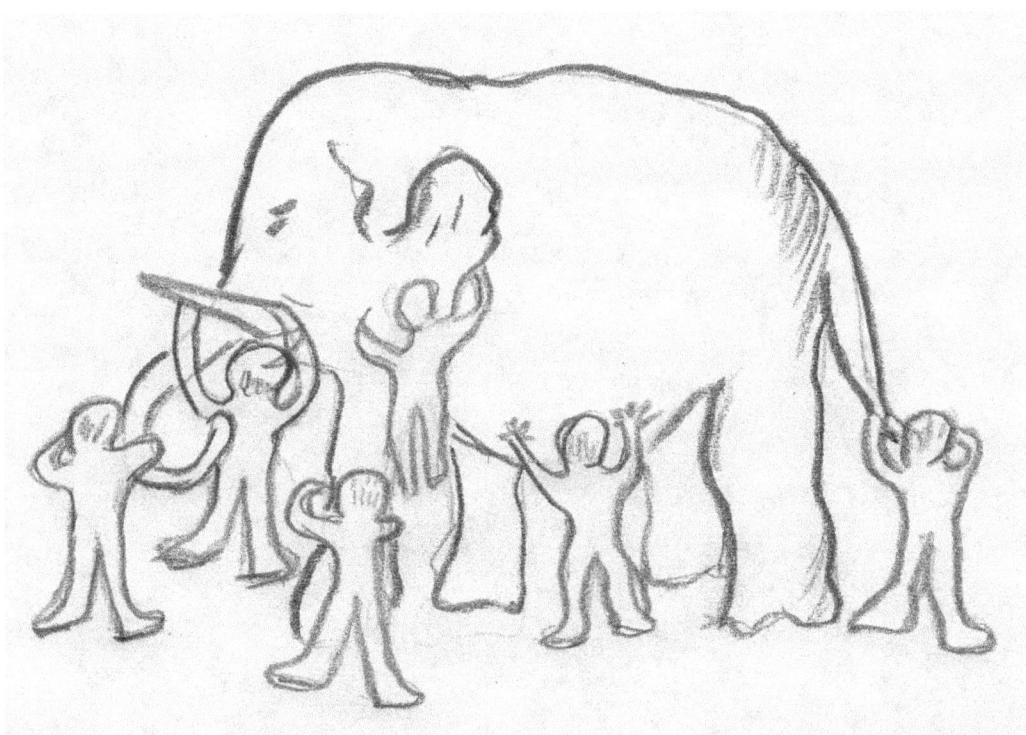

People with different interest and background may view properties such as neuroplasticity in a variety of ways. It is almost like the old story from India about the six blind men and the elephant (created as a poem by John Godfrey Saxe. (Artwork by Zahra Akhavi).

They all came to different results from their examination. "A wall!" "A snake!" "A spear!" "A tree!" "A fan!" "A rope!" They told the prince: "We are sorry. But we cannot agree on what an elephant is like. We each touched the same animal. But to each of us, the animal is completely different." The prince spoke gently, "The elephant is a very large animal. Its side is like a wall. Its trunk is like a snake. Its tusks are like spears. Its legs are like trees. Its ears are like fans. And its tail is like a rope. So you are all right. But you are all wrong, too. For each of you touched only one part of the animal. To know what an elephant is like, you must put all those parts together."

Section 1
Basics of Neuroplasticity

Neuroplasticity is just one of many fascinating functions of the brain. Other complex and important brain functions are the memory functions and the capacity to process a large amount of data. Neuroplasticity is responsible for memory, learning new skills and re-routing information after damage to the nervous system. Neuroplasticity is of vital importance for the development of the brain into a highly organized network of nerve cells, for learning new skills and restructuring and re-routing information.

The existence of neuroplasticity means that parts of the nervous system are not hardwired and that many functions of the central nervous system are not static. There are, however, some features that are difficult to change indicating that some circuits in the brain and the spinal cord cannot be changed or are hard to change. Examples are sexual preferences, some forms of handedness, long-term memory and personality.

The ability of the nervous system to change its functions is mainly based on the ability of synapses to change their efficacy. Synaptic plasticity is a key feature of neuroplasticity that controls neural connectivity by external as well as internal experience [112].

Neuroplasticity has been studied extensively in the sensory cortex, and Weinberger calls it "physiological memory" [36].

Anatomical connections in the brain and the spinal cord are only functional if the synapses that connect the axons of the pathways to their target cells can be activated by the activity that arrives at the synapses in question. The functionality of connections, therefore, depends on the efficacy of the synapse that connects an axon to its target cell.

Changes in synaptic efficacy can open and close connections in the brain and the spinal cord and thereby alter functional connections without changes in the neuroanatomy of the connections.

The strength of functional connections is related to the efficacy of the synapses that connect the axons to their target cells. That means that activation of neuroplasticity can control functional connections in the brain and the spinal cord. Connections in the central nervous system (brain and the spinal cord) and their strength are now the subjects of extensive studies and a new specialty, "connectivity" has developed in the field of neuroscience [190].

Activation of neuroplasticity also involves a change in the synthesis of proteins in nerve cells is a part of some forms of plastic changes [623]. Long-term potentiation (LTP) and long-term depression (LTD), which is associated with many functions of the brain, especially memory, are also involved in changes in function that occur as a result of activation of neuroplasticity.

In this section, Chapter 1 describes the basic properties of neuroplasticity highlighting the beneficial aspects of neuroplasticity in the central nervous system and its role in learning new skills and memory and for re-routing information after trauma. Chapter 1 also covers the role that activation of neuroplasticity plays in many diseases such as chronic neuropathic pain, severe forms of tinnitus and for creating the symptoms of spasticity and some forms of muscle spasm. Chapter 2 describes the anatomical and physiological basis for neuroplasticity. These topics are further explored in the chapters that follow.

What is Neuroplasticity?

Abstract

1. Neuroplasticity is a property of some parts of the central nervous system; it only becomes evident when activated.

2. Activation of neuroplasticity can alter connections (change connectivity) in the brain and the spinal cord by changing the efficacy of the synapses that connect an axon to its target cell.

3. Activation of neuroplasticity can control "connectivity" by changing the strength of connections through changes in synaptic efficacy.

4. Expression of neuroplasticity is necessary for normal postnatal development, and it plays a role in compensating for age-related changes; it is necessary for learning new skills and for adapting to changing demands.

5. External events, such as deprivation of sensory input, changes in demands, novel sensory stimulation, overstimulation, can induce expression of neuroplasticity. Physical or mental training can also activate neuroplasticity.

6. Internal events, such as the activity in neural structures and insults to nerves and the central nervous system structures, can cause expression of neuroplasticity.

7. Some functions are easy to change while others are difficult to change; some functions cannot be changed at all through neuroplasticity (hard-wired).

8. Examples of hard-to-change functions are sexual preference, personalities, long-term memory and some forms of handedness.

9. Plastic changes occur more easily and are more extensive during early postnatal development (critical period), but plastic changes can also be induced in the adult nervous system.

10. Expression of neuroplasticity can have beneficial effects, and it can have harmful effects and cause symptoms of disease ("Plasticity disorders").

11. Symptoms and signs of disorders that are caused by expression of "maladaptive" neuroplasticity are the phantom limb syndrome, chronic neuropathic pain, tinnitus, and different kinds of hyperactive motor disorders.

12. Activation of neuroplasticity is a contributing factor in many other diseases such as some forms of mood disorders, fibromyalgia and probably also some disorders with poorly defined pathology such as the chronic fatigue syndrome.

13. Activating neuroplasticity together with presenting stimuli that can induce plastic changes are now studied for use in the treatment of plasticity disorders such as chronic neuropathic pain, tinnitus and the effect of ischemic stroke.

Introduction

The basis for neuroplasticity includes changes in synaptic efficacy, changes in protein synthesis in nerve cells, and in some situations, morphological changes regarding axons, dendrites, and synapses. Elimination of entire cells through programmed cell death also occurs especially during the first years of life. Dormant synapses can be unmasked (made to conduct) and functioning synapses can become masked (dormant).

Neuroplasticity has similarities with learning, but it also has important differences. Learning (memorizing) relates to memory and what is learned must be recalled voluntarily and can be forgotten. In contrast, skills that are learned through expression of neuroplasticity are always available. A skill to pronounce unfamiliar words that has been acquired through activation of neuroplasticity is a skill that is always available, like the ability to do physical tasks such as bicycling, which when learned, is always available.

Once neuroplasticity was discovered, the concept of the customizable functionally dynamic central nervous system became popular; it is now assumed that many connections in the brain are plastic, but there are also connections that are not easily changed, "hard wired" [504].

Much less attention was given to such brain functions that were difficult (or impossible) to change ("hard-wired").

This chapter provides an overview of the fundamental properties of neuroplasticity and the anatomical and physiological basis for plasticity of the central nervous system. The chapter also discusses how neuroplasticity can be activated and it describes the mechanisms that are involved in the expression of neuroplasticity in general.

Neuroplasticity is a property of the nervous system

Neuroplasticity is a property of the central nervous system, and neuroplasticity must be activated to become apparent. Activation of neuroplasticity has many different effects. Correct postnatal development of the central nervous system requires activation of neuroplasticity. Successful recovery from injuries to the nervous system such as stroke depends on activation of neuroplasticity, but activation of neuroplasticity also plays important roles in recovery from many other forms of bodily injuries and for adaptation to the use of prostheses of various kind. Learning a new skill is dependent on activation of neuroplasticity.

Changing the strength of connections (synaptic efficacy) is the most common mechanism for affecting functional changes, but elimination and creation of new synapses are also parts of the repertoire of neuroplasticity as is the elimination of entire cells through programmed cell death. The changes in synaptic strength and efficacy are more reversible than changes in synaptic morphology.

It has been shown in many studies that the functions of many parts of the central nervous system (brain and spinal cord) and their connections, in fact, change regularly because of activation of neuroplasticity [596]. This means that both the function of individual parts of the brain and their interconnections are dynamic.

Many studies have confirmed that neural functions can change during the entire lifetime in response to environmental or internal factors.

Earlier, the emphasis had been on the beneficial effects of activation of neuroplasticity consisting of its role in learning new skills, memory and in recovery from trauma to neural tissue such as occurs in ischemic strokes. The importance of the beneficial effects of activation of neuroplasticity is apparent in the connection with everyday life.

Most nerve cells in the spinal cord and the brain have both inhibitory and excitatory input. A cell, therefore, becomes inhibitory when inhibition dominates and it becomes excitatory when excitation dominates. Activation of neuroplasticity can change the balance between inhibition and excitation in cells by changing the efficacy of excitatory and inhibitory synapses differently. Therefore, changing synaptic efficacy can make a cell that is excitatory becomes an inhibitory cell or vice versa. This means that activation of neuroplasticity can make wide changes in neural processing.

Some functions that are difficult to change

The most recent view of the central nervous system is that the degree of synaptic plasticity can vary widely and that some parts are malleable to a great extent while the function of other parts is stable. Although many functions and the interconnections between many parts of the nervous system are highly plastic, some parts are indeed very stable and could accurately be regarded as being "hard-wired." Examples are the long-term memory function, sexual preferences, personality, and handedness. This means that there are many circuits in the brain that are difficult to change. A person's character also seems to be rather stable.

Complex behavioral functions such as personality, empathy [48] aggression and giving without expecting a return (altruism) are other examples of human behavior that seems relatively stable during lifetime suggesting that it depends on stable synapses, or synapses the efficacy of which is difficult to change. In fact, much of our behavior seems to be stable during a lifetime. This means that many synapses seem to be stable and not plastic.

The fact that some functions such as sexual preference, addiction, long-term memory and handedness are difficult to change shows that the efficacy of some synapses cannot be changed or are difficult to change. Long-term memory must rely on synapses that are stable and which do not change their efficacy as is evident from failed attempts to erase memories such as for the treatment of the posttraumatic stress disorder (PTSD). All of these functions must depend on complex neural circuits that are not, or are no longer, malleable. It must, therefore, be assumed that the synaptic efficacy of some neurons is fixed, or can become fixed and not reacting to environmental influence such as sensory input.

Sexual preferences are perhaps the clearest example of functions that are very difficult to change. That sexual orientation appears to be "hard-wired" is indicated by the failure of the many attempts that have been made to change a person's sexual preferences. Very little is known about the neuroscience of sexuality, and it is in fact not known what specific features of the nervous system make a person become attracted to members of the opposite gender, which is regarded to be normal or by members of the same gender, which is regarded by many people to be abnormal.

People who are extreme left-handed often find it impossible to learn to write with their right hand indicating that the involved synaptic transmission has limited flexibility.

The function of synapses that are hard to change has not been studied to the same extent as synapses that are easy to change and which is the basis for plastic changes together with changes in protein synthesis.

Storing information (memory) requires changes in the efficacy of synapses similar to what is induced by activation of neuroplasticity. After being altered for storage of information, the same cells are becoming stable and not changeable making permanent storage of information possible.

Neuroplasticity is involved in making a person an addict and when addiction has become established these same neural circuits become virtually irreversible.

Neuroplasticity induced as a compensation for loss of function

After damage to specific parts of the spinal cord and the brain, the induced plastic changes may be too great and symptoms, such as spasticity and other forms of spasm, may result in overcompensation for lost functions. Reduced functions through trauma of pathology may be improved by plastic changes that increase the gain in neural circuits of the brain, but such changes in the gain can be overdone causing hyperactive disorders. This is believed to be the basis for symptoms such as those of spasticity.

Effect of not activation certain parts of the central nervous system

Another aspect of neuroplasticity is related to the consequences of not activating certain regions of the brain and spinal cord. Studies have shown that if a part of the cerebral cortex of one sense (for example, the auditory cortex) does not receive signals during the critical period, it may be taken over by other senses such as vision [265].

Activation of neuroplasticity

Both external and internal events may activate expression of neuroplasticity. Deprivation of input is perhaps the strongest promoter of plastic changes in sensory systems, but insults, such as trauma, inflammation, and compression or irritation to sensory nerves, are also frequent causes of expression of neuroplasticity. Novel sensory stimulations and overstimulation may also promote expression of neuroplasticity, and it may affect the balance between inhibition and excitation. Injuries to the central nervous system, such as from strokes and trauma, may also cause expression of neuroplasticity [297]. Age-related morphological and chemical changes might likewise promote expression of neuroplasticity.

There are factors that promote plastic change, and there are factors that can make it more difficult to activate neuroplasticity.

Activation of neuroplasticity mainly causes changes in synaptic efficacy, which can increase or decrease excitability depending on whether it acts on inhibitory or excitatory synapses. Activation of neuroplasticity can change the balance between inhibition and excitation in cells. Neuroplasticity can re-route information by an unmasking of dormant synapses thereby opening normally closed connections or masking of active synapses thereby closing normally conducting pathways.

Changes in the efficacy of synapses can change the strength of functional connections in the central nervous system (brain and spinal cord). Changes in synaptic efficacy are the main ways that activation of neuroplasticity can change the motor and sensory functions. Elimination and creation of new synapses are also parts of the repertoire of neuroplasticity as is the elimination of entire cells through programmed cell death.

Synapses are key components in neural networks

We are now beginning to gain some understanding about the basic structure of neural networks. Synapses that provide the connections between elements of the central nervous system are integral parts in very complex networks. Schlee used the hub structure of airline route maps to describe the network of brain structures that are involved in creating the symptoms of tinnitus.

Activation of neuroplasticity by external sources

Signals coming from outside and entering the brain through our senses or from inside the body can activate neuroplasticity as can events that occur in the spinal cord or the brain. Deprivation of sensory input is perhaps the strongest activator of neuroplasticity, but frequent stimulation with the same stimuli can also activate neuroplasticity.

The "kindling phenomenon" (in rats) studied by Goddard [218] was one of the first published reports that indicated that the function of the adult nervous system could be changed by external factors (electrical stimulation of the amygdala).

Thus, Goddard was one of the first scientists to show that certain brain functions changed after repeated electrical stimulation of a structure in the brain. Goddard showed that electrical stimulation every day of the amygdala in rats first gave no visible reactions, but after doing it every day for 4-6 weeks, it evoked seizures.

Goddard thought that the phenomenon he observed in the animals he studied was similar to lighting a fire and he called it kindling. Similar reactions have later been shown to occur in many other parts of the brain [693]. This phenomenon is what is now known as neuroplasticity.

Deprivation of sensory input

Deprivation of sensory input is a strong activator of neuroplasticity, but also novel stimulation is a strong activator of neuroplasticity. An early demonstration of the effect of activation of neuroplasticity involved animal experiments where Patrick Wall showed that when signals from the body to a segment of the spinal cord are cut off, connections to nerve cells in that segment might be activated by signals from distant segments [697]. Before such deprivation of input, these signals could not activate the cells in question. These cells in the segment that had been deprived of signals from the body became responsive to signals from branches of sensory fibers that entered at far away segments of the spinal cord. These studies illustrate the great power of deprivation of input which often occurs after trauma, including amputations, and that is often the driving force for activation of neuroplasticity.

Deprivation of sensory input that occurs in children who are born deaf prevent some parts of the brain to become activated in a normal way. The extreme of such abnormalities may be that other axons that carry information from other senses invade the idle regions of the brain such as of the cerebral cortex. An example of that was shown in animal studies where the auditory cortex was deprived of its normal input and then became invaded by axons from the visual system [265].

Physical exercise

Other examples of activation of neuroplasticity by external factors are physical training which is an effective means to promote neuroplasticity that can compensate for the loss of function and reduce the symptoms associated with injuries to the nervous system.

Neuroplasticity may also be promoted using artificial (electrical) stimulation of different central nervous system structures.

Other causes of activation of neuroplasticity

While deprivation of input is perhaps the strongest promoter of plastic changes in sensory systems, insults, such as trauma, inflammation, and compression or irritation to sensory nerves, are also frequent causes of expression of neuroplasticity. Novel sensory stimulations and overstimulation may also promote expression of neuroplasticity, and it may affect the balance between inhibition and excitation. Injuries to the central nervous system, such as from strokes and trauma, also cause expression of neuroplasticity [297]. Age-related morphological and chemical changes might also promote expression of neuroplasticity.

Effects of activation of neuroplasticity

Activation of neuroplasticity changes the strength of connections in the brain and spinal cord by changing the efficacy of the synapse that connects an axon to its target cell. This means that neuroplasticity can control connectivity in the brain and the spinal cord.

Most nerve cells in the brain and the spinal cord have both excitatory and inhibitory input. Changes in synaptic efficacy do not affect inhibitory and excitatory synapses to an equal extent. Activation of neuroplasticity, therefore, often changes the relationship between excitation and inhibition, most often shifting it towards excitation. In extreme, it can cause inhibitory neurons become excitatory neurons or *visa verse*.

A few published studies have shown that temporal integration can change as a result of expression of neuroplasticity [212, 442, 666]. On the cellular level, increased temporal integration makes input more efficient, and trains of impulses with lower frequency may activate cells that normally required higher frequency input.

Activation of neuroplasticity can cause morphological change by the creation of new anatomical connections (sprouting of axons and dendrites), elimination of existing connections, or by altering synapses morphologically or by the elimination of nerve cells (programmed cell death).

While most plastic changes involve changes in synaptic efficacy and thus, are reversible, changes caused by activation of neuroplasticity may also cause structural changes in the brain.

Donald Hebb, a Canadian psychologist, in 1949 presented a hypothesis that postulated that lasting (morphological) changes could occur if it caused a presynaptic cell to persistently fire on the postsynaptic cell [250].

This principle later became known as "neurons that fire together, wire together." This is a form of activity-dependent synaptic plasticity. Hebb's principle is assumed to be the basis for associative learning, also known as Hebbian learning.

Neural reorganization through activation of neuroplasticity

Our understanding of the reorganization of neural structures that may occur from activation of neuroplasticity comes from animal experiments that have shown that the auditory [278, 661] as well as the somatosensory sensory cortex may reorganize when deprived of input [695].

Re-mapping of the cerebral cortex

The cerebral cortex and many other structures have maps of the body and its movements. These maps are important for a person's perception of "self." The maps are normally updated constantly.

The changes in the function of the cerebral cortex that are induced by abnormal sensory input causing sensory dysfunction are accompanied by extensive changes in subcortical structures that result in the reorganization of sensory systems extending from the periphery to the sensory cortices. This means that the dysfunction that occurs after injuries to sensory organs, sensory nerves, and the spinal cord and amputations can be regarded as a disease of reorganization of large regions of the central nervous system.

It has been shown that regions of the cerebral cortex that are adjacent to the areas that are deprived of input expand to occupy the deprived cortical areas [295, 415, 695]. Studies have shown that the functions of many parts of the brain and spinal cord and their connections, in fact, change regularly and that many neural functions are thus dynamic [597].

Extensive use of some functions such as the fingers by playing a musical string instrument causes re-mapping of the somatosensory cortex with an increased representation of the area that represents the fingers that were heavily used [165].

Most studies of the effect of activation of neuroplasticity have concerned the input and output of specific structures of the brain such as thalamic or cortical nuclei. It is becoming increasingly evident, however, that brain functions, including symptoms of diseases such plasticity diseases, do not depend on the neural activity in any one structure, but involve several structures at one time. Connections and the strength of the connections have been found to play important roles in the expression of the beneficial neuroplasticity as well as in the symptoms of neuroplasticity diseases and other expressions of maladaptive neuroplasticity.

Harmful neuroplasticity

It is only recently that it has become evident that plastic changes in the central nervous system can have harmful effects causing symptoms and signs of disease by turning functional neural networks into dysfunctional networks.

Neuroplasticity can be harmful; it is involved in creating the symptoms of many common diseases, such as chronic neuropathic pain [461], some forms of tinnitus, spasticity and several less frequently occurring disorders [261, 450].

We call such harmful neuroplasticity "maladaptive neuroplasticity" and the diseases that results are called "plasticity diseases." Examples are the chronic neuropathic pain, some forms of tinnitus, spasticity and some forms of muscle spasms. The existence of harmful neuroplasticity is the dark side of neuroplasticity.

More recent studies have indicated a much wider role of activation of maladaptive neuroplasticity and that there is evidence of involvement of this form of neuroplasticity in the creation of the symptoms and signs of diseases such as a wide range of neurological diseases. Many of the changes that occur during aging may also be related to activation of maladaptive plasticity.

Maladaptive plasticity may be involved in some forms of muscle spasm, fibromyalgia and perhaps the chronic fatigue syndrome and it may also be involved in creating conditions such as different forms of dementia including Alzheimer's disease, possibly in connection with activation of the immune system [496].

Dysfunctional neural networks and altered connections may also be involved in many other forms of dementia and age-related changes [596].

Substance dependence and craving

There is evidence that maladaptive neuroplasticity is involved in creating various forms of substance dependence. Such dependencies have different forms including addictions that are associated with euphoria and distinct withdrawal symptoms when terminated. Some people will include the sense of craving that most people experience about food and drinks as a form of addiction.

Some opioids such as heroin can create addiction with withdrawal symptoms while the semi-synthetic opioids (hydrocodone, oxycodone, hydromorphone), used as painkillers involves a minimal risk of creating addiction with withdrawal symptoms [273] but may in certain people create a sense of (strong) craving with a desire to continue administration. These experiences are all created by a release of dopamine into the reward network including the nucleus accumbens.

Intake of any of the many different opiates that are now available for pain control does not pose a risk for organ damage or bleeding as is the case for many other kinds of pain medications. However, administration of any of various opiates that are available is life-threatening because they suppress respiration in large dosages. Because of the effect of tolerance of opiates that reduces their pain-relieving effect after long time use people may increase the dosage to a level that suppresses respiration, that without intervention leads to death.

Creation of diseases

Pathological synaptic functions (synaptopathic [359]) are key features of many plasticity disorders and may play a role in other diseases also. There are other ways that activation of neuroplasticity can become harmful, about which little is known.

Examples include diseases such as fibromyalgia and myofascial pain perhaps chronic fatigue syndromes and possibly Alzheimer's disease to mention a few [461].

The immune system is plastic

It is not only the nervous system that can change its function. Also, the adaptive immune system is plastic, and it can "learn."

There is evidence that the immune system plays an important role in diseases such as chronic neuropathic pain and perhaps also in dementia possibly also in diseases such as the chronic fatigue syndrome and fibromyalgia.

Like neuroplasticity, the immune system can respond in a way that is beneficial to a person, namely by eliminating an intruder such as bacteria or virus. It can also respond unfavorably by eliciting autoimmune reactions. This is why the immune system, like neuroplasticity, should not be too strong and not too weak. The optimal strength is such that it does not create too many autoimmune diseases but strong enough to defend the organism from most intruders.

This is also the reason that our immune system seems imperfect: It does not ward off all intruders or eliminate all forms of cancer cells, and it involves a certain risk of inducing autoimmune diseases.

The role of neuroplasticity in childhood development

In the past, it was assumed that brain functions changed very little after birth except for degenerative processes associated with aging. This changed some 50 years ago when it was shown that sensory stimulation was necessary for the normal development of the sensory nervous system [714]. Not only sensory functions, including pain, are now known to be influenced by environmental stimuli and internal activations [324, 334], but also activation of motor systems are vital for normal childhood development [428] [336].

The earliest indication that proper sensory stimulation is important for the maturation of sensory nervous systems came from studies of the visual system in kittens, by Torsten Wiesel [714].

Wiesel showed that deprivation of adequate stimulation during early age prevented the animals from ever gaining normal vision on the eye that was deprived of normal stimulation early after birth.

These findings were applied to humans, and it became evident that appropriate stimulation after birth was necessary for normal childhood development [614].

Many studies have confirmed that neural functions can change in response to environmental factors especially during the so-called sensitive period of life [714].

The sensitive period

Neural functions are more easily changed in early childhood during a period that is known as the sensitive (critical) period.

Activation of neuroplasticity is necessary during the first two years of life for the development and organization of the nervous system that was laid down before birth and guided by genetic (inheritance). Activation of neuroplasticity cannot correct or modify the genetic programs that control the prenatal and postnatal development, but activation of neuroplasticity after birth can modify the development of the nervous system in individual persons ("mid-course correction").

The study by Wiesel and Hubel [714] in cats was one of the first studies that showed the existence of critical periods during which development was guided by sensory input and that adequate sensory input was necessary for the development of normal sensory functions. Wiesel and Hubel also found that the deficits from early visual deprivation were largely preserved and only little recovery occurred after opening the eyes of the animals [715]. Additionally, they found that monocular and binocular deprivation had a different effect on the morphology and function of cells in the lateral geniculate nucleus (LGN) and the primary visual cortex.

While few cells in the primary visual (striate) cortex could be activated from the monocular deprived eye, many cells could be activated from binocularly deprived eyes although the response of many of the cells was not normal [716]. This was an unexpected finding, and it illustrates the complexity of the expression of neuroplasticity from early deprivation of input.

It means that the effect of deprivation of input to one eye depends on the input to the other eye. Bilateral morphological abnormalities were found in the LGN, but there were no observed morphological changes in the cerebral cortex.More recently studies with humans have been possible through the introduction of auditory prostheses (cochlear implants), which allows the effect of input to the auditory system at different ages to be studied after such input has been established through cochlear implants [324, 334, 613, 663]. Studies in humans have confirmed the results of animal studies that have shown that appropriate sensory input is necessary for normal development of the (sensory) nervous system.

Early studies concerned young individuals, but later, many studies have brought evidence that the function of the mature nervous system can be changed within wide limits through the expression of neuroplasticity, see [334, 415, 559, 661, 697].

Cochlear implants

Studies of children who had cochlear implants show that the critical period for hearing is the first 3-4 years after birth [334]). Sharma [616] has shown that the difference in the development of a component of the auditory Event-Related Potentials (ERP) that is assumed to have cognitive importance is related to the time after birth when congenitally deaf children begin to receive input to their auditory system (Figure 1.1). In these studies, the latency of a component of the auditory evoked potentials, the P1 component, was used as an indicator of maturation of the auditory system.

Figure 1.1 shows the effect of cochlear implants performed at different ages; before 3.5 years of age, between 3.5 and 6.5 years and after 7 years of age.

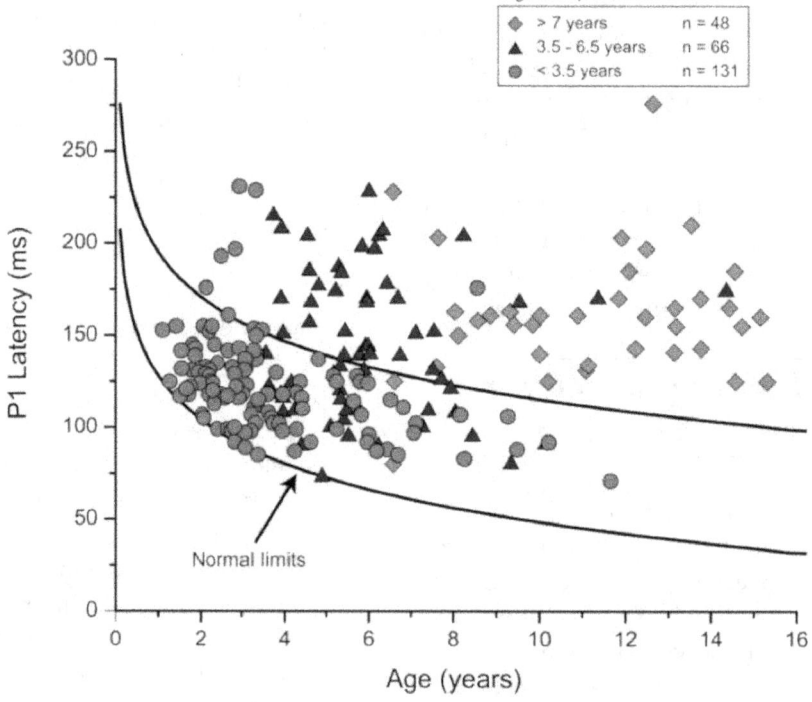

Figure 1.1. P1 latencies as a function of chronological age for children with cochlear implants. The solid lines are the 95% confidence limits for normal hearing children. P1 latencies for children implanted before age 3.5 years (early-implanted group) are shown as circles. P1 latencies for children implanted during the time of 3.5 and 6.5 years (middle-implanted group) are shown as triangles. P1 latencies for children implanted {Sharma, 2006 #3749} after age seven years (late-implanted group) are shown as diamonds. The results show clearly that the best recovery of useful hearing occurs when cochlear implants are applied early, and after 3.5 years, the recovery is not nearly as good as when implanted earlier. (Data from Sharma, A. and M.F. Dorman, 2002, [616][614].

Activation of neuroplasticity from internal factors

It is not only sensory stimuli that can activate neuroplasticity but also internally generated signals can activate neuroplasticity. An example of that is spontaneous activity in nerves, or, rather the absence of driven neural activity. Such absence of normal neural activity is assumed to be responsible for the abnormal reactions to severance of motor nerves that has been shown to cause muscle spasm. For example, Kreutzberg showed that the integrity of motoneurons depend on the integrity of their (efferent) axons [336].

Neurons that are not part of a neural network and receive appropriate input have been shown to lose their integrity in both adult and juvenile animals [20, 571]. Thus, morphological changes occur in the nerve's target cells after transection of their nerves [166, 336]. This is an indication that spontaneous activity in nerves is important for maintaining the integrity of the target neurons.

Studies of motoneurons in the embryonic chick have shown that being deprived of input is not the only factor in the death of neurons (Rubel 2002). In this study, it was shown that loss of motoneurons after transection of the spinal cord (to eliminate descending input to motoneurons) did not occur until after the completion of the major period of the naturally occurring death of motoneurons has been completed [500].

Effects on functional changes in connections

Activation of neuroplasticity can cause re-routing of information in the central nervous stem (spinal cord and brain). Anatomical studies can only provide information about which pathways are available, but physiological studies are required to determine if neural pathways are open to traffic, thus being functional.

The reason that morphological connections may not be functional is that the synapses with which they make contact to a target cell are ineffective (not conducting), or because the input is not able to exceed the threshold of the target neuron due to insufficient temporal integration.

Whether or not input from an axon to a nerve cell will activate its target cell so that an action potential is generated in the cell's axon depends on many factors.

The input to the cell, adequate presynaptic activation and especially the efficacy of synapses are some of these factors. Sensitization and the availability of neural transmitters and protein synthesis and protease activity are also important factors as are the balance between inhibition and excitation and the resting membrane potential that combined whether a target cell will respond or not.

Re-routing of information

Non-conducting (dormant) synapses are present in all parts of the central nervous system, and the strength of the synapses that conduct varies. This cause functional connections to have different strength and the strength of a connection is controlled by neuroplasticity. Consequently, most parts of the brain can be functionally rewired to different degrees by changing the efficacy of synapses that is under the control of neuroplasticity.

Unused connections are a form of redundancy of the nervous system that can be utilized when required, such as in response to a change in demand or after injuries.

Re-routing of information through activation of neuroplasticity can take many forms. For example, re-routing the pathways from the vestibular apparatus in the inner ear can result in abnormal sensations of various kinds; a person may vomit from excessive head motion that stimulate the vestibular apparatus. This is a sign of the activation of regions of the central nervous system that are not normally activated by the vestibular system but which have anatomical (normally unused) connections to many parts of the brain.

In addition to changes in connectivity between different regions of the central nervous system, specific regions change their internal organization as a part of the activation of neuroplasticity. Thus, the shaping of the receptive fields of cortical neurons that constantly occurs in response to the state of vigilance and learning [162] involves functional reorganization of many neural circuits.

The changes in the function of the cerebral cortex that are induced by abnormal sensory input causing sensory dysfunction are accompanied by extensive changes in the function of the subcortical structures [68] that result in the reorganization of sensory systems extending from the periphery to the sensory cortices.

This means that the dysfunction that occurs after injuries to sensory organs, sensory nerves, and the spinal cord and amputations can be regarded as a disease of reorganization of large regions of the central nervous system [696].

Remapping the central nervous system

Re-mapping of cortical areas through the expression of neuroplasticity is a complex process involving specific channels within the thalamocortical pathways initiated by sensory stimulation. It includes increasing the strengths of synaptic synapses that are conducting or unmasking of dormant synapses.

Such synapses can cause extension of the sensory activation areas by opening or strengthening of functional connections to adjacent neurons. Such widening of response areas is also known as "lateral spread." It is similar mechanisms as those that cause re-routing of information by opening connections to regions of the brain that are not normally activated. These dynamic changes may "crystallize" into long-lasting or permanent changes by learning-induced neuroplasticity.

Unmasking of dormant synapses may also explain the results of studies of the somatosensory representation in the cerebral cortex by Merzenich and colleagues [295] who were some of the first to publish experimental studies demonstrating widening of the cortical representation of the skin through altered input. When they had amputated a finger, the cortical space devoted to that finger became deprived of input and shrunk.

The cortical space devoted to sensory input from adjacent fingers expanded into that space. Stimulation of the skin of the middle finger, for example, would generate activity in the region formerly devoted to the index finger [415]. Similar phenomena have been observed in motor cortices and auditory cortices [559].

Studies of a person who was a string player and who used certain fingers more extensively than other fingers showed that the part of the somatosensory cortex devoted to those fingers became larger than expected based on what it was in individuals who use their fingers in a normal way. This is an example of how activation of neuroplasticity can alter the organization of a portion of the nervous system [165].

Similarly, Braille users develop observable changes in the organization of their somatosensory cortex [651].

The use of the mirror box mentioned for treating phantom sensations after amputations mentioned in Chapter 5 is another example of externally activated neuroplasticity [543]. In this case, the purpose has been to treat a condition induced by lack of appropriate updating of cortical maps of a person's body.

Frequent use of motor systems can make reflexes stronger and easier to elicit. Even the simplest of the components of the motor system, the monosynaptic stretch reflex shows the effect of neuroplasticity. The strength of the stretch response can increase and decrease as a result of behavioral manipulations (such as the presentation of a reward) [728].

Chapter 2

Anatomical and Physiological Bases for Neuroplasticity

Abstract

1. Plastic changes in the nervous system can occur because of changes in synaptic efficacy (unmasking of dormant synapses or masking of efficient synapses), the creation and elimination of synapses, and by sprouting or elimination of axons and dendrites.

2. Altered protein synthesis and protease activity in nerve cells are other forms of plastic changes.

3. External and internal events such as deprivation of sensory input, changes in demands, novel sensory stimulations and overstimulation can induce expression of neuroplasticity.

4. Internal events such as different kinds of insults to nerves and central nervous system structures can cause expression of neuroplasticity.

5. Expression of neuroplasticity is facilitated by activation of the acetylcholine system of the forebrain (the nucleus of Meynert) and by activation of the noradrenaline-serotonin system of the locus coeruleus.

6. Activity in the nucleus of the solitary tract (innervated by the vagus nerve) has a similar facilitatory effect on plastic changes.

7. GABA and other neurotransmitters play a role in the expression of neuroplasticity.

8. The NMDA receptor function is important for the expression of neuroplasticity and NMDA receptor antagonists, such as Ketamine, hamper activation of neuroplasticity.

9. Expression of neuroplasticity can cause changes in processing by altering the balance between inhibition and excitation.

Introduction

The anatomical and physiological basis for neuroplasticity has been studied extensively, and many of the general properties are now known. It is known, however, that changes in synaptic efficacy plays an important role in the functional changes of various parts of the central nervous system but also changes in protein synthesis and creation and elimination of synapses play important roles in the creation of the flexibility of the central nervous system.

While most plastic changes involve changes in synaptic efficacy and thus, are reversible, changes caused by activation of neuroplasticity may in fact also cause structural changes in the brain. Hebb (1949) [250] postulated that when many neurons fire at the same time, it may change the morphology in such a way that the neurons will connect morphologically together. This principle later became known as "neurons that fire together, wire together." This is a form of activity-dependent synaptic plasticity.

This chapter provides an overview of the anatomical and physiological bases for neuroplasticity of the brain, and it discusses how neuroplasticity can be activated. Specifically, the mechanisms involved in the expression of neuroplasticity and the physiological and anatomical basis for expression of neuroplasticity are discussed. The fact that there are two kinds of neuroplasticity, good and bad, is emphasized. The role of neuroplasticity in compensating for deficits and adapting to changing demands is discussed, and its ability to create signs and symptoms of the disease is discussed in detail. How to evaluate the effect of activation of good neuroplasticity, whether it is purposeful in signaling a disease or trauma, and whether it is also beneficial to a person are all questions that are discussed in this chapter.

Activators of neuroplasticity

Sensory stimulation or sensory deprivation are important activators of neuroplasticity. The strongest activator of neuroplasticity is a deprivation of sensory input, and reduced or absent motor activity can also activate neuroplasticity. Incoming sensory information is integrated into existing brain circuitry that drives behavioral output and may activate neuroplasticity. Heavily processed sensory information communicated through the classical sensory pathways (using the ventral thalamus and sensory cortices) is important for activating neuroplasticity. There is also a possibility that less processed information traveling in the non-classical sensory pathways (using the dorsal-medial thalamus) can activate neuroplasticity.

The neural circuits involved in activating neuroplasticity are similar to those involved in learning involving the synaptic plasticity in the amygdala [563], the auditory cortex and prefrontal cortex (PFC). In some of these studies, using recordings of the theta and alpha (electroencephalographic, EEG) power [255]), the functional connectivity between hippocampal, cortical and striatal regions has been correlated with functions of various kinds such as memory retrieval in humans.

Such studies have provided evidence that synchronization of cell firing across memory-related neural circuits may enable association between stimuli encoded in different parts of the brain. Disrupting brain derived neurotrophic factor, (BDNF) expression, on the other hand, has been shown to alter the theta power of the EEG that originates in the hippocampus and the prefrontal cortex, and decrease the phase synchrony of the theta rhythm between these areas. This has been shown to reduce late LTP, and it impairs fear extinction [257].

Other studies have linked specific patterns of synchronized cell firing, in particular, theta rhythmic activity, to neuroplasticity and memory mechanisms [91]. (For a review see [586]).

Glutamate and the NMDA receptors play an important role in the expression of neuroplasticity. Ketamine, a non-competitive antagonist of the NMDA receptor, blocks NMDA receptor-mediated neuroplasticity.

These neural transmitters, together with serotonin and acetylcholine, are important players in the dynamic regulation of sensory processing. Other studies have shown that the β-adrenergic system of the locus coeruleus together with the GABA and NMDA receptor systems have positive effects on regulation of ocular dominance neuroplasticity. Other studies have focused on deregulated glutamate neurotransmission [511].

Biology of critical periods

The existence of critical periods in humans has also been confirmed, which means that the sensory stimulation that occurs before a certain time in the life of children is more effective in changing the functions of the nervous system than input that occurs later in life. This confirmed by the results of studies of the performance of cochlear implants. These studies have shown that cochlear implants that are applied early in life serve better than those implanted in older individuals confirming that neuroplasticity is more pronounced in the young individual than the older organism ([334] and Figure 1.1).

The initiation and closure of a critical period are driven by the maturation of the inhibitory circuitry in the cortex [309]. The shift to a predominantly inhibitory activity culminates in the consolidation of neuronal circuits through curtailing development of new synapses and pruning of existing ones. Although the role of inhibition in the initiation of the critical period is still elusive, it probably mediates neuroplasticity by altering the composition of NMDARs [308] and facilitating LTD.

The extracellular environment is important for visual cortical plasticity, particularly perineuronal nets (PNN), which consist of chondroitin-sulfate proteoglycans (CSPGs). Inhibition has been shown to play a role in the ocular dominance shift. With age, GABAergic parvalbumin-expressing interneurons (PV cells) will eventually be encased by PNNs, thus marking the end of the critical period.

Control of neuroplasticity

Neuroplasticity is regulated by genetic, epigenetic and external factors. External promotors of neuroplasticity are the deprivation of sensory input, overstimulation, and novel stimulation.

NMDA receptor-mediated neuroplasticity is affected by factors such as stress and by drugs such as antidepressants. Similarly, the noradrenergic influence from locus coeruleus has been shown (in rats) to be important for modulating synaptic plasticity during critical periods for developing odor preferences. Acetylcholine and noradrenaline are the two major neuromodulators of plastic changes where the functional changes involve the interplay between neural circuits in the thalamus and primary sensory cortices.

The cholinergic basal forebrain system that includes the nucleus basalis also comprises GABA, calcium-binding proteins, and inhibitory neuropeptides and these could also play a role in cortical plasticity. These forebrain structures are altered in Alzheimer's disease.

Internal factors that can promote neuroplasticity include the cholinergic system of the forebrain (the nucleus of Meynert). Well-documented studies have demonstrated the importance of the cholinergic system of the forebrain regarding neuroplasticity. The nucleus of Meynert, also known as the basal nucleus is a prime source of cholinergic activity, and the activity of this nucleus promote activation of neuroplasticity [36, 317]. Neuroplasticity can thus be facilitated by electrical stimulation of the nucleus of Meynert (nucleus basalis).

The effects in the entorhinal, and perirhinal cortex and hippocampus may also play a role in controlling neuroplasticity. Both muscarinic and nicotinic acetylcholine receptors play a role in neuroplasticity including encoding of new memories. Acetylcholine may enhance encoding by increasing the strength of afferent input relative to feedback, contributing to theta rhythm oscillations, activating intrinsic mechanisms for persistent spiking, increasing the modification of synapses.

Nucleus of Meynert

The nucleus of Meynert receives input from the central nucleus of the amygdala, the locus coeruleus, and structures that are important for memory and memory consolidation; thus, most likely important for activation of neuroplasticity. This system influences the immune system, memory, learning and disorders of aging such as dementia including Alzheimer's disease.

The cholinergic anti-inflammatory pathway has recently been shown to play a wide and important role in the body's immune defense (see Appendix C). These systems are most likely affected by many factors including neuroplasticity.

The cholinergic system of the nucleus of Meynert in the brain facilitates plastic changes in the cerebral cortex. Electrical stimulation of that nucleus at the same time that a stimulus aimed at eliciting plastic changes is presented enhances the induced plastic changes [36] [316]. Such "pairing" of stimuli is now being developed for clinical use in treating severe tinnitus and chronic neuropathic pain. Stimulation of the vagus nerve only requires minimally invasive surgical procedures It was later shown that electrical stimulation of the vagus nerve has similar effects as stimulation of the nucleus basalis [168].

These effects may be different in different brain structures. High acetylcholine (ACh) levels enhance the magnitude of afferent input to cortex through action at nicotinic receptors. High ACh also suppresses the magnitude of feedback excitation in cortex via presynaptic inhibition of glutamate release.

It is also known that adrenergic substances promote consolidation of memory - a demonstration of how neuroplasticity can be enhanced [180]. The administration of substances such as corticosteroids, benzodiazepines, and barbiturates can have the opposite effect.

Most pharmacological treatments of dementia including Alzheimer's disease focus on compensating for a decreased function of the nucleus of Meynert by increasing acetylcholine levels. Activation of the nucleus of Meynert also influences the immune system, memory, learning and disorders of aging such as dementia including

The vagus nerve

More recently, the role of the vagus nerve in activation of neuroplasticity has become apparent. The target of the afferent fibers of the vagus nerve is the nucleus of the solitary tract and axons from cells in that nucleus reach many different structures in the brain. (The role of the afferent part of the vagus nerve is discussed in detail later in this chapter).

While the vagus nerve has lived a quiet life for many years – suddenly neuroscientists are now falling over each other to study the nerve and its function, the reason being that animal studies have shown that electrical stimulation of the vagus nerve has similar effects as stimulation of the nucleus of Meynert, namely promoting plastic changes [404] [169].

The basis for that is that neural activity in the vagus nerve that reaches cells in the nucleus tractus solitarius, subsequently activate cells in the locus coeureleus (norepinephrine) and the nucleus of Meynert, thus stimulating the cholinergic system of the brain.

Through its target, the nucleus of the tractus solitarii (NST) the vagus nerve connects to many structures in the brain, among others the nucleus of Meynert [404] (see Figure 2.1).

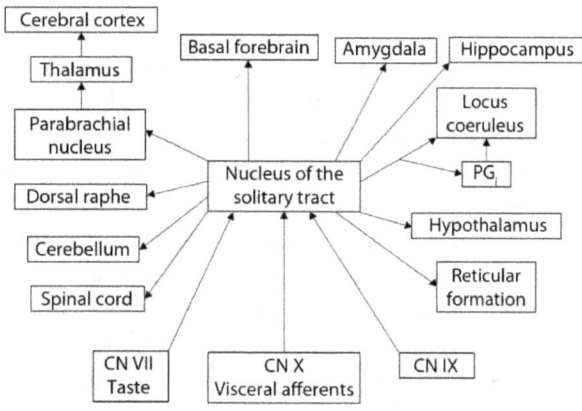

Figure 2.1 Connections from the NST nucleus, the cells of which are the target of afferent fibers in the vagus nerve. LC: Locus coeruleus, NTS: Nucleus tractus solitarius, PGi: Para gigantic nucleus. Modified from [404]. (Artwork by Monica Javidnia).

Activity in the nucleus of the solitary tract (innervated by the vagus nerve) has a similar facilitatory effect on plastic changes as that of the nucleus of Meynert because of connections from cells in the nucleus of the solitary tract to cells of the nucleus of Meynert. This means that neural activity in the afferent part of the vagus nerve can have similar effects as electrical stimulation of the nucleus of Meynert.

Under normal circumstances, signals from the organs in the abdomen (the gut) and the heart may influence neuroplasticity through the vagus nerve that innervate these organs.

The vagus nerve connects to many structures in the brain

The vagus nerve connects to many structures in the brain (see Figure 2.1and 2.2), and it plays an important role in memory.

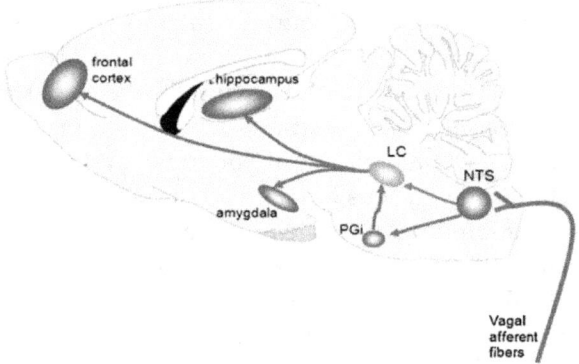

Figure 2.2 The vagus nerve plays an important role in neuroplasticity including memory. Pgi: Para-gigantocellular nucleus, LC: Locus coeureleus, Pgi is a source of cholinergic substances that can modulate many brain functions. (From McIntyre, 2012).

The fact that the afferent fibers of the vagus nerve terminate on cells in the nucleus tractus solitaries the cells of which project to many regions of the brain make it possible to achieve widespread actions of electrical stimulation of the vagus nerve (for details see Chapter 8). More recently the effect of stimulation of the vagus nerve on the ability to facilitate plastic changes has led to studies of the possibility to reverse maladaptive neuroplasticity.

Activation of nicotinic cholinergic receptors can provide anti-inflammatory effect, but it can also impair the body's ability to fight infections as occurs in traumatic brain injuries (TBI).

The vagus nerve normally modulates the immune system. The vagal immune reflex provides cholinergic anti-inflammatory response. Activity in the vagus nerve promotes plastic changes through its ability to activate the nucleus of Meynert. This makes electrical stimulation of the vagus nerve a convenient way for neuromodulation (Figure 2.3). In that way, electrical stimulation of the vagus nerve may open a way to treat disorders of memory and it may make it possible to erase memories such as would be beneficial in treatment of post-traumatic stress disorders (PTSD).

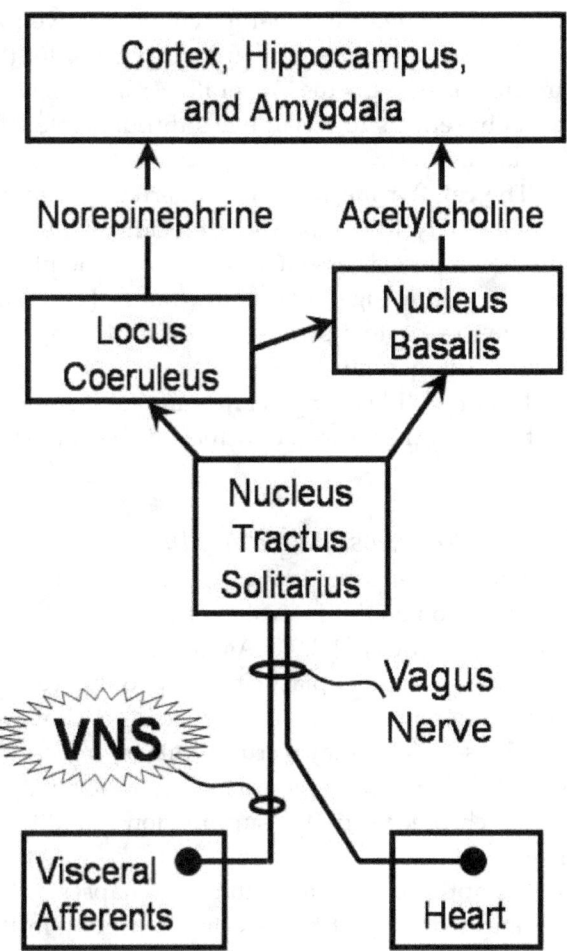

Figure 2.3 Neuromodulation pathways involving the vagus nerve. Activity in the vagus nerve activates cells in the nucleus tractus solitarius, subsequently activate cells in the locus coeruleus (norepinephrine) and nucleus of Meynert, (acetylcholine) (From [169]).

The observation that electrical stimulation of the (left) vagus nerve promote activation of neuroplasticity has led to studies where "pairing" of sensory stimuli and electrical stimulation of the vagus nerve is being developed for clinical use in treating severe tinnitus and chronic neuropathic pain [169, 404].

This principle of reversing maladaptive neuroplasticity by pairing electrical stimulation of the vagus nerve with sensory stimuli such as sound for alleviating tinnitus that was believed to be caused by maladaptive neuroplasticity have been studied in animals [316] and more recently in people with tinnitus [169].

The hypothesis that activity in the afferent part of the vagus nerve can modulate neuroplasticity has received support from studies of attempts to reverse the remapping of the cortex that is associated with tinnitus.

Stimulation of the vagus nerve can be done by placing electrodes on the nerve where it travels in the neck, thus requiring minimal surgical exploration. Stimulation of the vagus nerve is, therefore, a more attractive method for facilitating neuroplasticity in humans than using the techniques of deep brain stimulation for stimulation of the nucleus of Meynert.

Deep brain stimulation (DBS)

It is commonly experienced that the beneficial effect of deep brain stimulation that is used to inactivate specific structures in the basal ganglia or the thalamus for treatment of movement disorders or pain decreases with time. This reduced efficacy over time may be a result of expression of neuroplasticity because the stimulation is regarded as a novel stimulation. The expression of neuroplasticity then tends to reverse the effect of treatment.

Neuroplasticity and learning of motor skills

Motor skill learning plays a fundamental role in many aspects of our lives, without which it would be impossible to master a piano piece, learn bicycling or learn how to hit a tennis ball. Many jobs require many different motor skills that all have to be learned. Motor skill learning comprises the acquisition of movement sequences and is characterized by executing movements faster and more accurately with practice.

It has been proposed that motor skill learning can be divided into separable acquisition stages with an early 'fast' phase, characterized by rapid and considerable learning improvements, and a later 'slow' stage, in which a nearly asymptotic level is reached and further improvements are gained only slowly (For a review see [586]).

It is thought that interactions between cortico-thalamic-striatal and cortico-thalamic-cerebellar structures and the limbic system are essential to successfully build a motor memory trace.

These networks seem to be active during different time points of motor learning and, within each of them, specific associative-premotor and sensorimotor networks are activated.

When starting to learn a motor skill, the movement is often disjointed, poorly controlled and executed with considerable variation and immense attention. Once learned, however, the skill is retained for a long period with minimal decay. Acquisition, consolidation, and retention of motor skills require activation of neuroplasticity in different brain areas. However, molecular mechanisms driving and supporting motor learning, as well as the underlying synapse plasticity remain to be fully elucidated.

The primary motor cortex (M1) seems to play a crucial part in fast motor learning. Rodent studies have shown that motor learning can induce recruitment of neurons in the primary motor cortex (M1) and modulate synaptic efficacy through LTP and LTD. These results are supported by human studies, which also suggest that LTP-like plasticity in the M1 is involved in motor learning. While LTP-like effects are reversed after a period of motor learning, LTD like effects were shown to be either enhanced or unchanged [567].

Motor skill learning requires the involvement and integration of several cortical and subcortical regions. Motor learning can modulate functional connectivity of the cortical motor network, and early skill learning has been shown to lead to enhanced inter and intra-hemispheric coupling [653]. These investigators found greater connectivity between frontal regions and cortical motor regions in the early stages of learning. No changes in functional connectivity were observed in the previously learned experience. These results demonstrate that the functional connectivity of the cortical motor network is modulated with practice and suggest that early skill learning is mediated by enhanced inter-regional coupling.

Rodent studies suggest that BDNF is required for induction of neuroplasticity related to motor learning. Furthermore, it has been proposed that the Val66Met BDNF gene polymorphism reduces experience-dependent neuroplasticity of the human motor cortex and influences motor skill learning [322] [198], although the functional implications of this polymorphism regarding motor learning are still unclear [403].

Other studies have shown that increased spine density is accompanied by an expansion of the movement related neuronal ensembles, as well as an induction of excitatory neuron activity. After the learning process, the overall spine density gradually returns to basal levels through selective elimination [111].

The cellular mechanisms underlying synaptic plasticity in the M1 remain to be elucidated. *De novo* protein synthesis is essential for most of the plastic changes following motor learning [21] and inhibition of protein synthesis in the M1 impedes motor learning in rats [373].

Motor skill learning is an example of some of the benefits that can be achieved by physical training.

The role of homeostatic plasticity

The proper functioning of the mammalian brain relies on a joint interplay of homeostatic and Hebbian plasticity [179]. As such, homeostatic forms of synaptic plasticity not only reduce synaptic strength during elevated excitability conditions but also play a crucial role in preventing loss of information by increasing synaptic strength during chronic activity suppression conditions [691].

Synaptic scaling of excitatory synapses is the most studied form of homeostatic plasticity in the central nervous system. It is involved in the stabilization of neuronal networks and synaptic strength in the brain.

It is interesting that these two opposing phenomena likely cooperate at the molecular level by regulating effectors at the synapses [741]. Recently, disruptions in homeostatic plasticity have been associated with brain disorders such as autism spectrum disorder, schizophrenia, epilepsy, Alzheimer's, and Huntington's diseases [179].

Cellular and molecular mechanisms of synaptic plasticity

Activation of neuroplasticity causes both anatomical and function changes as we have discussed in Chapter 1. Synaptic plasticity is now widely accepted to be the most important part of the systems that are engaged in neuroplastic activation.

All the functions of neuroplasticity depend on precise control of synaptic functions [516]. Presynaptic plasticity involves alteration of neurotransmitter release tonus or dynamics, while postsynaptic plasticity usually encompasses alterations in receptor number, availability or properties [739] [359].

Expression of neuroplasticity depends on the availability of specific neural transmitters. The relative abundance of glutamate, acetylcholine, and GABA has been shown to contribute to the sculpting the receptive field of the cortical cells of the cerebral cortices and to the establishment of the balance between excitation and inhibition [701].

For example, long-term neuroplasticity that relates to memory (such as LTP and LTD) appear to derive from persistent stimulation of synapses at the high or low frequency, respectively [482]. Persistent stimulation triggers ion influx through NMDARs that, in turn, determines the rate of exposure of AMPARs through posttranslational modifications at the postsynaptic density.

Short-term synaptic plasticity is independent of protein synthesis and relies on modification of the already existing proteins. For longer-lasting changes, local translation in response to stimulation that uses the local machinery is crucial [1] [658]. However, this can only last for several hours, suggesting that transcriptional changes are required for maintaining long-lasting plasticity, such as LTP and LTD [14].

Change in efficacy of synapses

Change in synaptic strength (efficacy) is an important component of expression of neuroplasticity [335, 586, 596]. Recent studies have unveiled the basis for the system wide modifications that may occur in many parts of the brain and the spinal cord as a result of changes in synaptic efficacy brought about by activation of synaptic plasticity.

Some of the early studies on dynamic synaptic efficacy that were done in the spinal cord in the context of pain research [697] demonstrated that synapses that normally were too weak to cause their cells to fire could be activated after deprivation of input. Dr. Wall [697] coined the term "dormant synapses" to describe synaptic connections that are effectively blocked due to high synaptic thresholds or too low strength.

The opening of dormant synapses has been described as "unmasking" of synapses.

The changes described in these early studies caused cells in the dorsal horn of the spinal cord to respond to input from dermatomes from which they normally did not respond. Wall [697] hypothesized that many synapses exist anatomically but are masked. An abnormal event such as deprivation of input or intense stimulation may unmask them. These early results were followed by an extensive literature discussing how masking and unmasking contribute to the re-routing of information (for a review see [586]).

It is only recently that it has become evident that the ability to change synaptic efficacy varies widely among synapses in the brain. Some are very easy to change whereas the strength of other synapses is very difficult to change. Little is known about what factors are responsible for these difference in the ability to change synaptic strength through activation of neuroplasticity [586]).

Many factors can cause short-lasting or long-lasting increases or decreases in the strength of many kinds of synapses. This is known as short-term or long-term potentiation (LTP) and long-term depression (LTD) respectively.

Synaptic plasticity is a complex process that involves, among other molecules, glutamate and brain-derived neurotrophic factor (BDNF). Glial cells are important components of the process of regulation of synaptic connectivity [171, 174].

Both LTP and LTD are involved in many brain functions, particularly those concerning memory. Studies of LTP in hippocampus slices in rats or guinea pigs show that LTP is best invoked by stimulation at a high rate [581]. The effect may last from minutes to days and glutamate's binding to the NMDA receptor has been implicated in LTP [493].

Change in synaptic morphology

Synapses undergo processes of assembly and disassembly during postnatal development and aging. These processes are related to activity-dependent neuroplasticity [217].

Despite extensive research efforts, relatively little is known about the dynamic processes that govern creation and elimination of synapses. The factors that determine the size of synapses are incompletely known.

In postnatal brain development, however, a recent study has shown that neuroplasticity involved in the elimination of synapses is related to glutamate receptor-mediated synaptic plasticity such as long-term depression (LTD) [605].

Several hormones that are associated with the digestive system such as peptin and leptin are also involved with control of synapse morphology [245, 279]. The hormone Leptin is known to be involved in fat storage and energy homeostasis. Recent studies have shown that Leptin can also modify the structure and the function of synapses throughout the central nervous system. Leptin seems to have the potential to enhance cognitive functions through its ability to modulate cellular processes involved in learning and memory such as dendritic morphology, glutamate receptor use and activity-dependent synaptic plasticity [279].

Programmed cell death

Programmed cell death (in contrast to causes such as injuries and asphyxia), is an event believed to depend on the expression of neuroplasticity [303]. Programmed cell death is important in postnatal development where it can be affected by neural activity such as that evoked by sensory stimulation [498]. Programmed cell death is a structural (anatomical) process that involves changes that can be detected using known techniques of anatomical studies.

Change in protein synthesis and protease activity

Rubel and colleagues have shown that insults to the nervous system, such as deprivation of input, can change protein synthesis in the target cell [623]. This is yet another expression of neuroplasticity. These investigators showed that the changes occur rapidly and that the change in protein synthesis is related to presynaptic impulse activity. Local regulation of protein synthesis is a key process allowing for focal physiological responses in many cell types. This is especially relevant for larger and polarized cells, showing that these cells can quickly respond to the local cues [658].

Degradation of proteins by a proteasome is an important regulator of neuroplasticity [675]. Injuries to the nervous system or changes in the input to nerve cells may affect various proteases.

Proteases of the caspase and calpain families have been implicated in neurodegenerative processes. Their activation can be triggered by calcium influx and oxidative stress [107].

The substrates of caspases and calpains are localized in pre- and postsynaptic compartments of neurons. Changes in protease activity can affect the way neurotrophins regulate synaptic plasticity [371]. Neurotrophins are assumed to be involved in synaptic plasticity. The synthesis, secretion, and action of neurotrophins are regulated by electrical activity in the nervous system [591].

Sprouting of dendrites and axons

Studies of pain have shown evidence of outgrowth of new connections in response to an expression of neuroplasticity. For example, some studies indicate that Aδ synapse fibers of the spinal cord can sprout from a lamina deep within the dorsal horn into more superficial laminae where C-fibers normally terminate (lamina II of the dorsal horn). These immature filaments of emerging nerves may make synaptic contacts with cells that are typically activated by noxious stimuli [158, 326, 730].

Sprouting may explain symptoms, such as allodynia (pain from normally innocuous stimulation), that often occurs after peripheral nerve injuries, but allodynia may also be explained by changes in synaptic efficacy. In peripheral nerves, sprouting causes the creation of neuroma that is pain sensitive. For example, studies in animals indicate that expression of neuroplasticity in the auditory system may promote outgrowth of new connections possibly causing symptoms such as tinnitus [470].

Effects on glial cells

Recently it was shown that glial cells are important regulators of synaptic connectivity [171] and thus involved in the process of neuroplasticity. There are signs that glial cells may be involved in creating symptoms of many diseases such as tinnitus [594] [335] and some forms of chronic neuropathic pain. (Chronic neuropathic pain is a pain condition where neuroplasticity plays an important role [461]). Opioid tolerance is another example of the importance of plastic changes in the spinal cord and the brain.

Functional changes from activation of neuroplasticity

Activation of neuroplasticity affects many parts of the central nervous system, and it causes many different kinds of changes. Change in synaptic strength has a wide range of effects on the functions of many neural systems including re-routing of information. These changes are graded and regulated, mainly by the cholinergic system but also other systems can affect activation of neuroplasticity.

Connectivity

Recent studies of brain connectivity have revealed many features of neuroplasticity [190]. The fact that it is now possible to study the behaviors of large systems has brought forth many novel results.

Many connections between neurons are not functional because stimulation delivered through such connections are not sufficient to excite the target cell. Synapses that are ineffective, due to insufficient temporal summation or overly high thresholds prevent EPSP from reaching a sufficient amplitude to cause the neuron to fire.

Changes in synaptic efficacy are the most prevalent mode of connectivity alteration in the brain. This means that neuroplasticity can change neural connectivity in the brain; connectivity is now regarded as an important factor in normal brain functions as well as in many neurological diseases. The strength of the synaptic signal can be modified by cellular processes such as that of cell-adhesion molecules [53, 174].

The nervous system modulates connectivity depending on the activity of cells that receive inputs from their surroundings [396] or internal sources. The modulations may be in the form of changes in transmitter release probability causing the strength of synaptic transmission to change without changing the function of the synapse synapses, or by changes in the excitability of nerve cells, where inhibitory neurons play an important role [405].

Structural modifications that affect connectivity may be related to the emergence or disappearance of dendritic spines [167] or synapses [390].

Re-routing through changes in synaptic efficacy)

Figure 2.4 illustrates how activation of neuroplasticity can re-route information in neural networks. The same signal is sent simultaneously to both A and B cells. Since cell A is not sufficiently excited, the entire network that follows it will not receive the original signal. Only the neural network connected to neuron B will receive this information.

Altering the function of nerve cells through increased synaptic efficacy, a proliferation of synapses or through decreased thresholds could make it possible for the same input to elicit an EPSP that could exceed the threshold of the target cell marked A in Figure 2.4.

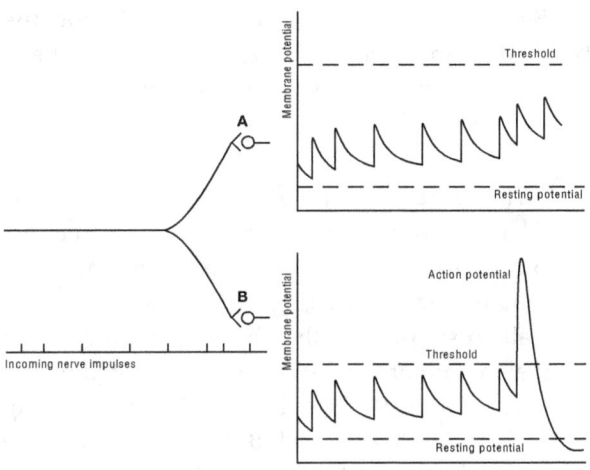

Figure 2.4. Illustration of how the same input to two neurons, each representing a separate pathway, causes one of the neurons (B) to open and the other (A) to remain unresponsive.

Making a cell that can normally not be activated functional (by unmasking it) can open a path that is normally closed (A in Figure 2.5) and thereby create new functional routes where information can travel to neuronal populations that normally do not receive such information.

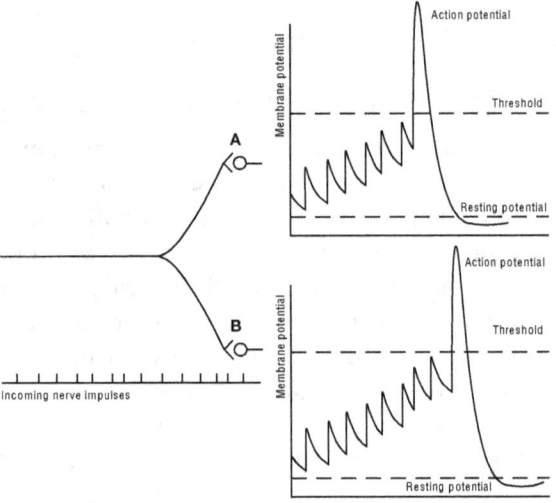

Figure 2.5. Re-routing by a change in impulse frequency.

Similar changes may be the basis for the observed changes in connectivity that have been described in some forms of tinnitus [592, 594] and in aging [596, 597].

Activity-induced re-routing

Changes in the way a nerve cell fire can affect which cells are activated. Increased firing rate such as occurs in burst firing (Figure 2.6), can also make both cells respond and thereby, allow information to travel in both of the pathways represented by the two cells (A and B). It is known that burst firing occurs in pathologies and it may explain some pathological changes that may occur in connection with re-routing in the central nervous system.

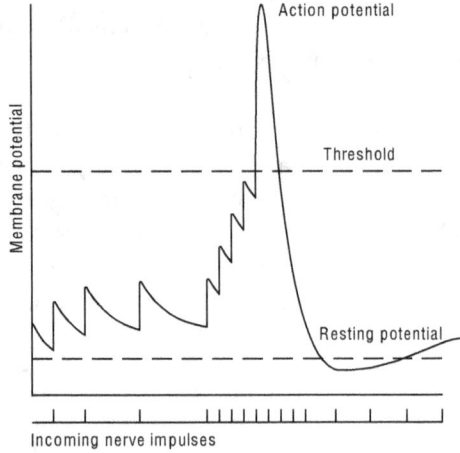

Figure 2.6. Hypothetical description of the effect of burst activity on the excitation of a cell.

The effect of a change in the input from continuous firing to burst firing is an example of how a change in input can make normally non-responsive cells respond and thereby opening new connections. Change from sustained activity to burst activity, is often seen in slightly injured nerves.

Impulses with short intervals, such as occur in burst activity, may generate EPSPs of sufficient amplitude to reach the threshold of a target neuron that normally was not activated by sustained activity (Figure 2.6). Changes in synaptic efficacy, changes in temporal integration or changes in the threshold of neurons can have the same effect. Changes in the relationship between inhibition and excitation can also make neurons respond to an input to which they normally do not respond.

Activity-induced plasticity

The extent of neuroplastic change in synapses that may occur is dependent on the level of presynaptic activation and the efficacy of a synapse, which in turn is influenced by that synapses history of activation. These historical patterns include activity-dependent synaptic plasticity, long-term potentiation (LPT), and long-term depression, (LTD).

Some of the anatomical and physiological bases for activity-induced neuroplasticity are expressed in Hebb's principle although that principle was first hypothesized in the context of learning before the neuroscience was known. Hebb's principle states [250] that neurons that are activated together may establish morphological connections. This indicates that increased neural connectivity is directly related to, and caused by neural activity. The concept is often summarized as "neurons that fire together, wire together." Also, an improvement in synaptic efficacy occurs when presynaptic inputs and postsynaptic activity are synchronized.

Hebbian plasticity

A Hebbian plasticity is a form of synaptic plasticity which creates positive feedback loops of activity-dependent changes in synaptic strength, that, in turn, cause perturbations in the stability of neuronal networks. Hebbian plasticity triggers long-lasting activity-dependent changes in synaptic strength resulting from both LTP and LTD.

These durable forms of plasticity require correlated precise and strong firing of the pre- and post-synaptic neurons specific to active input, and therefore are thought to facilitate the empowerment of particular synaptic connections [691].

Activity-dependent synaptic plasticity (Hebbian plasticity) involves regulation of ion channels in the membrane of the postsynaptic cell resulting in changes in membrane the potential of the cell.

The finding that changes occur in many auditory nuclei [162, 317], and in the cerebral cortex after deprivation [212] or by oversaturation [666] of auditory input implies that experience-dependent neuroplasticity (Hebbian plasticity) is more anatomically diffuse than earlier believed.

Studies in the rat have shown widespread changes in the molecular composition, and cellular morphology throughout the brainstem occur after modifications of auditory input [277].

These findings have implications for the treatment of hearing deficits through artificial stimulation (cochlear and brainstem implants) but are relevant to the study of the effects of novel stimulation (or absence of stimulation) in general.

Jenkins and colleagues [295] demonstrated how stimulation of the somatosensory system could change the way that body parts were mapped on the somatosensory cortex.

Are there plastic and non-plastic synapses?

It was shown in Chapter 1 that some functions are stable and not changeable through activation of neuroplasticity (hard-wired). Examples are the long-term memory, sexual preferences, personalities and some forms of handedness. The neural networks that control these functions are assumed to have synapses the efficacy of which cannot change. There is also evidence that synapses that are easy to change can be altered so that they become difficult to change. This is assumed to occur in memory circuits.

Initially, in early childhood development, the entire brain and spinal cord may be plastic, but through environmental and internal processes some parts may become hard-wired.

Acquiring new memory information requires synapses that have a great degree of plasticity, but then attain great stability to keep the information for a long time.

To complicate matters further, the contemporary view of nervous system functions is that some functions can be changed through activation of neuroplasticity, but once changed, the neural circuits become stable and show signs of being hard wired. This is particularly the case for creating a long-term memory. Memories require neuroplasticity to form, but the plastic synapses may have to become stable for the memory to be retained in the long term.

Therefore, it seems as there are two kinds of synapses, one the efficacy is easy to change and one that is hard to change, causing "hard-wired" neural networks. When first acquired, memories seem fragile for a short period, after which they become stable and gain the ability to last a long time [13].

It is relatively easy to activate memory, but after consolidation, some memories become very difficult to change or forget. It seems that the process of consolidation of memory induces a process that limits the plasticity of the synapses involved. Establishment of memories require synaptic plasticity but after a memory has been consolidated the degree of plasticity of some synapses seems to become very low.

The hypothesis that the degree of synaptic plasticity in memory circuits of the brain can change is supported by recent studies that suggest that memories are reconsolidated many times. Memories become labile during learning and rigid during consolidation. If learning happens to occur during retrieval, that newly learned information will become part of that memory during reconsolidation.

That memories go through rigid and labile phases implies that synaptic plasticity of a given network is variable. The identification of the process of memory reconsolidation has explained why memory storage is dynamic, and it has supported the hypothesis that the degree of synaptic plasticity if variable.

Is it that the factors necessary for maintaining synaptic plasticity are absent during memory consolidation or do some basic properties of the synapses in question change during memory consolidation? What about protein synthesis, which has also been shown to be plastic - can that remain plastic after memories have consolidated?

Although much of the molecular biology of neuroplasticity involving synaptic efficacy and synthesis of proteins in nerve cells is known, little is known about the molecular mechanisms that are responsible for maintaining a stable function or transforming a plastic function into a stable function.

Perhaps there is no specific action that causes synapses to become stable, other than the absence of a mechanism to cause them to adapt. Functional connections in the brain and the spinal cord depend on synapses being able to conduct the neural activity. If synapses can change from being plastic to being stable, it also explains which kinds of new connections in the brain can be established and why such connections can become permanent or at least very difficult to change.

Maladaptive neuroplasticity

It has been shown recently that maladaptive neuroplasticity plays important roles in creating the symptoms and signs of many different diseases. The most common diseases caused by activation of maladaptive neuroplasticity in the brain and the spinal cord are the chronic neuropathic pain, muscle spasm after spinal cord injuries (spasticity) and severe tinnitus [461] [444, 451]. Several factors can promote these processes; stress is one and another is inflammatory processes.

There is a growing body of evidence that indicate that maladaptive neuroplasticity together with activation of the immune system are involved in diseases such as fibromyalgia [487] and the chronic fatigue syndrome [113, 469]. Genetics (predisposition) is also involved in most of these processes.

There is increasing evidence that synaptic dysfunction (synaptopathy [359]) is a key factor in many neurodegenerative disorders including many forms of dementia. The contributions of neuroplasticity in the aging process may explain why some age-related neural deficits are influenced by a person's lifestyle. It has been suggested that the brain-derived neurotrophic factor (BDNF) that plays an important role in synaptic plasticity, synaptogenesis and synaptopathy may also play a role in forms of dementia such as Alzheimer's disease perhaps in connection with an effect of the immune system [372].

The fact that the risk factors for dementia are similar to the risk factors for cardiovascular diseases are important to consider when the pathology of these diseases is considered [55].

It has also been suggested that symptoms of diseases, such as Alzheimer's disease and other forms of dementia, may be explained by specific changes in connectivity in the brain [597]. Again, genetics (predisposition) is involved in most of these processes.

Sensitization

Sensitization can occur in the peripheral parts of the nervous system or the central nervous system and affect many neurological diseases. Sensitization is involved in pain and hyperactive disorders such as tinnitus and it can occur peripherally or centrally [461].

Peripheral sensitization in pain

Nociceptor sensitization can be caused by frequent repeat activations that reduce the threshold for depolarization that is needed to elicit an action potential in the afferent axon or by secretion of noradrenaline from sympathetic nerve endings located close to the receptor. Vanilloid receptors that are found in C fibers are important for this kind of sensitization.

Prostaglandins (PGE2), serotonin, bradykinin, epinephrine (EP), adenosine, and nerve growth factor (NGF) that act on receptors in the afferent axon can also promote sensitization at the receptor level [68]. Exposure to heat, capsaicin, or acidity can cause such peripheral sensitization (Figure 2.7).

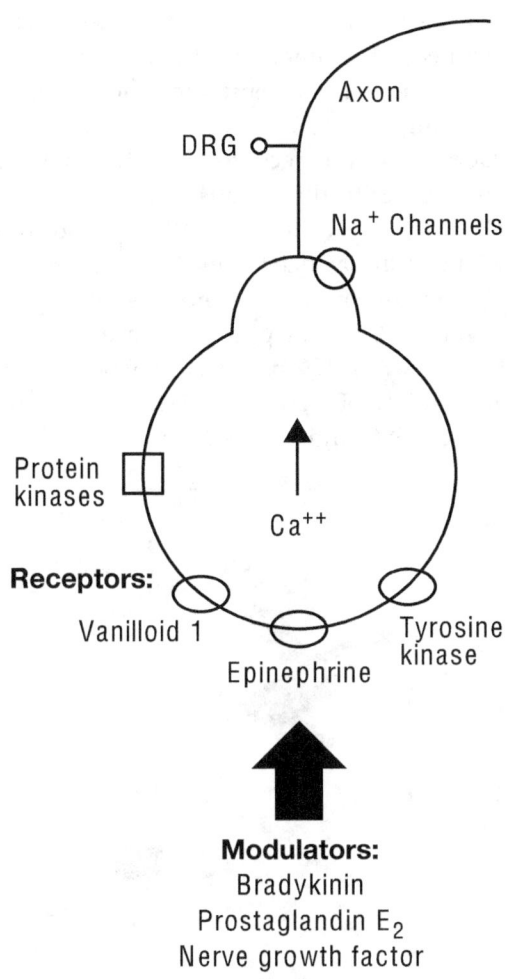

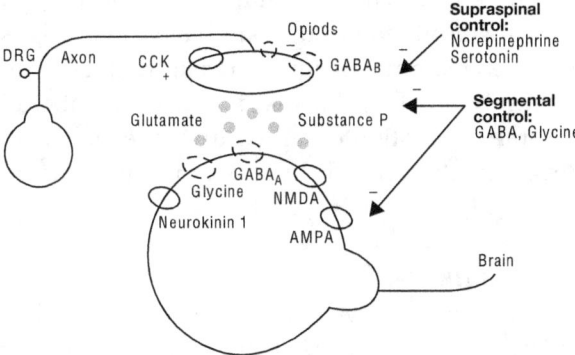

Figure 2.8 Nociceptive stimulation of a cell in the dorsal horn. Receptors and factors involved in central (spinal cord) sensitization. DRG: Dorsal root ganglia; NMDA: N-Methyl-D-aspartic acid (Based on [68] Artwork by Monica Javidnia).

Several receptors are involved in central sensitization, but the N-Methyl-D-aspartic acid (NMDA) receptor [68] (Figure 2.8) is especially important for sensitization to repeated noxious stimulations such as from heat and capsaicin. Vasoactive peptides, such as calcitonin, gene-related peptide (CGRP), substance P (SP), and neurokinin A, may also promote sensitization [68].

The NMDA receptor is involved in central sensitization to pain impulses [729] (Figure 2.8) [68] and triggers a cascade of events involving calcium. These events play an important role in creating the "wind-up" phenomenon. The release of SP and glutamate from intense, sustained noxious stimulation can cause a removal of the magnesium blockade of the NMDA calcium channel and EPSPs that last tens of seconds and [68].

Figure 2.7 Factors involved in peripheral sensitization. DRG: Dorsal root ganglia (Based on Bolay and Moskowitz, 2002 [68] (Artwork by Monica Javidnia).

Central sensitization of pain circuits

Central sensitization is evident from studies of pain [68, 731] [422] and studies of other hyperactive disorders such as tinnitus [210, 292, 455]. Central sensitization can occur at the level of the first neuron in the dorsal horn (Figure 2.8) (or the trigeminal nucleus) where cholecystokinin (CCK) enhances transmission of noxious stimulation while opioids and gamma-aminobutyric acid (GABA), cause decreased transmission by enhancing inhibition [68].

Temporal integration

A wind-up phenomenon is a form of exaggerated temporal integration where the response to stimulation is abnormally affected by a preceding stimulation. Central sensitization is involved in the wind-up phenomenon that has been studied in connection with pain [673, 729]. The wind-up phenomenon, an example of neuroplastic changes in central processing [68] is believed to be caused by repetitive firings of C fibers [673], and it changes the way neurons, such as the wide dynamic range neurons (WDR), respond.

Studies of temporal summation of painful electrical stimulation to the skin have shown signs of changed temporal integration in individuals with pain disorders [442]. This is similar to the altered temporal summation observed in connection with neuroplasticity related hyperactivity in sensory systems [212, 666].

The dopamine pathway

Local inhibitory circuits may act as key regulators of synaptic changes during motor learning, memory consolidation and retrieval [111].

Moreover, it has been proposed that the mesocortical dopaminergic pathway connecting the VTA with the M1 is essential for successful motor skill learning [266].

Dopamine D1 receptors (D1Rs) have been shown to be critically involved in LTP induction, and D2 receptors (D2Rs) mediate spine addition in the M1 [230]. It has been suggested that dopamine receptor activity influences motor skill acquisition and synaptic LTP via phospholipase C signaling [556]. The cAMP/PKA pathway may be involved in the acquisition of new motor skills [537]. (For a review, see [586] and Figure 2.9).

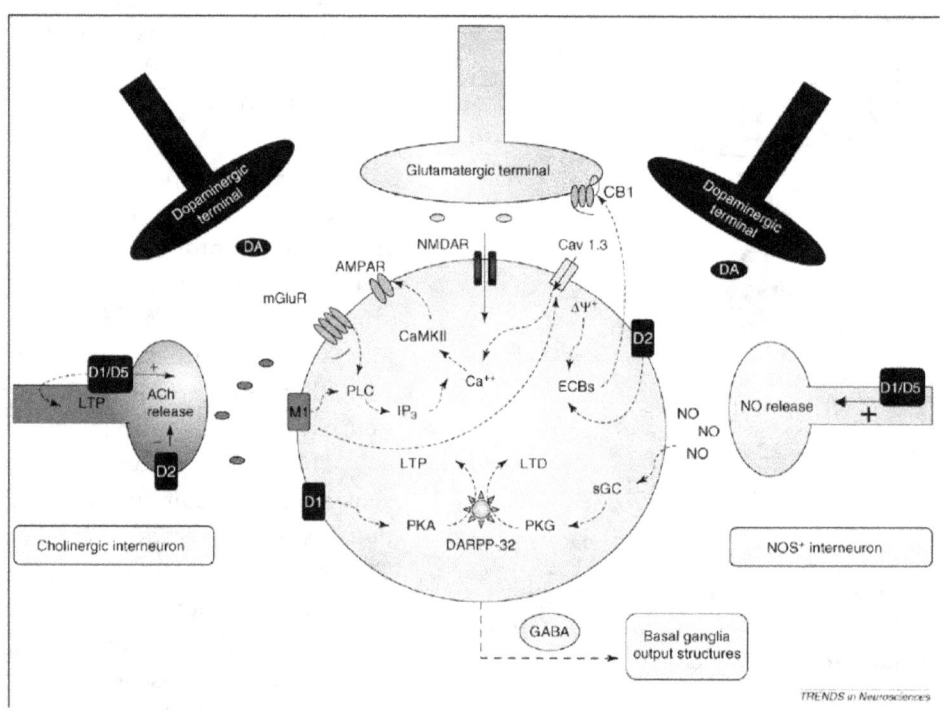

Figure 2.9 Dopamine-mediated regulation of corticostriatal synaptic plasticity.
CaMKII, Ca 2+ –calmodulin-dependent kinase II; CB1, cannabinoid receptor 1; IP 3, inositol 1,4,5 trisphosphate; PKG, protein kinase G; sGC, soluble guanylyl.

The striatum plays an important role in neuroplasticity

The caudate nucleus and the putamen are often referred to collectively as the striatum or neostriatum. The striatum receives glutamatergic and dopaminergic input from many sources. It coordinates cognition, motor and action planning, decision-making and motivation and it is a part of the reward system.

The striatum plays important roles in disorders such as addiction, Parkinson's disease and bipolar disorders of various kinds and it represents the main input into the basal ganglia. Neurons projecting from the striatum receive a large convergence of afferents from all areas of the cortex and transmit neural information to the basal ganglia output structures. Corticostriatal transmission is essential in the regulation of voluntary movement, in addition to behavioral control, cognitive function and reward mechanisms.

Section 2
Beneficial Effects of Activation of Neuroplasticity

The beneficial effects of expression of neuroplasticity can be divided into three main groups:

1. Makes the nervous system adapt to changing demands throughout life.

2. Re-routing of information. Necessary for normal postnatal development

3. It can compensate for a loss of function and reorganize the nervous system to replace lost functions.

Many of the functions of the spinal cord and the brain are plastic. This makes it possible to learn new skills, adjust excitability of reflexes, and change the routing of information in the spinal cord and the brain. Neuroplasticity also makes it possible to change how sensory stimuli are processed.

Proper activation of neuroplasticity is important for childhood development. An adequate input to the sensory nervous systems during the first years of life is essential for normal development of the sensory nervous systems, and if not provided, the normal function of the sensory systems cannot be achieved after what is known as the critical period has elapsed [615] [324]. The question about the importance of the critical period has been the object of much research, particularly in the auditory and the visual systems where the development of auditory prostheses (cochlear and cochlear nucleus implants) have been studied extensively. Kral (2013) [334] further elaborated on the topic of the critical period, suggesting that the most important developmental effect of experience is the maturation of "naïve cortical networks" into those that are capable of categorization [334].

This section describes how neuroplasticity may provide benefits to a person.

Chapter 3

Adaptation to Changing Demands

Abstract

1. New skills that has been learned through activation of neuroplasticity such as bicycling, how to pronounce unfamiliar words, singing, etc. do not need to be recalled, are always available. This is in contrast to memorized matters which have to be recalled and can be forgotten.

2. Neuroplasticity can make the nervous system adapt to changing demands such as in adaptation to prostheses (cochlear and cochlear nucleus implants and different kinds of limb prostheses).

3. Pathologies that have been caused by injuries to the nervous system such as occurs after ischemic strokes or other kinds of changes in the function of the nervous system may be compensated for by redirecting information to intact structures by inducing expression of neuroplasticity.

4. Physical training is an important means for inducing beneficial neuroplasticity that can alleviate the symptoms of some plasticity diseases.

5. Alleviating the symptoms of diseases caused by activation of bad (maladaptive) neuroplasticity is now being studied for treating of plasticity disorders.

Introduction

The ability of the nervous system to adapt to changing demands by activating neuroplasticity is present throughout life, but it is most prominent in childhood. That the ability to reorganize the nervous system is greater in the immature nervous system than in the mature nervous system was first demonstrated in the classical studies by Wiesel and Hubel [714] who discovered existence of "critical periods" where the nervous system can most easily be molded by input to the organism [324, 334, 615]. Some investigators have called this form of neuroplasticity "environmental regulation of nervous system development" [571].

The efficiency of this process varies among different persons, and it takes considerably longer time with increasing age. For example, above the age of 60 years, recovery from a loss of vestibular function is normally incomplete while a 20-year-old person who loses vestibular function will recover good function within weeks. The lack of efficiency of neuroplasticity is responsible for much of the decline of vestibular functions such as posture control and proprioception associated with old age.

Adaptation to the use of prostheses

The proper use of prostheses of any kind requires adaptation of the nervous system. What is often known as "learning" is in fact caused by activation of neuroplasticity. Adaptation to artificial limbs includes reprogramming of the motor system. This occurs during training, and it is maintained without the needs of being recalled. Training is an effective means to activate neuroplasticity to acquire proper adaptation to the use of prostheses and activating the nucleus of Meynert facilitate this process. Activity in the afferent fibers of the vagus nerve can also promote and facilitate neuroplasticity because the target cells in the nucleus of the solitary tract project to the nucleus of Meynert. This means that structures in the gut where receptors that are innervated by the vagus nerve are located can influence neuroplasticity.

The ability to change the function of the brain and the spinal cord is greater in young individuals than in adults, and there are some changes that can be made in the brain of young individuals that cannot be made in adults.

Studies of children who had cochlear implants show that the critical period for hearing is the first 3-4 years after birth [615]. The critical period for vision has been reported to be 2-3 years [253] (see Chapter 1).

Any facilitation of the ability to make plastic changes would naturally be welcome in that it will reduce the need for physical therapy and other forms of training that are required for optimal use of prostheses.

The findings that activity in the afferent part of the vagus nerve can facilitate activation of neuroplasticity may in the future lead to methods that use electrical stimulation of the vagus nerve as a practical way of speed up adaptation to the use of many kinds of prostheses.

Recovery from traumatic brain damage and strokes

Trauma of various kind and ischemic strokes cause damage of various degrees to specific regions of the brain. Activation of neuroplasticity is the main basis for the recovery of motor and other functions that occur during days and months after the loss of the function of brain tissue. Re-routing of information to and from regions of the brain that has been rendered non-functional to intact regions that may perform the same functions as those that have lost normal function are the most important benefits from activation of neuroplasticity after brain damage.

It has been known for many years that physical and cognitive training can speed up these plastic changes in motor and cognitive functions through activation of neuroplasticity.

Recent animal studies have indicated that electrical stimulation of the vagus nerve improves recovery of motor functions after experimentally induced stroke by making physical training more effective [315]. Animal experiments have shown that electrical stimulation of the vagus nerve paired with forelimb use can recovery from experimentally induced brain injuries from ischemic stroke faster by facilitating plasticity [532].

Other beneficial effects of expression of neuroplasticity

Not all beneficial effects of neuroplasticity have been fully explored. For example, the finding that auditory stimulation can slow age-related hearing loss [722] might be a sign that activation of neuroplasticity is involved in creating this kind of hearing loss. The same may be the case for the "toughening" of ears regarding susceptibility to noise-induced hearing loss. James Miller discovered this paradoxical phenomenon in 1963 [420] [99, 420].

The use of electrical stimulation of the cerebral cortex to enhance the effect of training is another example of the beneficial effect of expression of neuroplasticity explored recently [134]. The mechanisms of the beneficial effect of sound exposure on age-related hearing loss may be similar to that of sound exposure that can reduce noise-induced hearing loss (NIHL) ("toughening of the ear") [721]. That effect may be caused by changes in the central nervous system and mediated through activation of neuroplasticity.

The extensive efferent innervation of outer hair cells [646] may also be involved in some of these mechanisms because this innervation of outer hair cells makes it possible to control the function of the outer hair cells through descending neural activity. This means that input from the central nervous system, can affect the mechanical properties of the ear.

In Chapter 7 we discuss recent studies that indicate that induction of neuroplasticity can reverse harmful plastic changes that cause tinnitus and how that effect can be enhanced by electrical stimulation of the vagus nerve.

Chapter 4

Postnatal Development

Abstract

1. The central nervous system is not fully developed at birth.

2. The last part of the nervous system to develop is the from part of the cerebral cortex and that is not fully developed until the age of 18-22 years.

3. Elimination and creation of new synapses are extensive during the first few years of life. There is a net loss of synapses and nerve cells in the brain during that time.

4. Some of the early changes may be controlled by programs that are established before birth.

5. During the later parts of the childhood development expression of neuroplasticity plays a fundamental role, and for development to proceed normally, sensory input is required as is the use of the motor systems.

Introduction

Perhaps the greatest advantage from neuroplasticity is its role in the postnatal development. The nervous system of a newborn child is relatively immature compared to that of many newborn animals. (Newborn foals, for example, can walk on their first day and so can calves). In contrast, the immature nervous systems of newborn children organize and adapt according to needs established by inputs from the environment [300]. It is also noteworthy that the brain is not fully developed until the age of 18-22 years.

Exposure to environmental signals is critical for the normal development of the nervous system and establishing of the normal neural functions including that of sensory functions. The classical studies of ocular dominance by Wiesel and Hubel [714] demonstrated the importance of visual input for normal development of the visual nervous system.

Postnatal deprivation of auditory sensory input causes neural degeneration of the cerebral cortex in a layer-specific manner but can be partly avoided by electrical stimulation of the auditory nerve in the cochlea [334].

These findings have been confirmed and extended in many later studies, (see for example [571]) confirming that adequate stimulation is necessary for the normal functional and anatomical development of many parts of the nervous system.

Normal postnatal development

Normal postnatal development requires a programmed expression of neuroplasticity that is influenced by external events, and by internal neural activity. Some of these changes are programmed (genetic guidance), and some are caused by expression of neuroplasticity evoked by sensory input [334] and most likely also by motor activity.

During the first years of life, a considerable pruning of nerve cells (programmed cell death) and synapses occur in the brain and the spinal cord. These processes may be regarded a form of plastic changes in the function of many neural circuits induced by external or internal events or the changes may be programmed.

Studies of the auditory system have shown that programmed cell death, the formation of new connections or elimination of connections [100] and changes in synaptic efficacy are all parts of the normal postnatal development of the central nervous system [579].

It has also been shown that children with autism spectrum disorders have more nerve cells and more densely packed neurons in the brain than people who do not have autism. This is regarded to be caused by a failure in the pruning process that normally occurs in early childhood as a part of the "midcourse correction".

The auditory system is anatomically organized according to the frequency of sounds, and such frequency maps exist throughout the auditory system including the various auditory regions of the cerebral cortices (see [459]). It is assumed that these maps are the result of the frequency selectivity of the basilar membrane of the cochlea causing excitation of the sensory cells in a way that is related the frequency of the sounds that reach the ear. It is also assumed that the resulting tonotopic organization of the nervous system together with the frequency tuning of individual nerve cells is important for proper processing of auditory information.

A cochlear implant does not generate the same frequency maps as the normal cochlea, and the nervous system must, therefore, go through appropriate re-organization to make it possible to discriminate sounds through the use of cochlear and cochlear nucleus implants. Since the frequency maps created in the auditory nervous system are important for discrimination of sounds such as speech sounds, the nervous system must reorganize after implantation of such auditory prostheses to achieve a mapping of the central nervous system is by the activation that the cochlear implants provide.

It is not known if the normal frequency maps are created in response to sound stimulation during postnatal development, or are independent of sound stimulation. (Deaf animals that have been deprived stimulation of the auditory nerve have only a rudimentary cochleotopic organization in brainstem nuclei [251] and the auditory cortex according to some studies [243]). This may explain why adaptation to cochlear implants is different in individuals who were born deaf and those who became deaf after hearing experience.

Little is known about the role of neuroplasticity in the development of motor skills. The basics of walking, for example, is programmed in the spinal cord (locomotory control pattern generator), but dexterity and other manual skills require adaptation to demands and depend on learning; it, therefore, requires the expression of neuroplasticity.

The development of subtle facial expressions from the massive face-wide movements of young children may be a sign of the postnatal organization that involves the severing of functional connections within the facial motonuclei. The mass movements occur because of functional connections between the neural network that controls movements of mimic muscles in the face.

Older children, in whom some of the anatomical connections from early childhood are no longer functional (synapses becoming dormant), can control these muscle groups independently. These connections that become dormant during postnatal development may become activated during adult life because of for example disease processes. The synkinesis that is present in people with hemifacial spasm, or after recovery from facial trauma, are signs of abnormal functional connections between innervations of groups of the mimic muscles.

The enhanced ability to activate neuroplasticity in children can also make their central nervous systems more vulnerable to injuries and pediatric neurological disorders [303]. Impaired plasticity may lead to symptoms and signs of various kinds where cognitive impairments play import roles. Excessive activation of neuroplasticity may lead to maladaptation of various kinds.

These matters are extremely complex, and the expression of abnormalities depends on many factors such as genetics, epigenetics and environmental factors of various kinds and have not until recently attracted much attention.

Effects of errors in postnatal development

Errors in the normal postnatal development may cause abnormalities in various kinds of neural functions. Failure to block synapses and inadequate pruning of the nervous system may play a role in developmental disorders of many different kinds such as schizophrenia and autism [386, 447]. Similar errors may cause disorders that can manifest later in life such as neurodegenerative disorders including Alzheimer's and Huntington's diseases.

Whether programmed cell death is entirely genetically controlled or, more likely, controlled by a combination of environmental and internal factors, has been debated, especially as it regards disorders such as autism [386]. There are critical periods regarding vulnerability to insults from environmental factors that can interfere with normal postnatal development [555] just as there are critical periods regarding the necessity of sensory input for normal postnatal development.

It was recognized early that input to a cell during early postnatal development is important for adequate protein synthesis within the cell [80].

Studies in the avian auditory system have shown that changes in auditory receptors cause changes in neurons in the auditory brainstem [74] and alter protein synthesis in these neurons [623].

Rapid changes in protein synthesis, ribosome production, and ribosomal RNA has been demonstrated to occur in the chick cochlear nuclei [623] after ablation of the cochlea.

The hypothesis that synaptic input to these neurons is important in regulating their protein synthesis and metabolism was supported by the finding that administering of a neurotoxin (Tetrodotoxin, TTX) causes similar changes as ablation of the cochlea and changes in protein synthesis seem to be the earliest cellular sign of reduced input to nerve cells [276]. Also, protease activity is beginning to become recognized as an important factor in regulating the activity of nerve cells [675].

Importance of sensory stimulation for normal postnatal development

Auditory input is necessary for normal childhood development of the auditory nervous system [334]. It has been documented in animal studies that absence of input to the auditory system, such as that occurs in congenital deafness, can cause anatomical and functional abnormalities in the primary auditory cortex, altering postnatal development [324]. Inadequate stimulation probably also interferes with other aspects of childhood development of the nervous system.

Reduced sensory input can affect normal childhood development of sensory systems. For example, hearing loss due to middle ear pathologies that often occur in childhood decreases sound transmission to the cochlea. This can result in impaired language development because of lack of (or reduced) input to the central nervous system during the postnatal development.

Development of the perception of "self."

Many factors are involved in the creation of the perception of "self." Loss of a body part such as from amputation of a limb affects the perception of "self." The brain keeps maps of the body, the position of body parts and movements of the body.

These maps are important for the perception of "self", and they are constantly updated by sensory input from all parts of the body and the environment. Input from the motor system including proprioceptive systems also contributes to the creation and updating of the maps related to the perceptions of "self." If that does not occur correctly, severe disturbances of normal neural functions may result. Deprivation of sensory input is a common cause of failure to properly update these maps.

Establishment of perception of "self" is a complex process with components involved. There are indications that for example oxytocin may enable activation the neuroplasticity necessary for acquiring a generative model of the emotional and social "self" [123] [191].

Development of social attachment

Pair bonding between mates, parental (both maternal and paternal) care toward offspring and the influences of the social environment on those behaviors have been well described. It develops early in life, and some understanding of the neuroscience of that process has been achieved [539]. Development of these features requires activation of neuroplasticity, and that is associated with liberation of molecules such as oxytocin, dopamine, and vasopressin. Oxytocin plays an important role in creating and forming a person's socio-sexual behavior.

Plasticity in the maternal brain

Activation of neuroplasticity in the parts of the brain that regulates maternal mental capacity and caregiving concerns many neural circuits including the nuclei of the amygdala, the dorsal anterior cingulate cortex (dACC), the ventral (vACC) and the prefrontal cortex (PFC). Extensive processing occurs in the amygdala, insula, ventral striatum, and in structures that are related to the cortical executive function (dorsolateral prefrontal cortex, DLPFC). Empathy is associated with the medial prefrontal cortex (MPFC), precuneus, superior temporal sulcus circuits (Figure 4.1).

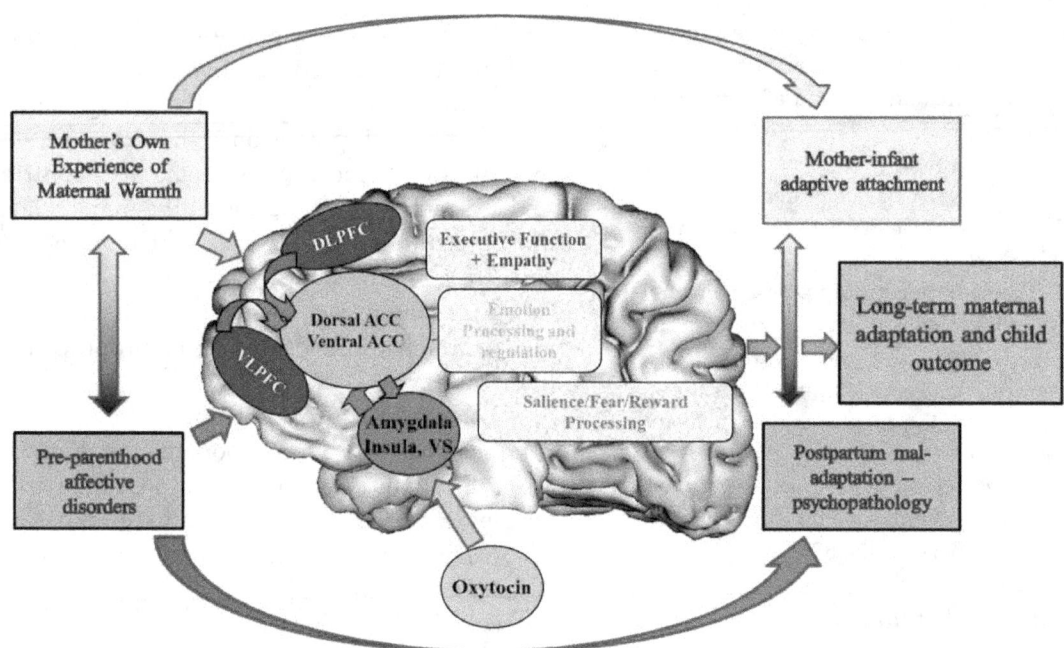

Figure 4.1. Schematic illustration of neural circuits that regulate maternal mental capacity and caregiving outcomes including the amygdala, the dorsal anterior cingulate cortex (ACC), the ventral ACC. The picture shows how salience/fear/motivation processing involves the amygdala, the insula, the ventral striatum (VS) working with the cortical executive function, the ventrolateral prefrontal cortex (VLPFC), the dorsolateral prefrontal cortex (DLPFC). Circuits involving empathy, the medial prefrontal cortex (MPFC), the precuneus, the superior temporal sulcus are also shown. From [318] (adapted from **Moses-Kolko et al., 2014**).

Oxytocin

Oxytocin and vasopressin are released from the pituitary gland into the blood circulation. Oxytocin has many functions that are related to reproduction; it regulates peripheral functions such as the milk letdown reflex and uterine contractions in females as well as vasoconstriction and water retention in both males and females. Oxytocin is perhaps best known for its use to induce uterus contractions in a pregnant woman.

Oxytocin and vasopressin are also released throughout the brain to regulate a variety of complex social behaviors including social recognition, mating, bonding, parenting, and social buffering [667]. Thus, it has been shown that positive social interaction such as physical contact is associated with oxytocin release.

Oxytocin reduces amygdala and HPA axis reactivity to social stressors (demonstrated by the inhibitory arrow in Figure 4.1), and as such it is an important mediator of the anxiolytic and stress-protective effects of positive social interaction ("social buffering").

Oxytocin influences the function of the amygdala, specifically it augments the gain in the amygdala and attenuates sensory precision in the hypothalamus. As a mediator of successful reproduction oxytocin plays a crucial role in establishing a normal socio-sexual behavior not only affecting the reproductive system but also in other parts of the brain.

Female offspring of monkeys [240] that experience stress and anxiety during early postnatal days tend to display poor maternal care behavior later on in life.

Parental care mediates the effects of environmental adversity on the development of the nervous system and, therefore, early postnatal experiences may subdue the genetic predispositions [408] [155].

Oxytocin mediates a top-down modulation, and it may play a role similar to other modulators of NMDA receptor function—not only in the cerebral cortex but also in the autonomic nervous system and associated subcortical regions of the brain.

Acquisition or learning of hierarchical models may depend upon oxytocin dependent selection of cues with interoceptive associations or significance in the environment.

Oxytocin, dopamine and vasopressin

Figure 4.2 shows some similarities and some differences between the effects of oxytocin and vasopressin in the rat.

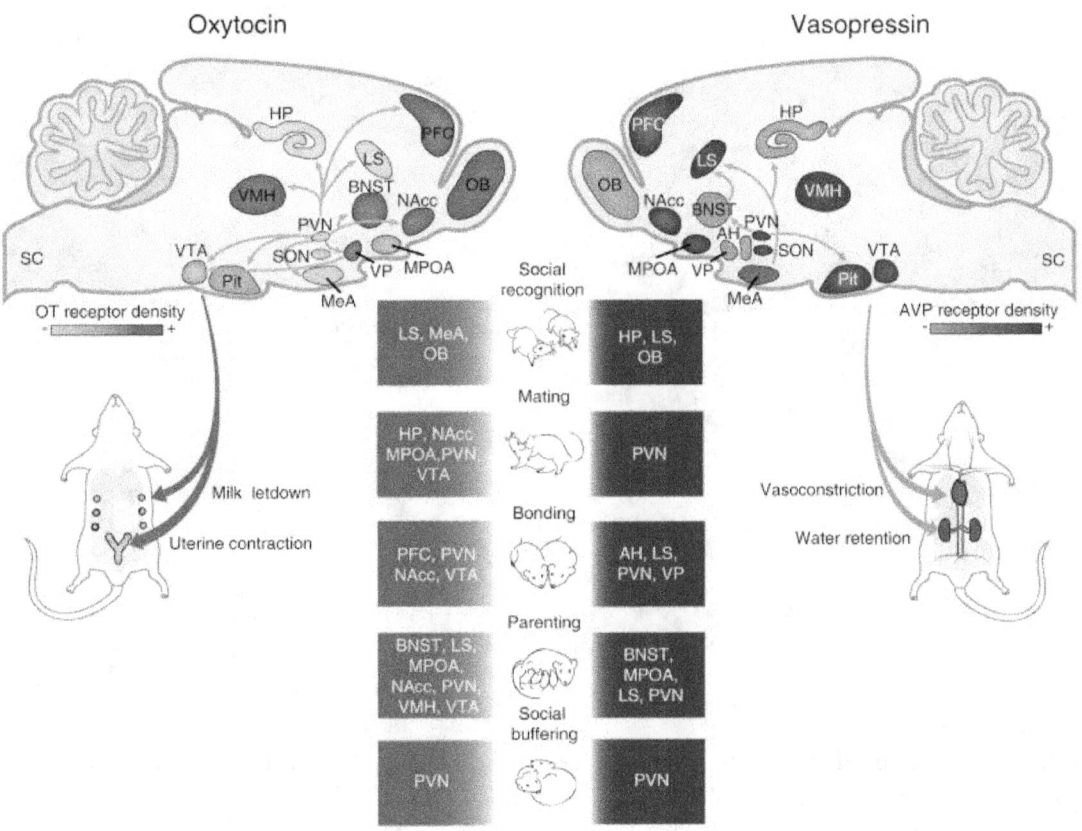

Figure 4.2 Schematic drawings of sagittal brain sections of a rodent (the prairie vole) showing the anatomical locations of oxytocin cells (OT, left) and vasopressin cells (AVP, right) and their projections to selected brain regions that are regarded to be important in social behaviors. The distribution and regional density of OT receptors and AVP receptors in the brain ([667]).

Abbreviations: AH, anterior hypothalamus; BNST, bed nucleus of the stria terminalis; HP, hippocampus; LS, lateral septum; MeA medial amygdala. MPOA, the medial preoptic area of the hypothalamus; NAcc, nucleus accumbens; OB, olfactory bulb; PFC, prefrontal cortex; Pit, pituitary gland; SON, supraoptic nucleus; VMH, ventromedial hypothalamus; VP, ventral pallidum; VTA, ventral tegmental area.

The anatomical basis for the similarities between the role of oxytocin in modulating the precision of signals produced within an organism, especially in the gut and other internal organs and the role of dopamine in modulating proprioceptive signals are depicted in Figure 4.3. This figure also illustrates some of the similarities and differences between the actions of oxytocin and dopamine.

Comparative anatomy of Oxytocin and Dopaminergic systems

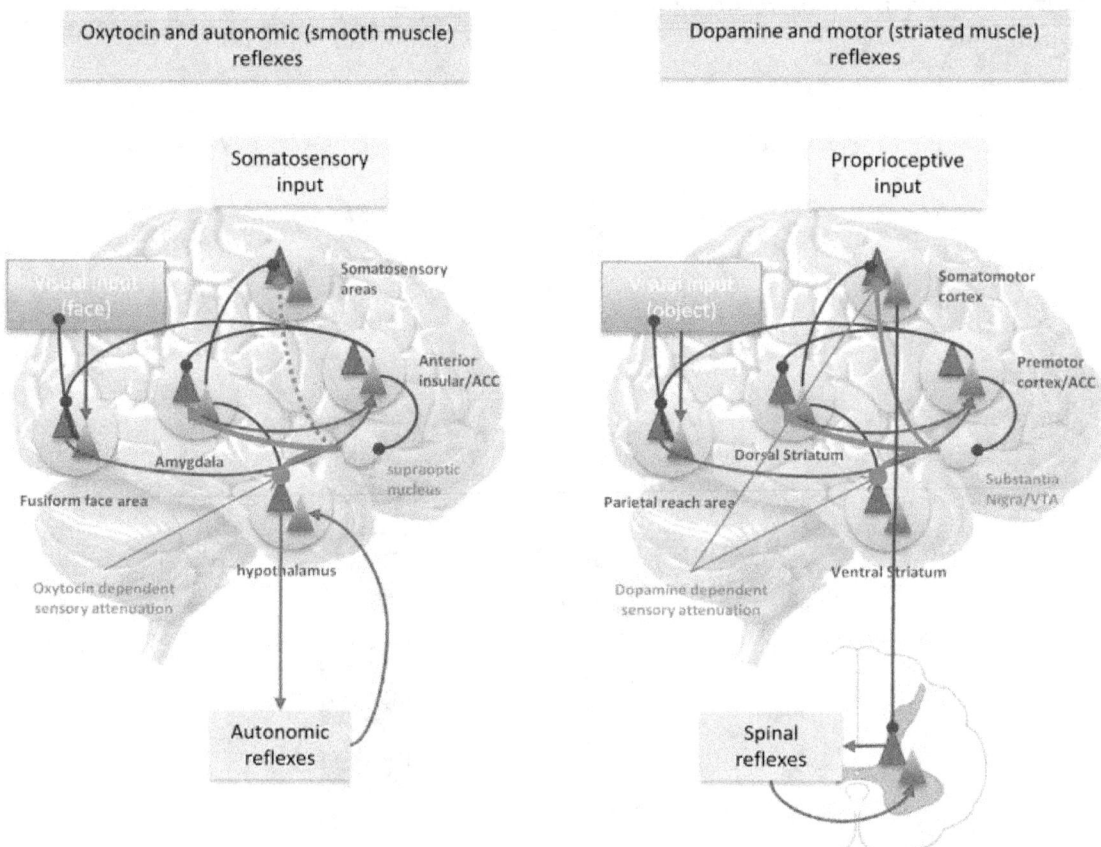

Figure 4.3 The overall architecture depicted here emphasizes the similarity between the effect of oxytocin and dopamine regarding opposing neuromodulatory roles. From: [539].

The actions of oxytocin have many similarities with the actions of dopamine [539]. Dopamine has the same complementary effects as oxytocin in the dorsal and ventral striatum, mediated by D1 (go pathway) and D2 (no-go pathway) receptors, respectively. Deficits of oxytocin may lead to a failure of interoceptive processing, while deficits of dopamine (for example in Parkinson's disease) compromise proprioceptive processing and the initiation of action.

Vasopressin has a similar effect as oxytocin (left-hand side of Figure 4.3) [667] and those of dopamine (right-hand side of Figure 4.3). Oxytocin augments the gain in the amygdala and attenuates sensory precision in the hypothalamic region.

Oxytocin augment the gain in the amygdala and attenuate sensory precision in the hypothalamic region. For dopamine, the same complementary effects are illustrated in the dorsal and ventral striatum, mediated by D1 (go pathway) and D2 (no-go pathway) receptors, respectively.

Deficits in oxytocin and dopamine

It has been suggested that deficits of oxytocin lead to a failure of interoceptive processing, while deficits of dopamine (for example in Parkinson's disease) compromise proprioceptive processing and the initiation of action) ([539]).

Melatonin

Melatonin is a hormone secreted primarily by the pineal gland but also other organs contribute such as the gut, retina, and leukocytes produced melatonin. Melatonin is involved in circadian rhythms, it is controlled by light and secretion increases when it is dark. It does not induce sleep but it signals when it is time to sleep. Melatonin is involved in sleep disturbances, especially because it is suppressed by light [62].

In some people, especially elderly persons, the pineal gland may not secrete adequate amounts of melatonin and taking melatonin as a supplement may help such people to sleep.

Melatonin is an antioxidant; it boosts the immune system, and it has been shown to decrease the risk of some cancers such as breast cancer [564]. Melatonin also has some effects on mood disturbances. Melatonin has a beneficial effect on memory deficits and possibly other symptoms in Alzheimer's disease and other dementias [18].

The role of the insular lobe

The insular cortex holds a primary position in interoception and is thought to mediate the integration and associative learning that underlies higher level interoceptive inference [130]. The prefrontal cortex (e.g., anterior cingulate and ventromedial prefrontal region) can then integrate the ensuing representations as part of hierarchical inference that underlies emotional awareness, regarding that the brain works as a prediction machine [611].

Section 3
Harmful Effects of Plastic Changes "Plasticity Disorders."

Historically, the search for the cause of a disorder of the nervous system has been focused on finding morphological or chemical abnormalities. In the past, it was assumed that diseases were caused by malfunction of a specific region of the brain. One of the first scientists to find an adverse effect of plastic changes was Goddard. He delivered electrical current to the amygdala of rats daily. At first, there were no visible reactions, but after 4-6 weeks of treatment, the electrical current began to evoke epileptic seizures [218]. Goddard likened the reaction he saw to the lighting of a fire, and he called it a "kindling" reaction. Later, it was shown to occur in many other parts of the brain [693].

We know today that systemic malfunction is often the cause of disease. The symptoms and signs of many disorders of the nervous system are caused by changes in the function of some circuits in the brain or the spinal cord and not caused by morphological or chemical abnormalities as earlier believed.

The role of network dysfunctions in neurological disorders has recently been recognized, and there is now a consensus that network dysfunctions are related to many disorders of the sensory and the motor systems. The list of such disorders seems to increase as more research is done. Bad neuroplasticity (maladaptive neuroplasticity) can explain the changes in the function of specific neural circuits are caused by

Chronic neuropathic pain is an example of how harmful neuroplasticity can create dysfunctional neural networks in the brain by disrupting default-mode network dynamics (DMND).

Phantom sensations are typical signs of maladaptive neuroplasticity in sensory and pain systems. Chronic neuropathic pain is a typical phantom sensation as are many forms of severe tinnitus.

Maladaptive neuroplasticity is an important component in the cause of the sensations of pain. In these diseases sensations, sound, and pain are referred to a different location of the body than that where the neural activity that causes the pain is generated [475].

Phantom sensations are sensations that are created by neural activity in the brain without the contributions from neural activity from sense organs. It is now believed that altered connections are responsible for these systemic malfunctions. Recent studies indicate that changes in connections between different parts of the brain are involved in age-related changes [42, 596] and in causing symptoms of many diseases.

Phantom sensations may be created in connection with cortical sensory reorganization [399]. Some of the symptoms of these pathologies can be explained by incorrect mapping in structures of the brain. It has been shown that this can be corrected by the use of appropriate visual sensory input, such as using a "mirror box" [544] that also has been described for treatment of some forms of phantom limb pain [106].

The phantom limb syndrome is one of the clearest examples of adverse sensations that are a result of activation of neuroplasticity causing abnormal neural activity in the central nervous system while the sensations are referred to specific peripheral location. Phantom limb sensations consist of pain, paresthesia and other abnormal sensations.

Typical symptoms and signs of disorders that are caused by expression of maladaptive neuroplasticity are a chronic neuropathic pain, some forms of tinnitus, spasticity and different kinds of hyperactive motor disorders.

Neuroplasticity is involved in creating the symptoms of other diseases such as fibromyalgia [487], and probably also diseases such as chronic fatigue syndrome.

Recent studies present evidence that maladaptive neuroplasticity may also play a central role in the creation of the symptoms of disorders such as whiplash, headaches, chronic pelvic pain syndrome and some forms of osteoarthritis, low back pain, epicondylitis, shoulder pain and cancer pain [496].

Even such sensory deficits as presbycusis (age-related hearing loss) have a central component [663] most likely caused by plastic changes. Hearing loss from noise exposure has earlier been ascribed to morphological changes in the cochlea, but studies have shown evidence of a central component of that hearing loss [397, 661].

There is now increasing evidence that more and more neurological diseases are associated with network malfunction, and these changes in function are brought about by activation of neuroplasticity. The cause of many congenital diseases such as autism and spina bifida seems to be established before birth and in fact early in pregnancy.

In addition to causing the distinctive symptoms of a disease activation of maladaptive neuroplasticity can cause many adverse effects through changes in the processing of sensory information causing symptoms such as hyperpathia, allodynia, hyperacusis, etc.

Since symptoms of "plasticity disorders" are not associated with morphological changes that can be detected by present clinical diagnostic methods, the disorders have not received the attention deserved. No tests have yet been designed that can detect and measure the changes in the brain that cause plasticity disorder such as chronic neuropathic pain, some forms of severe tinnitus, spasticity, the phantom limb symptoms and other neurological disorders. That activation of neuroplasticity can cause symptoms and signs of disorders of the nervous system have therefore received less attention than morphological abnormalities. Also, research has been driven by what could be seen and what could be measured, and that is one of the reasons for the lack of research efforts regarding disorders such as pain and tinnitus.

Traditional imaging methods such as MRI are not suitable for studies of such changes in function and methods to determine the strength of functional connectivity is now a valuable tool in studying pathological signs of network dysfunction. Methods that can determine the strength of connections are beginning to emerge in research connections, and these methods may, therefore, become parts of the clinical diagnostic methods in the future.

Inducing expression of neuroplasticity is an effective means for treating some disorders of the nervous system. Training is the most common form of intervention that causes expression of neuroplasticity, but also hypnosis has its action through activation of neuroplasticity. It has now become evident that these actions to activate neuroplasticity can be made more effective when supplemented by different forms of electrical stimulation of the nervous system.

However, more effective methods are needed for treatment of plasticity disorders such as chronic neuropathic pain and severe tinnitus. Finding a beneficial treatment for plasticity disorder such as chronic neuropathic pain and tinnitus and perhaps also diseases such as fibromyalgia and the chronic fatigue syndrome may be within reach through neuroscience research [379, 487, 496] and specifically through the development of methods for reversing maladaptive neuroplasticity. Especially electrical stimulation of the vagus nerve is now studied extensively especially for reversing the neuroplastic changes that are involved in plasticity disorders.

In this section, we will discuss some specific disorders for which there is evidence that neuroplasticity may play a major role. The first part of this section (Chapter 5) is a general discussion of how activation of neuroplasticity can cause symptoms and signs of the diseases we call "plasticity diseases." The role of the immune system is also discussed in this chapter.

The two following chapters will discuss chronic neuropathic pain (Chapter 6) and severe tinnitus (Chapter 7) in more detail. The final chapter, Chapter 9, covers maladaptive neuroplasticity regarding the phantom limb syndrome, spasticity and some forms of muscle spasm.

Chapter 5

Neuroplasticity as a Cause of Symptoms and Signs of Diseases

Abstract

1. In this book, we will use the term plasticity disorders to describe disorders where activation of neuroplasticity causes the signs and symptoms of diseases.

2. The abnormal neural activity that causes symptoms and signs is a result of activity in dysfunctional networks in the spinal cord or the brain, brought about by activation of maladaptive neuroplasticity.

3. The symptoms are phantom sensations such as pain, tingling, and other abnormal sensations and abnormal muscle activity.

4. Phantom sensations are caused by activity in the central nervous system that occurs without input from sensory receptors.

5. Chronic neuropathic pain, severe tinnitus, phantom limb syndrome, and spasticity are common plasticity disorders.

6. There is now strong evidence that activation of maladaptive neuroplasticity is the root cause of several other diseases such as fibromyalgia, and possibly also the chronic fatigue syndrome.

7. It is possible that maladaptive neuroplasticity is involved in many other disorders such as whiplash, headache, chronic pelvic pain syndrome and some forms of osteoarthritis, low back pain, epicondylitis, shoulder pain and cancer pain.

8. Commonly used diagnostic methods cannot identify the pathology of plasticity disorders which are mainly functional. The symptoms of plasticity disorders are often cryptic not directing attention to a specific anatomical location.

9. The pathology of plasticity disorders is functional and there are no morphological or chemical abnormalities that can be identified by clinical tests.

10. Plasticity disorders are difficult to treat successfully but functional changes are likely to be reversible and, therefore, it may become possible to alleviate pain and tinnitus and other plasticity disorders without conventional treatment using medications or surgery.

11. Many plasticity disorders are preventable.

   a. The risk of getting chronic neuropathic pain can be reduced by effectively treating acute pain.

   b. Physical exercise, and intake of supplements such as vitamins and omega 3 fatty acids can decrease the risk of many neurological diseases.

   c. Inflammation is involved in many neurological diseases and that can be reduced by reducing the intake of sugar and other carbohydrate.

   d. The likelihood of giving birth to a child with spina bifida or autism can be reduced by the mother taking folic acid before and during pregnancy.

Introduction

Historically, the search for the cause of a disorder of the nervous system has been focused on finding morphological or chemical abnormalities. Now we know that the symptoms and signs of many disorders of the nervous system are caused by changes in functions. That is not directly a result of morphological or chemical abnormalities, but rather there is evidence that activation of maladaptive neuroplasticity is the main cause of symptoms of many neurological disorders.

The term plasticity disorder is used for diseases where activation of neuroplasticity causes the main symptoms. This form of neuroplasticity is known as maladaptive neuroplasticity in contrast to neuroplasticity that is beneficial or purposeful. The term maladaptive neuroplasticity has mainly been used to describe changes in the organization of neural circuits that are not beneficial, thus bad neuroplasticity.

There is now evidence that the phantom limb syndrome, chronic neuropathic pain, some forms of severe tinnitus and spasticity are caused by activation of maladaptive neuroplasticity. There is also evidence that the primary cause of the symptoms of other diseases such as fibromyalgia, and various kinds of muscle spasm is caused by activation of bad forms of neuroplasticity, thus maladaptive neuroplasticity. Activation of neuroplasticity can also affect and contribute to different other kinds of neurological diseases. Re-routing of sensory information in the dorsal horn of the spinal cord contribute to the cause to the cause of allodynia and hyperpathia.

These conditions are associated with abnormal connections between somatosensory circuits and pain circuitries in the spinal cord [326, 528, 529]. Phantom limb sensations [411] may be due to similar nervous system changes as may some forms of tinnitus [292]. These symptoms are believed to be related to activation of maladaptive neuroplasticity.

The symptoms and signs of some vestibular disorders are caused by re-routing of information. Thus, while information from the balance organ (inner ear) normally does not reach our consciousness, disorders of the auditory-vestibular nerve can cause information about movements of the head to reach consciousness and produce the sensation of dizziness and vertigo. An example of an abnormal sensation from that occurs as a result of activation of neuroplasticity is the sensation experienced from head movements after intoxication for example from intake of alcohol.

Phantom sensations

Phantom sensations are defined as sensations that are not elicited by stimulation of sensory receptors. The sensations are caused by neural activity in the brain or the spinal cord by activation of neuroplasticity. Therefore, these sensations are called phantom sensation.

There are two kinds of phantom sensations; one type involves meaningless sensory perception and the other, also known as hallucination, that invokes meaningful sensory perceptions such as music, speech or various kinds of visual experiences [81].

Meaningless sensory sensations that occur without any physical input to the sensory organs [292] are most common in the auditory system (tinnitus [458]) and the somatosensory system (tingling, pain, etc). Visual phantom sensations are rare and can consist of different forms of light sensations (phosphenes).

All senses are associated with some forms of phantom sensations but the pathology of phantom perceptions such as chronic pain and tinnitus have only been described recently through complex models [139].

The phantom limb syndrome is one of the clearest examples of sensations that are caused by abnormal neural activity in the central nervous system while the sensations are referred to specific peripheral location. A phantom limb syndrome is a form of dysesthesia that consists of sensations including tingling and pain that are referred to specific anatomical locations on an amputated limb [34, 185, 411]. A person who have has a body part amputated may perceive pain, tingling, itch, and other sensations as coming from a part of the body that does not exist such as an amputated limb.

Sensations such as tinnitus are caused by neural activity generated in dysfunctional networks created by maladaptive neuroplasticity. Some forms of pain (chronic neuropathic pain) are also phantom sensations that are generated by neural activity in a dysfunctional neural network. The changes in the function of neural circuits in the spinal cord or the brain that causes chronic neuropathic pain may have been created by physiological pain.

Some forms of paresthesia, vertigo and other vestibular symptoms are also phantom sensations that are caused by physiological abnormalities in the brain, and expression of neuroplasticity causes these functional abnormalities.

Even such sensory deficits as presbycusis (age-related hearing loss) have a central component [663] most likely caused by activation of neuroplasticity. Hearing loss from noise exposure that has earlier been ascribed to morphological changes in the cochlea has evidence of a central component of the hearing loss [397, 661].

Plastic changes can also affect and contribute to the symptoms of many other disorders, discussed in Section 4.

Fibromyalgia

Fibromyalgia (FM) is characterized by widespread chronic pain (tenderness in at least 11 of 18 pre-defined points), lasting at least three months, typically accompanied by fatigue and sleep disturbance. Many studies have supported the hypothesis that fibromyalgia is a central, widespread pain syndrome caused by a generalized disturbance in pain processing in the central nervous system {Napadow, 2014 #5664}.

Although 10-12% of the population worldwide experience chronic widespread pain, in the USA only about 2% (3.4% of women and 0.5% of men) meet the American College of Rheumatology (ACR) criteria for Fibromyalgia (FM).

While no single etiology has been identified for the condition, a unifying hypothesis that continues to receive increasing scientific support suggests that FM is a consequence of sensitization of the central nervous system [379] typically accompanied by fatigue and sleep disturbances.

The current concepts of the circuits in the brain that are involved in creating the symptoms of mood disorders and chronic neuropathic pain have similarities with the circuits that are assumed to be involved in creating the symptoms of fibromyalgia. There are similarities between fibromyalgia and chronic neuropathic pain; these diseases have in common that activation of maladaptive neuroplasticity plays a central role in both chronic neuropathic pain and fibromyalgia [379] (Figure 5.1 and 5.2).

Activation of maladaptive neuroplasticity can also cause other adverse effects in the form of changes in the processing of sensory information causing hyperpathia, allodynia, hyperacusis, etc.

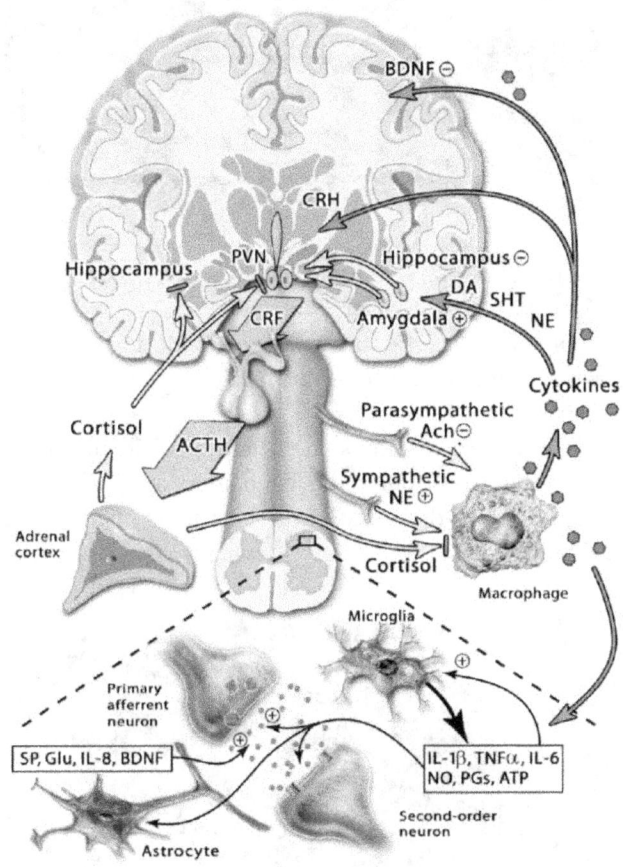

Figure 5.1. Mood disorders, fibromyalgia (FM) and neuropathic pain (NeP) may have shared systemic consequences. From: [379].

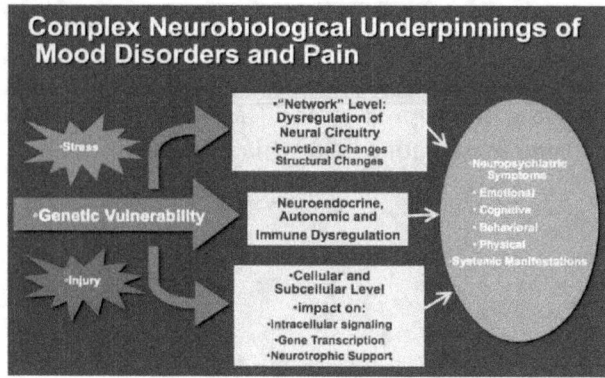

Figure 5.2. An integrated view of the shared neurobiological underpinnings of major depression (MDD), fibromyalgia (FM) and neuropathic pain (NeP). From: [379].

Figure 5.3 shows the anatomical locations of the structures that have been identified as being involved in the regulation of the symptoms of fibromyalgia.

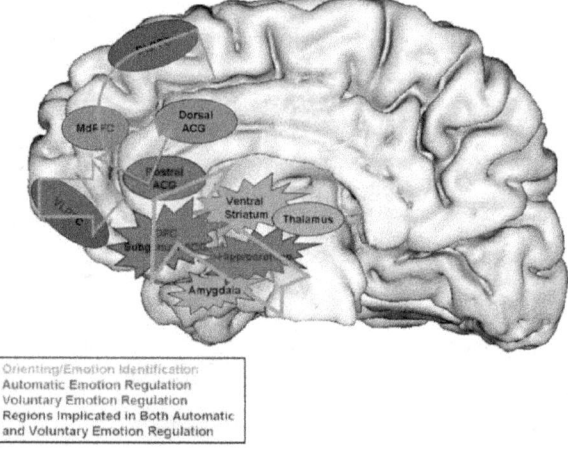

Figure 5.3. Cortical and subcortical areas involved in voluntary and automatic regulation of mood and the stress response. From: [379].

There are also connections between chronic neuropathic pain and depression, and between depression and fibromyalgia [487]. Clinical experience has earlier suggested the existence of these connections. Now, support for these hypotheses is beginning to come from neuroscience studies.

Other diseases where maladaptive neuroplasticity plays a role

Recent findings also support the hypothesis that maladaptive neuroplasticity contributes to the symptoms and signs of a wide range of other disorders including the chronic fatigue syndrome, low back pain, whiplash, headache, chronic pelvic pain syndrome and some forms of osteoarthritis, epicondylitis, shoulder pain and cancer pain [496].

These findings naturally open possibilities of effective treatments of many diseases including fibromyalgia which has been difficult to treat effectively [125] (see Appendix C).

Disorders caused by a failure in "mid-course correction."

It was mentioned in Chapter 1 that the brain undergoes major changes during the first few years of life. We called these changes "mid-course correction." Considerable evidence has been presented that if these changes do not proceed normally symptoms of a disease may occur. One such disease is autism or autism spectrum diseases.

Autism

Autism spectrum diseases is a term used to describe a pervasive development disorder characterized by profound social and verbal communication deficits. People with autism typically have a stereotypical motor behavior, and they have restricted interests and cognitive abnormalities.

There are indications that abnormalities in the ascending sensory pathways are parts of the pathologies of autism. The auditory system has two ascending pathways, known as the classical (lemniscal) pathway and the non-classical (extralemniscal). The classical pathways use the ventral thalamic nuclei the cells of which project to primary sensory cortices. The non-classical pathways make use of the dorsal and medial thalamic nuclei the cells of which project to secondary and association cortices, bypassing the primary sensory cortices. The cells in the dorsal and medial thalamus also project directly to cells in subcortical structures including the lateral nucleus of the amygdala [10, 97, 353].

The fact that the non-classical auditory pathways also receives input from other sensory systems such as the somatosensory system but the classical auditory pathways only receives auditory input was used in studies of the activity of the non-classical pathways.

In these studies, children and adults were asked to assess the loudness of sounds consisting of series of meaningless clicks (40pps at 65dB) presented unilaterally with and without electrical stimulation of the median nerve. The electrical stimulation was found to modulate the perception of loudness in young children but not in older children and adults [447]. The results were interpreted to show and abnormal interaction between the somatosensory and the auditory system occurred in young children but not in older children and adults.

Similar studies have found evidence that children with autism have stronger signs of involvement of the non-classical auditory pathway than children who do not have signs of autism and that adults with autism also have an abnormal cross-modal interaction indicating active non-classical pathways.

In children with autism electrical stimulation of the median nerve (activating the somatosensory system) affected the perceived loudness of the sound to a greater extent than was the cases in young children who did not have autism. Also, adults who had autism had a similar effect on the perceived loudness of sounds when the median nerve was electrically stimulated.

These results were interpreted to show that the non-classical auditory pathways were overrepresented in children with autism and that there were signs of involvements of the non-classical pathways in adults with autism [447, 449].

Below the age of 15 years, children who do not have autism have signs of involvement of their non-classical auditory pathways in listening to sounds [446], but adults have none or only weak representation of the non-classical auditory pathways [438].

Other studies using similar technique showed that some people with some forms of tinnitus had the same signs of interaction between auditory and somatosensory systems thus indications that the non-classical pathways were active in adults with some forms of tinnitus [438].

Recent studies have linked mutated genes to the pathology of autism causing dysregulation of activity-dependent signaling pathways in nerve cells [160]. Blocking of normally functional synapses and elimination of connections is a normal phenomenon in postnatal development.

There is evidence that the oxytocin system plays a role in autism [539]. Oxytocin contribute to modulation of neural circuits that are involved with social behavior, and since abnormal social behavior is the main part of the symptoms of autism, the oxytocin system plays an important role in creating the symptoms of autism [387].

As discussed in Chapter 4, oxytocin is a hypothalamic neuropeptide that affects social behavior. Oxytocin modulates synaptic neuroplasticity and adaptively modifies the neural circuits for social interactions such as nonspecific recognition, pair bonding, and maternal care [539].

Characteristics of plasticity disorders

Plasticity disorders such as chronic neuropathic pain and tinnitus have two components. One component is the sensation of pain as occurs in chronic neuropathic pain or the sound individuals with tinnitus experience. The other component of plasticity disorders is perhaps best described as suffering.

Many people cannot sleep and cannot do intellectual work because of the tinnitus or pain. The degree of suffering (or distress) is difficult to assess, and most assessments of plasticity disorder relate to the strength of the sensation of pain or the loudness of the sound in tinnitus ignoring the suffering component of these diseases. The suffering component is not directly related to the strength of the perceived symptoms such as pain and tinnitus. People with similar strength of pain or similar loudness of their tinnitus may suffer differently. The suffering component of these disorders often reduces the person's quality of life to a greater extent than what the perception of pain or tinnitus does.

The symptoms of plasticity disorders may be felt in different parts of the body rather than at the location of the pathology (which is the brain). This is also one of the reasons that plasticity disorders are challenging for the physician who treats these diseases, and it may cause difficulty in explaining the treatment for the patient.

For example, most forms of severe tinnitus are caused by pathologies located to the brain, but the symptoms are sounds that are distinctly referred to one ear or both ears. Patients with tinnitus, therefore, want some treatment of their ears and they often claim that there is nothing wrong with their brain.

Causes of plasticity disorders

Historically, the search for the cause of disorders of the nervous system has been focused on finding morphological or chemical abnormalities and then the development of treatments aimed at correcting these abnormalities. Now we know that changes in function cause the symptoms and signs of many disorders of the nervous system and that these changes are not directly caused by or related to morphological or chemical abnormalities as these variables are measured in people with plasticity disorders. Overdoing compensation for lost functions in specific parts of the spinal cord and the brain, such as may occur from trauma to the brain, including strokes, can lead to the creation of hyperactive disorders such as spasticity.

This may occur by increasing the gain in neural circuits in sensory and motor systems of the brain and the spinal cord.

This form of maladaptation is one way that neuroplasticity can become harmful, causing unwanted effects of expression of neuroplasticity such as hyperactivity. Some types of tinnitus and chronic neuropathic pain, phantom limb symptoms, and spasticity after spinal cord trauma, etc. are examples of pathologies where activation of neuroplasticity may have been caused by overdoing compensation of lost or reduced function.

Factors that are known to activate beneficial neuroplasticity such as deprivation of sensory input are also commonly the factors that activate maladaptive neuroplasticity.

The number of known factors implicated in the causes of the symptoms of plasticity diseases has grown and now including the action of factors such as brain-derived neurotrophic factor (BDNF) in addition to the action of maladaptive neuroplasticity.

This is a favorable development in that these factors can be affected by relatively simple means. BDNF can be increased by physical exercise and administration of innocuous agents such as Omega 3 fatty acids. The ratio of omega 6 and omega 3 is also of importance, and that can easily be affected by increasing intake of Omega 3 [630].

Overstimulation of sensory systems can cause injury to sensory receptor cells, such as the cochlear hair cells, resulting in elevation of the threshold of hearing. However, over-stimulation can also promote expression of neuroplasticity, and it is possible that overstimulation, with or without injuring sensory cells, can cause changes in neural processing through the expression of neuroplasticity. Neural deficits that earlier were associated with morphological changes in sensory organs may also have contributions from functional changes in the nervous system that are related to activation of neuroplasticity.

Pathology of phantom sensations

The abnormal neural activity that causes the phantom sensations may be a result of a maladaptive neuroplastic reorganization of the nervous system by activation of neuroplasticity or by the absence of normal sensory input.

The existence of phantom sensations demonstrates that sensations can be generated by activity in the central nervous system without peripheral stimulation and perceived as originating from a peripheral location.

The existence of the phantom limb syndrome is a clear sign that neural circuits in the central nervous system can produce sensations that are referred to specific anatomical locations on the body without any physical stimulus being applied to that location.

The sensory abnormalities that often follow amputations of limbs may be regarded as examples of compensatory actions in response to deprivation of somatosensory or proprioceptive input from the amputated limb, including changed visual perception of a missing body part.

The plastic changes that cause the symptoms of plasticity disorders include changed cortical representation (mapping) of the amputated limb and adjacent structures, and change in motor and sensory function [274].

Proprioceptive brain maps, encompassing the brain's awareness of a person's body are constantly updated based on input from the senses, particularly the touch and sight. Studies of upper limb amputees [274] found that almost all had an awareness of the amputated limb and that awareness could be altered by tactile stimulation of the stump and, to a lesser degree, by visual input. Tactile stimulation of the stump, or of the face, gave a dual perception of the anatomical location of the stimulation in half of the studied individuals. This dual representation was strongest with eyes closed as visual input could override this dual perception [274], but the awareness of the limb was not affected by visual input.

There is now evidence from studies of functional connections that many neurological disorders including age-related deficits are associated with the altered strength of functional connections. This is in contrast to earlier concepts that assumed that pathologies of the nervous system were limited to morphological or biochemical changes.

Disorders of sensory nerves may alter the information that reaches the nervous system resulting in symptoms and signs of abnormal processing of sensory information such as phantom sensations (tinnitus and paresthesia). Re-direction of sensory information in the central nervous system may cause allodynia (pain from normally innocuous stimulation) and sensation from activation of the vestibular system by head movements.

Many of the disorders that are caused by maladaptive neuroplasticity are associated with the altered strength of functional connections in the brain and the spinal cord. The changes can be due to an unmasking of synapses that can open connections that were not previously open thus making new parts of the central nervous system accessible for input or it can change the strength of connections. The changes in the strength of functional connections can occur rapidly because activation of neuroplasticity causes them. There is a consensus among scientists of neuroscience that network dysfunctions are related to many disorders of the sensory and the motor systems. Also, some disorders where memory is affected including various forms of dementia including Alzheimer's disease are in the same category.

Recent studies of connectivity have shown abnormalities in the functional connections between different structures of the brain in people with plasticity disorders such as tinnitus (Figure 5.4), but these techniques have not yet been adopted to clinical diagnosis.

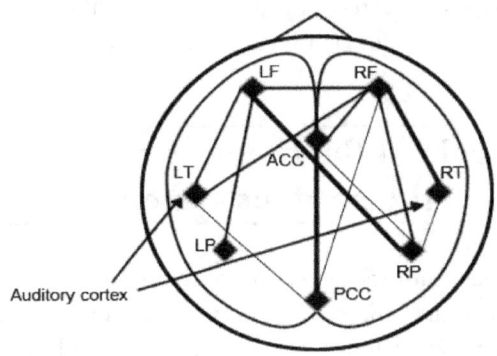

Figure 5.4. Illustration of connections in the brain of persons with tinnitus. The thickness of the lines shows the strength of the connections. (Modified from [138] Artwork by Monica Javidnia).

Another recent study of connectivity has shown that age-related changes in memory function are reflected in changes in connections between different structures of the brain [596] (Figure 5.5). This study demonstrated that there is a relationship between cognitive changes and changes in connectivity in the temporal lobe.

Quantitative studies of functional connections require specialized equipment and complex computations processing of the collected data, requiring resources that are not normally available in clinical settings. It also requires that the investigator has as certain mathematical knowledge.

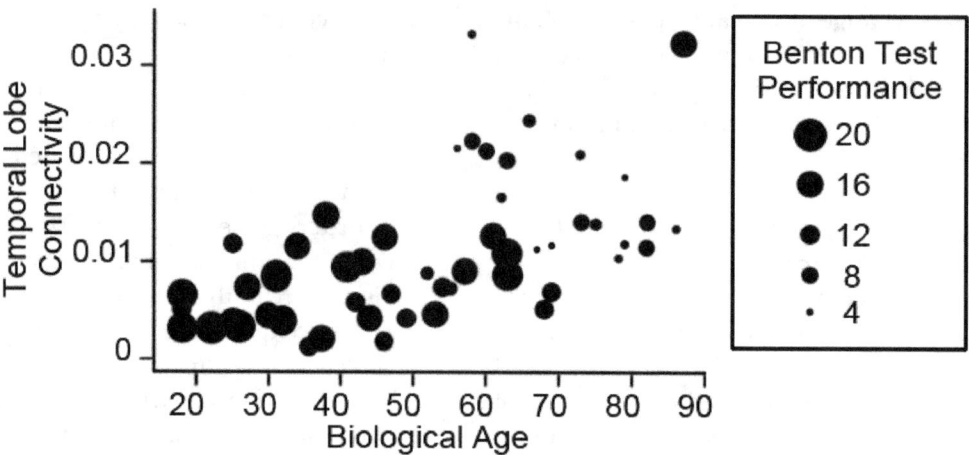

Figure 5.5 An example of determination of functional connections in the brain to study the pathologies of plasticity disorders (tinnitus). From: [596].

The role of the immune system on the nervous system

The immune system controls many brain functions, and the central nervous system controls the immune system. The immune system has two parts, the innate system, and the adaptive immune system. Both the innate and the adaptive immune systems are heavily involved in many neurological diseases. The immune system is involved in eliciting neuroplasticity, and it is thus involved in causing plasticity disorders such as chronic neuropathic pain. The immune system can modulate (increase or decrease) many forms of pain and treatment with immunoglobulin is now being studied. Parts of the immune systems are also indirectly connected to the hippocampus, mPFC, and amygdala, critical regions in fear circuitry that are affected by stress and estrogen (Figure 5.6).

The role of stress

Stress, pain, and depression all can lead to the excessive and untimely release of corticotropin-releasing hormone (CRH), adrenocorticotropic hormone (ACTH) and glucocorticoids. Sympathetic over-activity, combined with diminished parasympathetic tone, contributes to immune activation and release of proinflammatory cytokines (e.g., tumor necrosis factor alpha, TNF-α, and interleukins IL-1, IL-6) from macrophages and other immune cells. Inflammatory cytokines further interfere with monoaminergic and neurotrophic signaling. They may also downregulate central glucocorticoid receptor sensitivity, leading to further disruption of feedback control of the hypothalamic-pituitary-adrenal (HPA) axis and the immune system. In depression and pain states, disturbances of serotonin (5HT), norepinephrine (NE) and dopamine (DA) transmission may impair regulatory feedback loops that turn off the stress response, with a resultant compromise in the function of descending pain modulatory pathways (see Figure 5.6).

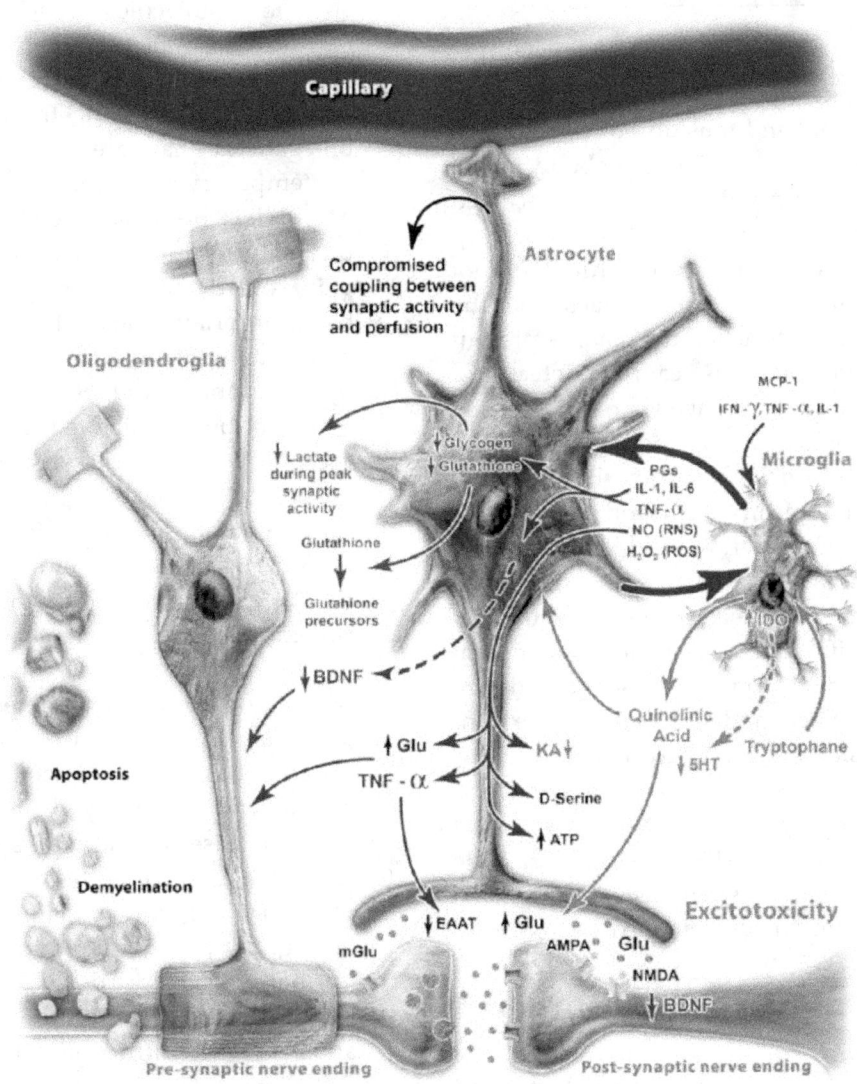

Figure 5.6. Microglia is the primary recipients of peripheral inflammatory signals as they reach the brain. Activated microglia initiate an inflammatory cascade by releasing cytokines, chemokines, prostaglandins and reactive nitrogen and oxygen species (RNS and ROS, respectively). Bi-directional exchanges between microglia and astroglia amplify inflammatory signals within the central nervous system (CNS). Cytokines including interleukin (IL)-1, IL-6, tumor necrosis (TNF)-α and interferon (IFN)- gamma induce indoleamine 2,3 dioxygenase (IDO), the enzyme responsible for degrading tryptophan, the primary precursor of serotonin (5-HT), into kynurenine, which is eventually metabolized into quinolinic acid (QUIN), a potent NMDA agonist and stimulator of glutamate (Glu) release. From: [379].

Elevated mediators of the inflammatory response, combined with excessive sympathetic tone may further have an impact on the processing of pain signals in the dorsal column of the spinal cord and the brainstem by contributing to activation of microglia and astroglia.

Activated microglia exchange signals with astrocytes and nociceptive neurons, amplifying pain-related transmission of glutamate (Glu), substance P (SP), adenosine triphosphate (ATP), brain-derived neurotrophic factor (BDNF), pro-inflammatory cytokines (IL-1, IL-6, IL-8, TNF-α, nitrogen oxide NO) and prostaglandins (PGs) [379, 517].

Diagnosis of plasticity disorders

Common for plasticity disorder is that traditional imaging techniques or biochemical blood test are normal and thus do not contribute a diagnosis of these disorders. This is probably one of the reasons that plasticity disorders have received less attention than deserved.

The symptoms of plasticity disorders are not associated with morphological changes and the pathologic changes in function that causes present clinical diagnostic methods cannot detect the symptoms. No clinical tests have yet been designed that can identify and measure the changes in the brain that cause plasticity disorder such as pain, tinnitus, and phantom limb symptoms. Plasticity disorders can therefore not be diagnosed and evaluated in a similar way as many other disorders.

There are methods used in research that can detect and quantify functional changes in neural circuits [140, 596, 597]. Some of these methods are still under development and may in the future be of value for diagnosing plasticity disorders.

Some of these methods such as magnetoencephalography (MEG) and electroencephalography (EEG) can provide information about the strength of functional connections in the brain and spinal cord.

Treatment of plasticity disorders

Chronic neuropathic pain does not respond well to treatment with conventional pain relievers including opiates.

There is some evidence that increased brain-derived neurotrophic factor (BDMF) may have a beneficial effect on plasticity disorders such as chronic neuropathic pain. BDNF increases after physical exercise. Intake of Omega 3 and especially decreasing the ratio of omega 6 to omega three has been shown to increase BDMF [630].

There are now large efforts by neuroscientists towards finding ways to counteract the various forms of maladaptive neuroplasticity and thereby modulate the symptom of many of plasticity disorder.

One example is the attempts to increase specific molecules such as brain-derived neurotrophic factor (BDNF), which can be accomplished by physical exercise and by intake of omega 3 and reducing the ratio of omega 6 and omega three as are now suggested based on contemporary research.

It has been assumed that the symptoms of plasticity disorder such as chronic neuropathic pain, severe tinnitus, and spasticity can be reversed by appropriately activating neuroplasticity. Such reversed activation of neuroplasticity occurs in hypnosis and acupuncture. These methods may be effective, but are looked upon with doubt – the accepted forms of treatment are presently pharmacological or surgical treatment. More recently other methods for reversing unwanted plastic changes are under development.

Selection of treatments for plasticity disorders is hampered by the lack of suitable (objective tests) to verify the efficacy of treatments. Because plasticity disorders lack detectable physical signs, diagnosis of these diseases must rely on the patients' description of their symptoms. Since the people with plasticity disorders have no visible signs of diseases (except spasticity and muscle spasm), it is tempting to conclude that they are not as severely ill as they claim. Lack of visible signs also gives persons with plasticity disorder less sympathy from friends and relatives. The fact that many plasticity disorders have two components adds to the difficulties that patients have in describing the symptoms of their disease adequately.

Treatment or prevention?

While treatments for many diseases have been developed during recent years there are still many diseases that lack effective treatments, and most treatments in use have side effects, and their efficiency varies. Many treatments have limited time of action (tolerance) that requires increased dosage after a certain of use.

The same time span has seen the development of effective prevention for many diseases. However, the focus has been on treatment both from the medical profession and from the public despite the many disadvantages of treatment and the many advantages of prevention. The reason that prevention has received little support may be that it lacks the immediate reward that (successful) treatment enjoys.

Chronic neuropathic pain is often caused by the transformation of acute pain that has not been treated effectively. The risk of acquiring chronic neuropathic pain can, therefore, be reduced by treating acute pain aggressively.

Here are a few other examples of the advantages of prevention of serious neurological diseases. Autism (autism spectrum disorders) and spina bifida have no known effective treatment and cause devastating effects and reduction in the quality of life for the person who has that disorder. These disorders can have catastrophic effects on an entire family. The results of recent studies indicate that administration of folic acid, a B-vitamin that has no known side effects, before and during pregnancy can reduce the risk of giving birth to a child with autism spectrum disorders [657]. These simple precautions almost eliminate the risk of giving birth to a child with spina bifida and reduce the risk of giving birth to a child with autism by at least 50% according to recent studies [657]. Similar advantages have been shown for other congenital defects such as cleft lip and palate [313].

More than 35 years ago it was shown that the risk of giving birth to a child with neural tube defects such as spina bifida could be almost eliminated by the mother taking folic acid before and during pregnancy [391], yet a recent study showed that only 30% of pregnant women (in Japan) took folic acid [330].

There are other advantages from supplements such as folic acid and other B-vitamins, which, for example, have beneficial effects on pain from peripheral nerve neuropathies such in the common diabetes neuropathy and from the effect of administration of certain cancer drugs.

It is unfortunate that there is a negative attitude to take supplements such as omega 3 and vitamins. These additives are remarkable by being inexpensive and essentially free of side effects. (A recent study found that using vitamin D as a supplement would provide a noticeable increase in the health of people in Germany, [751]). This is contrary to many pharmaceutical drugs used for the treatment of many diseases, in fact it is difficult to find any pharmaceutical drug that does not have some side effects, and many treatments have serious side effects.

The phantom limb syndrome

Phantom sensations are sensory sensations that have no bodily cause. A prime example is the phantom limb syndrome where a person perceives pain, tingling, paresthesia (itch), torsion, and other sensations as coming from a part of the body that does not exist such as an amputated limb. Phantom sensations are defined as perceptions that are not elicited by stimulation of sensory receptors. Phantom sensations occur in all senses. A prime example is the phantom limb syndrome where a person perceives pain, tingling, paresthesia (itch), torsion, and other sensations as coming from a part of the body that does not exist such as an amputated limb. A phantom limb syndrome is a form of dysesthesia that consists of sensations including tingling and pain, which are referred to specific anatomical locations on an amputated limb [34, 185]. It is obvious that these sensations are generated in the central nervous system without any input from receptors in the body part to which they are associated.

Creation of the phantom limb symptoms

Studies of upper limb amputees [274] found that almost all had an awareness of the amputated limb and that awareness could be altered by tactile stimulation of the stump and, to a lesser degree, by visual input. Tactile stimulation of the stump, or of the face, gave a dual perception of the anatomical location of the stimulation in half of the studied individuals.

It has been hypothesized that the phantom limb syndrome is related to maladaptive neuroplastic changes triggered by overstimulation that occurs during the surgical operations to amputate the limb in question. This hypothesis is supported by the finding of some studies have shown that the risk of phantom limb symptoms can be reduced by applying local anesthetics before surgery to the peripheral nerve that innervate the body part that is to be amputated [34]. However, other studies have produced contrary results ([407].

The importance of maps

All parts of the body are mapped on structures in the central nervous system. When the position of the limbs changes, the structures are re-mapped. This cannot be done for a structure that has been amputated. There is evidence that failure to re-map the amputated body part contribute to the phantom limb symptoms.

There are many reasons why pain and other sensations are referred to the maps of a limb that may persist after amputation. The main reason is that the brain still keeps a map of the amputated limb. This may cause pain and other sensations referred to the amputated limb.

The map of the amputated limb in the brain may also cause a distorted body image where the amputated limb may be stuck in an unpleasant position with its owner unable to move it. The mirror treatment described below can solve the problems by activating neuroplasticity. Such treatment can relieve the pain and odd sensations experienced after amputations [543]. Relieve of the phantom limb symptoms.

Ramachandran [542] reasoned that if someone were to lose their right hand in an accident, they may then have the feelings of the phantom limb syndrome because the input that normally would go from their hand to the left somatosensory cortex would have been stopped. By this reasoning, Ramachandran designed the mirror treatment that now bears his name and which is in general use to relieve some of the symptoms of amputated body parts. The mirror treatment described below has been shown to solve these problems for many patients including the pain by activating neuroplasticity.

The patient looks into the mirror on the side with the good limb and makes mirror symmetric movements. Because the patient who is being treated sees the reflected image of the good hand moving, it appears as if the phantom limb is also moving.

Through the use of this artificial visual feedback, it becomes possible for the patient to move the image (mapping) in the brain of the phantom limb, and to unclench it from potentially painful positions. Because this visual feedback elicits sensations that are related to the movement of a limb, Rogers Ramachandran [542] called this kind of treatment "synesthesia," although this is true only in the broadest sense of the term. It is a practical use of activation of neuroplasticity to reverse functional changes that are unwanted.

Other use of virtual reality

The success of the mirror method inspired a team of researchers at the University of Pool, UK [116] and the University of Manchester [481] in England to experiment with a technology called "immersive virtual reality" to combat the discomfort that is a part of the phantom limb syndrome [481]. The researchers reported that with this technique, phantom limb pain could be relieved by attaching the sufferer's real limb to an interface that allows them to see two limbs moving in a computer-generated simulation. This works on the same principle as the mirror box technique in that it "tricks" the somatosensory cortex by an illusion that supposedly activates neuroplasticity to changes the map of an amputated limb. This kind of development of treatment for phantom sensations inspired by the original work by Ramachandran [542] is in steady progress in many laboratories and clinics [116]. The mirror box is also of use in the rehabilitation of patients with hemiparesis (paralysis on one side of the body) due to stroke [19].

Chapter 6

Chronic Neuropathic Pain

Abstract

1. Chronic (central) neuropathic pain is a form of pathological pain that is not caused by stimulation of pain receptors. The pain sensation is, therefore, a phantom sensation.

2. Like other plasticity disorder, chronic neuropathic pain has two parts, the sensation of pain and a part that is best described as suffering.

3. Dysfunctional networks cause chronic neuropathic pain in the spinal cord and the brain created by activation of neuroplasticity.

4. The neural activity in such networks creates a sensation of pain, and the cause of the suffering that is are the two parts of the symptoms of neuropathic pain.

5. Chronic neuropathic pain often follows after ineffectively treated acute pain such as pain after trauma including that of surgical operations.

6. Stress of various kinds can promote the development of chronic neuropathic pain from acute pain.

7. The sympathetic nervous system is involved in some forms of chronic neuropathic pain.

8. Sensitization of nociceptors (peripheral sensitization) and central nervous system structures (central sensitization) plays an important role in creating the symptoms of chronic neuropathic pain.

9. Chronic neuropathic pain is often accompanied by allodynia (pain perception from normally innocuous stimulation of the skin), hyperalgesia (increased sensitivity to painful stimulation) and hyperpathia (an exaggerated reaction to light to moderate pain stimulation).

10. Chronic neuropathic pain is difficult to treat; it does not respond well to NSAID and opioid pain relievers.

Introduction

The term central neuropathic pain has been used to describe pain that is generated by neural activity in the brain without and physical stimulation can be detected. We will in this book use the tern chronic neuropathic pain.

Chronic neuropathic pain is one of several common diseases where activation of maladaptive neuroplasticity plays an important role in creating and maintain the symptoms. Chronic neuropathic pain is a form of pathological pain that causes enormous suffering, and it is a challenge to the physician with regards is fundamentally different from pain that is caused that of nociceptor elicited pain.

Pain is a self-experience that is subjective; it cannot be measured using objective methods, and the experience depends on the circumstances. Pain can cause many different reactions: it can activate the autonomic nervous system (affecting heart rate, blood pressure, sweating, etc), cause involuntarily muscle contraction (spasm), mood changes (fear, anxiety, depression), and it can prevent sleep.

While the acute (nociceptor based) pain has many advantages to a person, chronic neuropathic pain has no apparent benefits, but the disadvantages are many. The chronic neuropathic pain can ruin a person's life, causing affective disorders that often result in suicide. Pain in general also affects many body functions.

That chronic neuropathic pain is to a large degree preventable has not received the attention it deserves. Prevention is especially important in the light of the poor effect of treatment with pain medications such as opioids. There are indications that poorly treated acute pain causes many (perhaps most) forms of chronic neuropathic pain.

Common forms of pain are acute pain, chronic pain, somatic pain, neuropathic pain, and chronic neuropathic pain. This chapter will concern chronic neuropathic pain.

General aspects of pain

Somatic and visceral pain play important roles as a warning signal of diseases, and it plays a central role in diagnostics of many kinds of diseases and pain is therefore beneficial to a person. Some forms of pain are not purposeful and not beneficial to a person but cause suffering. Other forms of pain are a nuisance.

"The only tolerable pain is someone else's pain."
René Leriche, French surgeon, 1879–1955

The International Association for the Study of Pain (IASP) has defined different forms of pain. The term "physiological pain" is used to describe pain caused by stimulation of pain receptors (nociceptors) in normal tissue whereas the term "pathological pain" is used to describe the pain that occurs in association with pathologies with or without stimulation of pain receptors. Complex diseases such as fibromyalgia [487] are also often discussed under the heading of pathological pain see Appendix C). There is also evidence that the insula lobe is involved in creating the symptoms of pain diseases such as migraine [76].

The abnormal neural activity that causes symptoms of many forms of pain is not generated at the location where the symptoms are felt which can make the diagnosis of the disease difficult. The sensations of pain that are referred to a different location of the body than that where the neural activity that causes the pain is generated [475] (referred pain) is an obstacle in the use of pain for diagnostics of diseases.

Pain can initiate two different forms of vicious circles, a psychological and a physiological, that can amplify the effects of various forms of pain (Figure 6.1).

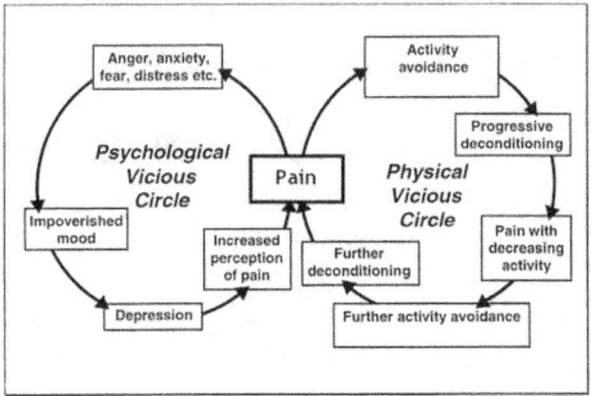

Figure 6.1 Two different possible outcomes of pain. (From a Google search.)

What is the chronic neuropathic pain?

Chronic pain is defined as pain lasting longer than six months that extends beyond the expected period of healing. Chronic neuropathic pain is pain that originates from the brain without any physical stimulus. This form of pain can arise from an initial injury such as a neck or back sprain or be due to an ongoing cause such as an illness.

Chronic neuropathic pain has two components; one is the sensation of pain, and the other is best described as "suffering." Chronic neuropathic pain is fundamentally different from pain that is caused by stimulation of nociceptors, and its neural substrate may be different from that of nociceptor elicited pain, it belongs to a group of disorders where maladaptive neuroplasticity plays an important role. The component of chronic neuropathic pain we call suffering have signs of affecting different parts of the brain than those involved with the sensation of acute pain that is caused by stimulation of pain receptors.

Chronic neuropathic pain is a typical phantom sensation. Phantom sensations are sensations that are not caused by stimulation of receptors by physical stimuli such as sound, touch or chemical agents. Phantom pain is similar to other phantom sensations such as some forms of tinnitus [292, 451].

The chronic neuropathic pain is a disease that is difficult to treat successfully; it does not respond well to conventional pain medications such as NSAIDs and opioids. It has been questioned whether it responds at all to administration of common opioid pain medications.

When treated with conventional pain relievers and no effect is experienced, a natural reaction is to increase the dosage of the pain medication that is administrated, and that can cause severe side effects including death from an over dosage. The use of opioid pain relievers is especially prone to overdosing which can cause death because large dosages of opioids can cause respiratory arrest.

Diagnosis of chronic neuropathic pain

Chronic neuropathic pain is not caused by stimulation of nociceptors but by neural activity generated in the central nervous system, the sensation of pain is referred to a peripheral location, and it may occur without any known cause. Chronic neuropathic pain, or stimulus-independent pain, is fundamentally different from pain that is caused by stimulation of nociceptors and the neural substrate (part of the nervous system that is involved) is different in these two types of pain. Chronic neuropathic pain is referred to specific regions of the body, although these regions may not contribute to the generation of the sensation of pain [531].

Clinical imaging studies such as MRI and conventional neurophysiologic tests do not reveal any noticeable abnormalities in persons with chronic neuropathic pain. A person's description of the symptoms is the only assessable measure of chronic neuropathic pain.

The use of an analog scale to describe a person's perception of the pain may be of some help, but the magnitude of the suffering from the pain does not correlate well with the perception of the pain. For example, a person who has psychological coping skills may suffer less from a very intense pain than a people without these skills. This disjoint renders such measures to be of limited value in assessing the severity of an individual's pain. This all makes it difficult to correctly diagnose chronic neuropathic pain.

Other features of chronic neuropathic pain

Referred pain

The regions of the body to which pain is referred often extend with time, thus a form of lateral spread of activation. It has been suggested that a peripheral nerve trunk is capable of sustaining a "flare" response similar to that observed in injured skin and other tissue [752] and thus cause an extension of the region from which pain sensation perceived.

Measurable abnormalities in chronic neuropathic pain

There are few measurable abnormalities in persons with chronic neuropathic pain. An exception is measures of temporal integration.

Temporal integration at threshold

Temporal integration of sensation and of pain has been studied by observing the threshold for stimulation of the skin with electrical impulses at different frequencies. When the strength of the electrical stimulation of the skin is increased, the first sensation that can be noticed is a weak tingling sensation. When the strength of the electrical impulses is increased further, at a certain strength, the sensation changes distinctly from a strong tingling to a painful sensation.

Comparing the threshold of just noticeable sensation and the threshold of painful stimulation for different frequencies of the stimulus provides information about the differences in the temporal integration for these to manifestations of electrical stimulation of the skin.

In a person who did not have pain, the threshold to painful stimulation decreased when the rate with which the stimuli were presented was increased (shorter intervals between individual impulses). This means that stimulation at a high rate was more effective in eliciting a sensation pain than impulses presented at a slow rate, thus with long intervals between the impulses (Figure 6.2A).

This means that transient painful stimulation, such as electrical stimulation, is normally subjected to temporal integration whereas the innocuous sensation from electrical stimulation has few or no signs of temporal integration (Figure 6.2A).

The situation is different for a person with signs of chronic neuropathic pain (Figure 6.2B); the threshold for tingling and pain are not noticeably dependent on the rate with which the stimuli are presented indicating little temporal integration. This means that there were no signs of temporal integration for pain in the person who had indications of chronic neuropathic pain.

Also, the pain threshold in the person with pain was lowered, and it became close to that of sensation (tingling) [442].

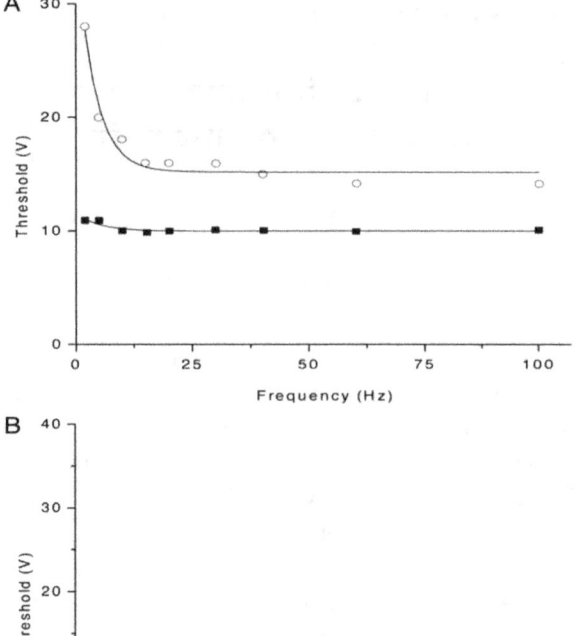

Figure 6.2 Measures of the temporal integration of sensation and pain in a person without pain (A) and in a person with signs of chronic neuropathic pain (B). The threshold of sensation (filled squares) and pain (open circles) in response to electrical stimulation with impulses applied to the skin of the forearm are shown as a function of the frequency of the stimulus impulses. The threshold for just noticeable tingling (filled squares) and the threshold for a pain sensation (open circles) are shown to illustrate temporal integration in an person without pain (From [442]).

Other symptoms caused by pain

Persistent, intense pain, activates secondary mechanisms both at the periphery and within the central nervous system that cause allodynia, hyperalgesia, and hyperpathia that can diminish normal functioning.

Hyperalgesia
The term hyperalgesia is used to describe an increased sensitivity to pain. It is a form of peripheral sensitization. Animal studies and studies in humans have supported the hypothesis that neural sensitization promotes the development of hyperalgesia [51].

Hyperpathia
Hyperpathia is a sign of central sensitization as characterized by state 3 of Doubell's classification of different states of the dorsal horn [158] (see above). The International Association for the Study of Pain's (IASP) definition of hyperpathia ist: "A painful syndrome characterized by an abnormally painful reaction to a stimulus, especially a repetitive stimulus, as well as an increased threshold."

Though hyperpathia has some survival importance, discouraging manipulation of injured tissue, in many situations, it offers no benefit to the organism. It is often regarded as pathology in itself and compounds the suffering of neuropathic pain. The pathophysiology of hyperpathia is unknown, but clinical experience shows that it can be alleviated by antidepressants that affect serotonin receptors. Amitriptyline and nortriptyline have been found to be the most effective antidepressants for treating hyperpathia.

How does chronic neuropathic pain develop?
It is now generally recognized that chronic neuropathic pain is mainly caused by poorly treated acute pain, together with stress and some unknown factors. This means that chronic neuropathic pain is to a great extent preventable by known means, namely by treating acute pain more effectively.

Threating acute pain such as pain from trauma (including surgery) efficiently may go against the general sentiment namely that pain relievers should be used sparsely for the treatment of acute pain because of fear of side effects such as stomach bleeding from ibuprofen and other NSAIDs and addiction from opioids.

Little attention is given to the risk of developing chronic neuropathic pain as a side effect of poorly treated acute pain on the form of promoting the development of chronic neuropathic pain.

When stimulus based pain lasts for some time, it can activate neuroplasticity that can result in a chronic neuropathic pain condition. This is one reason it is important to treat acute pain aggressively and eradicate all sensation of pain as soon as possible. This can be done using modern pain relievers such as NSAIDs and natural opioids (codeine, morphine) or semisynthetic opiates (oxycodone, hydromorphone etc.).

How can acute pain develop into chronic neuropathic pain?

Pain from injuries to peripheral nerves is especially powerful in initiating changes in the function of specific structures in the central nervous system through the expression of neuroplasticity. Persistent, intense pain causes changes in the periphery where upregulation of cyclooxygenase-2 and interleukin-1β-causes sensitizing of first-order neurons.

This may eventually sensitize second-order spinal neurons by activating NMDA channels, which in turn can send a signal to the immune system (microglia) to alter neuronal cytoarchitecture. The development of chronic pain is complex, and it may be different for the different forms of chronic pain. It is assumed, however, that activation of harmful neuroplasticity plays a major role in the initiation and maintenance of chronic neuropathic pain [536]. Plastic changes (expression of neuroplasticity) in the nervous system play some role in most pain conditions, it plays a dominating role in chronic neuropathic pain [30, 383, 731].

Activation of bad (maladaptive) neuroplasticity is assumed to underlie the mechanisms that make pain chronic [30, 176]. Many forms of chronic neuropathic pain may start with pain caused by activation of pain receptors (physiological pain), which, after some time, activate harmful neuroplasticity resulting in activity in central nervous system structures that are perceived as pain sensations.

Prostaglandins, endocannabinoids, ion-specific channels, and scavenger cells are all playing a key role in the transformation of acute to chronic pain [692]. In addition, stress and thereby the sympathetic nervous system play an important role in facilitating the conversion from acute pain to chronic neuropathic pain (Figure 6.3).

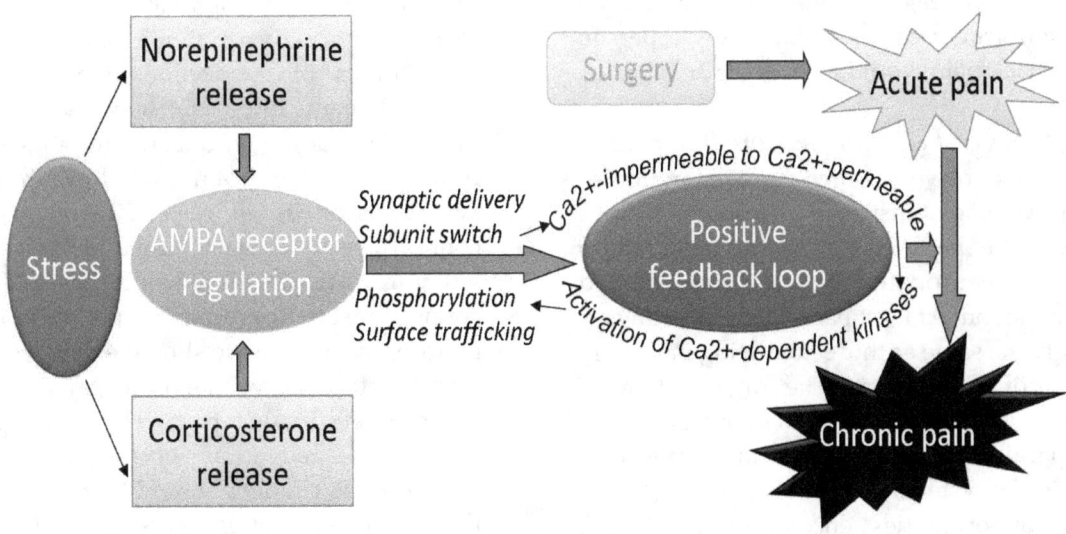

Figure 6.3 The role of stress in the development of chronic neuropathic pain. (From [363]. Courtesy of Dr. Feng Tao, 2015).

The transition between acute pain to chronic pain has been studied in people who had undergone surgical operations [109]. The authors of these studies concluded that there were five classes of hypotheses regarding the transfer of the postoperative pain to chronic pain, and these hypotheses propose that chronic pain results from:

1) persistent noxious signaling in the periphery;

2) enduring maladaptive neuroplastic changes at the spinal dorsal horn and higher central nervous system structures reflecting a multiplicity of factors, including peripherally released neurotrophic factors and interactions between neurons and microglia;

3) compromised inhibitory modulation of noxious signaling in medullary-spinal pathways;

4) descending facilitatory modulation; and

5) maladaptive brain remodeling in function, structure, and connectivity.

During the development of chronic neuropathic pain, several changes in brain anatomy have been observed [37]. Decreases in gray matter density and abnormal functional connectivity between nucleus accumbens and parts of the prefrontal cortex could predict the persistence of the pain.

This observation was taken to confirm that corticostriatal circuits are causally involved in the transition between acute pain and chronic pain [38]. Apkarian and colleagues found that abnormal white matter structures can predict how a person with lower back pain would recover [382].

Pathophysiology of chronic neuropathic pain

Despite extensive research, understanding of the pathophysiology of chronic neuropathic pain is incomplete. The pathways that are involved in severe chronic neuropathic pain are complex and poorly understood. At least parts of these pathways are probably the same as those mediating pain from stimulation of nociceptors. The organization of these pathways is dynamic and involves a high degree of parallel processing, including connections with autonomic systems and limbic structures.

These abnormalities encompass emotional, autonomic, and pain perception regions, implying that they likely play a critical role in the global clinical picture of CRPS.

Members of the Apkarian laboratory have shown that the volume of gray matter in the brains of the same persons who had persistent pain decreased over the year [247]. They showed that brain activity could be used to predict whether a subject recovered or experienced persistent pain.

Recently studies of connectivity in the brain have brought an understanding of some of the network abnormalities that are present in people with chronic neuropathic pain. These changes involving altered functional connectivity in certain parts of the brain may be the root of symptoms such a pain and other cognitive functions that are associated with chronic neuropathic pain and which cause reduced quality of life.

Chronic neuropathic pain is an example of how harmful neuroplasticity can create dysfunctional neural networks in the brain by disrupting default-mode network dynamics (DMND). During the chronic stage, however, neural activity shifts to circuits relating to emotion. [247]. Reward circuitry is active during both acute and chronic stages.

These observations are another example of a revised understanding of how different brain regions are activated and confirm the contemporary understanding that connections in the brain are dynamic and that many different regions may be involved in a specific task.

It has been suggested that the nuclei in the loop created by ascending and descending connections between the thalamus and cortex play an important role in chronic neuropathic pain through creating thalamocortical dysrhythmia [367, 700].

Studies of connections (connectivity) have revealed many important aspects of neurological diseases including chronic neuropathic pain. Most functions of the brain including those causing symptoms of disease depend on many functional connections between anatomically different structures of the brain. Studies of functional connections in the brain in people with chronic neuropathic pain have shown extensive changes in many structures of the brain in a person with chronic neuropathic pain. These changes can be related to activation of neuroplasticity, and therefore the changes should be reversible without the use of medications or surgery. It is therefore important to understand how the structures that are involved in diseases are connected.

Altered processing of nociceptive information at the spinal segmental and supraspinal levels are involved in chronic neuropathic pain [731], and both peripheral and central sensitization are most likely play important roles in creating the symptoms of many forms of chronic neuropathic pain [68, 380]. Deprivation of input or overstimulation can cause such plastic changes of the nervous system.

There are signs that the emotional brain may somehow be involved. One of the signs of that is the high prevalence of depression and suicide. The general decrease in a person's quality of life that often accompany chronic neuropathic pain are all signs of a general change in the function of the central nervous system. The complexity of the neural structures that are involved in chronic neuropathic pain may explain these complex expressions of chronic neuropathic pain.

Learning is assumed to underlie the mechanisms that make pain chronic [30, 176]. Neuropathic pain may start with physiological pain (pain caused by activation of pain receptors), which, after some time, activate harmful neuroplasticity resulting in activity in central nervous system structures that are perceived as pain sensations.

The role of the dorsal horn in chronic neuropathic pain

Changes in the processing in the dorsal horn can explain many of the symptoms of chronic neuropathic pain. Sensitization at the periphery as well as in the dorsal horn, the fifth cranial nerve (CN V) nucleus, and at supraspinal levels play important roles in the creation of chronic neuropathic pain [68, 731].

The changes in the function and the organization of the dorsal horn neural circuits can be caused by both external and internal factors that can cause expression of neuroplasticity.

Evidence has been presented that the processing of pain signals in the dorsal horn of the spinal cord (and the trigeminal nucleus) can operate in four main states [158]

State 1. The normal state. Stimuli activate low-threshold mechanoreceptors to produce innocuous sensations such as that of touch, vibration, pressure, warmth or cool. Receptors exist for all these modalities that have thresholds in unsafe ranges of stimulation.

These are called nociceptors. Activation produces localized pain sensations that are distinctly different from innocuous stimulation. Although painful, these sensations are not accompanied by any noticeable emotional engagement.

State 2. A functional re-organization of the dorsal horn (and the trigeminal sensory nucleus). This state is characterized by suppression of transmission of somatosensory information, and the ability of high-intensity stimuli to evoke a sensation of pain is reduced in this state.

A decrease in transmission of pain signals is caused by inhibitory influence on neurons in the dorsal horn. The source of the inhibition can be peripheral such as from activation of Aδ fibers, or supraspinal such as a part of "flight or fight" reactions mediated by the noradrenaline (NA)-serotonin descending pathways.

It is believed that these are the mechanism through which stimulation of skin receptors, hypnosis, suggestions, distraction and cognition suppress the perception of painful stimuli. The placebo effect may be caused by activation of similar neural circuits. Pharmacological agents such as opioids, α-adrenergic agents and GABA$_A$ antagonists (bicuculline) can also promote the expression of state 2 of the function of the dorsal horn pain circuits.

State 3. Increased excitability and decreased inhibition of dorsal horn sensory cells that sensitizes these cells to innocuous sensory stimuli. In this mode of function, low-intensity input, which is normally harmless, generates a sensation of pain (allodynia) and exaggerated pain experience that outlasts the duration of noxious stimulation (hyperpathia). Central sensitization causes hyperpathia.

Mononeuropathies may promote the changes that occur in stage 3 [735], and the extension of existing nociceptive receptive fields of dorsal horn neurons may occur through activation of ineffective (dormant) synapses [264].

State 4. Changes occur in the morphology including deaths of cells, degeneration or atrophy of synapses, a creation of new synapses and modification of the contacts between cells and synapses.

Aβ fibers that usually terminate in layers III-V of the horns of the spinal cord may invade the territory of C fibers (lamina II) and make synaptic contact with cells that are innervated by C fibers [158]. Innocuous sensation carried by the Aβ fibers is passed on to pain pathways, creating the phenomenon of allodynia.

The role of central sensitization

There is considerable evidence that the wide dynamic range neurons (WDR) neurons play a major role in the central sensitization including an increased sensitivity to C-fiber input. Activation of neuroplasticity causes increased the efficacy of excitatory synapses or a decreased efficacy of inhibitory synapses [731].

The "wind-up" phenomenon is related to central sensitization, and it is assumed to develop when C-fibers discharge in response to sustained high-frequency stimuli [480]. This causes the WDR neurons to increase their response progressively after each stimulus. Peptidergic fibers (in nervi nervorum) that contain SP, calcitonin and other peptides may be involved in the creation of sustained neural activation that causes pain sensation to persist beyond the duration of the tissue damage. Diffusion of substance P (SP) in the spinal horn may change the function of WDR neurons so that they become hyperactive.

The WDR neurons undergo neuroplastic changes in their function induced either by lowered inhibitory input from large diameter myelinated nerve fibers or increased excitatory input from C fibers as may occur in mononeuropathies [735]. That would explain why mononeuropathies are associated with changes in the firing pattern of WDR neurons (Figure 6.4).

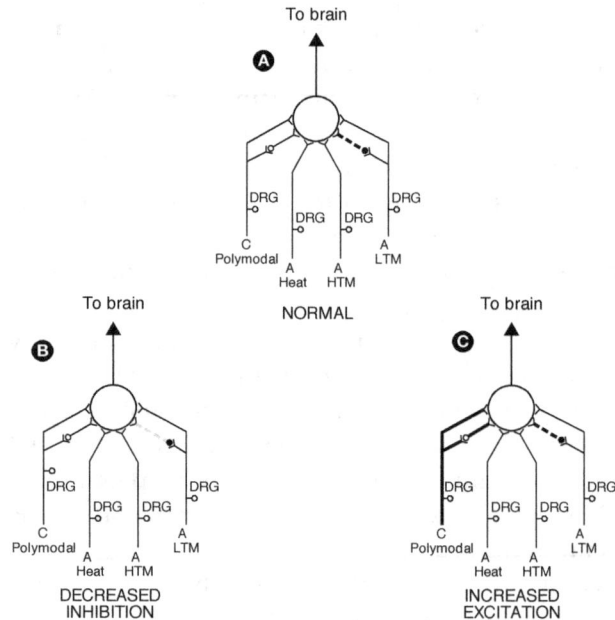

Figure 6.4 WDR neurons showing different states:

A: Normal situation

B: Decreased inhibitory input from LTM receptors through Aβ fibers.

C: Increased excitatory input from polymodal receptors through C-fibers. (Adapted from [528].

One such change in the function of WDR neurons includes an increase of the maximal firing rate of WDR neurons, and that may unmask normally inefficient synapses of their targets. Increased discharge rate or abnormal neural activity such as burst activity that replaces a "smooth" train of nerve impulses may cause re-routing of pain signals. This may be the basis for establishing functional connections between somatosensory circuits and pain circuits [115] and such abnormalities in the function of WDR neurons may, therefore, explain the cross-modal interaction expressed as allodynia.

Role of NMDA receptors

Sustained and transient activation of C-fiber nociceptors can induce central sensitization involving NMDA receptors [68]. Central sensitization may last as long as several weeks after it has been induced and the stimuli that caused the expression of neuroplasticity has been terminated. The threshold of WDR neurons may be further lowered by prostaglandins and nitric oxide synthesis.

Neurotransmitters involved

Glutamate plays an important role in damage to nerve cells that may be involved in creating pain. Excitotoxicity and other effects of glutamate can cause permanent damage to cells. Frequent stimulation of pain pathways thus damages their neurons more quickly. As we have discussed earlier, nerve damage provides an opportunity for maladaptive neuroplasticity, which is most undesirable, particularly in the dorsal horn and the trigeminal nucleus. Activation of the NMDA (glutamate) receptor is permissive for the release of SP in the dorsal horn [366].

The NMDA and neurokinin receptors are involved in chronic neuropathic pain [729], and that has suggested that NMDA receptor antagonists such as the experimental drug MK 801, would be effective in the treatment of chronic neuropathic pain. So far, however, attempts to modulate or affect the effect of glutamate that is found throughout the central nervous system has yielded little success.

The NMDA receptor antagonist MK 801 has been available for many years, but the success in using it in the treatment of pain has not materialized, mainly because of its hepatoxicity. Intravenous administration of Ketamine, another NMDA receptor antagonist has been shown to have some beneficial effect on such pain [643]. These drugs have considerable psychiatric side effects that have prevented their adoption. The universality of glutamate receptors across the central nervous system thwarts attempts to selectively regulate specific glutamate systems responsible for pain without causing a wide range of harmful side effects.

Symptoms related to activation of the sympathetic nervous system

The sympathetic nervous system plays a major role in many pain conditions such as Reflex Sympathetic Dystrophy (RSD) and, causalgia. The terms RSD and causalgia have been used as general descriptions of pain that involve the sympathetic nervous system. The new term "complex regional pain syndrome" or CRPS Type I has replaced the term RSD recently. The symptoms of CRPS Type I follow noxious events and include spontaneous pain and possibly allodynia and hyperpathia.

Skin edema and abnormal sudomotor (sympathetically activated sweat glands) activity in large regions of the body [585] are often components of CRPS I.

CRPS II may include allodynia, hyperpathia, and skin edema in areas not broad enough to be characteristic of CRPS I [413, 585].

Recent studies have shown that CRPS is associated with morphological changes in the brain. Geha and collaborators showed that gray matter morphometry and white matter anisotropy in people with CRPS differed from those of matched controls [207]. Atrophy has been shown to be present in the right insula, right ventromedial prefrontal cortex (VMPFC), and right nucleus accumbens people with CRPS and there were changes in the left cingulum-corpus callosum bundle. White matter connectivity in these regions showed signs of re-organization consisting of changes in branching patterns and altered connectivity of the VMPFC. Connections to the insula increased but connections to the basal ganglia decreased. The observed regional atrophy correlated to pain intensity and duration but the strength of connectivity between specific atrophied regions related to anxiety.

Pain conditions that are directly related to sympathetic neural activity are known as sympathetically maintained pain (SMP) [68].

Partial nerve injury can cause local nerves, both injured and uninjured, to express α adrenoceptors that allow the neurons to discharge in response to circulating epinephrine and norepinephrine.

Sympathetic afferent fibers enter the dorsal horn of the spinal cord, and their activity can modulate neural transmission in pain circuits of the dorsal horn. Sprouting sympathetic nerve fibers that project to the dorsal root ganglia (DRG) may also be involved in causing SMP.

The sympathetic nervous system gives some forms of chronic neuropathic pain their characteristics. Using lower back pain as a model, Apkarian and his colleagues have found an anatomical marker in the brain for chronic pain [381]. Recent concepts regarding the pathology of many forms of chronic pain involve learning and memory circuits in the brain.

During the chronic stage, however, neural activity shifts to circuits relating to emotion [247]. Reward circuitry is active during both acute and chronic stages. Recent studies have shown evidence of a strong involvement of the state of the motivational and emotional mesolimbic-prefrontal circuitry of the brain.

Affective symptoms in chronic neuropathic pain

Affective (mood related) symptoms such as depression often accompany severe pain, and these symptoms may be explained by the establishment of new connections in the pain pathways in the brain or spinal cord and other parts of the brain.

Normally, existing pathways may be amplified. The dorsomedial portion of the thalamus is likely to be involved providing subcortical connections to limbic structures such as the amygdala nuclei [353], the supplementary motor area, SMA, and prefrontal cortex. In these respects, chronic neuropathic pain has many similarities with other hyperactive sensory disorders such as tinnitus [93, 451] (Figure 6.5).

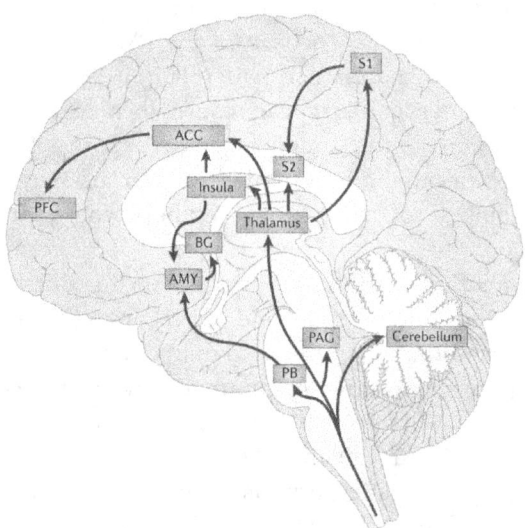

Nature Reviews | Neuroscience

Figure 6.5 Afferent nociceptive information enters the brain from the spinal cord. Nociceptive information from the thalamus is projected to the insula, anterior cingulate cortex (ACC), primary somatosensory cortex (S1) and secondary somatosensory cortex (S2), whereas information from the amygdala (AMY) is projected to the basal ganglia (BG). (Adapted from [90]).

Afferent spinal pathways include the spinothalamic, spinoparabrachio–amygdaloid and spinoreticulo–thalamic pathways.

Recent studies have shown evidence of a high involvement of the state of the motivational and emotional mesolimbic-prefrontal circuitry of the brain. Nociceptive inputs elicit plastic changes within this circuitry are involved in shifting the pattern of brain involvement from acute pain to chronic pain thereby making the pain less somatic and more mood-related [383]. Studies have also found that structures of the hippocampus, the insula and amygdala are involved in many forms of pain.

The insula is a complex and poorly understood structure. It has recently been associated with such complex functions as the identification of one's body or the "self." The techniques used to study the functions of these structures have been resting-state functional connectivity [39, 176].

These interconnections in the brain associated with chronic pain are the basis for the interaction between pain and other functions such as emotions and cognition (see Figure 6.5) and it is the basis for how several other brain functions can affect pain.

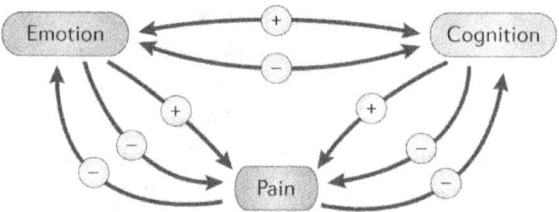

Figure 6.6 Feedback loops between pain, emotions, and cognition. Pain can have a negative effect on emotions and cognitive function. Conversely, a negative emotional state can lead to increased pain, whereas a positive state can reduce pain. Similarly, cognitive states such as attention and memory can either increase or decrease pain. Of course, emotions and cognition can also reciprocally interact. The minus sign refers to a negative effect, and the plus sign refers to a positive effect. (Adapted from [90]).

Deafferentation pain

Deafferentation pain is due to maladaptive neuroplastic changes caused by lack or reduction of normal sensory input. An extremely severe form of deafferentation pain is Anesthesia Dolorosa, which is characterized by constant severe burning pain and reduced or sensation to innocuous stimulation.

Anesthesia dolorosa occasionally occurs after injury to the nerves in the trigeminal system of the face [135, 392]. Anesthesia dolorosa may be a complication to the partial sectioning of the trigeminal nerve as a treatment for trigeminal neuralgia.

According to an expanded definition, anesthesia dolorosa may occur outside of the trigeminal system and may also occur after surgical sectioning of peripheral nerves or spinal nerve roots [506], although it has been claimed that anesthesia dolorosa is specific to the trigeminal system [659]. No known treatment has proven effective, although deep brain stimulation (DBS) recently has been found to provide some relief [135, 310, 491].

Deafferentation pain and phantom limb pain [475] are forms of chronic neuropathic pain. Nociceptor based pain conditions that endure may have a central component that is similar to chronic neuropathic pain, created by activation of maladaptive neuroplasticity.

Treatment of chronic neuropathic pain

Modern treatments of pain span a wide range of attempts to modify the function of the parts of the central nervous system that is involved in pain. We have already discussed some methods for treatment of chronic neuropathic pain. This book will only cover treatment of pain where it may relate to neuroplasticity. A more thorough description of the treatment of neuropathic pain may be found in clinically oriented books, and some information about various kinds of treatment may be found in [461].

Drug treatment of chronic neuropathic pain

Drugs that treat physiological pain effectively are not equally efficacious for all kinds of pain. Especially disturbing is the fact that most (if not all) pharmacological treatment of chronic neuropathic pain exhibit tolerance which means that their pain-relieving effect decreases with the time they are used. Most known pain relievers are only effective for a short period of use, usually less than 12 weeks.

The use of opioids in the treatment of chronic neuropathic pain has been controversial. Short-term studies have not provided clear evidence of efficacy in reducing the intensity of chronic neuropathic pain. Some investigators have reported significant efficacy compared with placebo, but the results of these results have been set in question because of small size, short duration, and potentially inadequate handling of dropouts [406] thus less tolerance than other studies. The efficacy of opioids as treatment of chronic neuropathic pain is, therefore, unclear.

Due to the tolerance effect the dosage must be increased after some time to achieve the same effect. This increases the risk associated with pain relievers such as opioids which can cause difficulties in breathing and even death. Non-steroidal anti-inflammatory drugs administrated in high dosages may have adverse effects on the stomach and the kidney.

A recent study emphasized that the beneficial effect of common pain relievers is short and that no beneficial effect seems to last more than 12 weeks due to the tolerance effect. There is an agreement between pain researchers that treatment for longer periods than 12 weeks are ineffective [109, 227]. While semisynthetic opioids have a very small risk of causing addition, they may cause craving that sometimes have been mistaken as addiction.

Of the NSAIDs, ibuprofen has the lowest risk of stomach bleeding [461]. Overdosage of some pain relievers can have serious consequences. For acetaminophen (Tylenol), intake of 4,000 mg over 24 hours has a high risk of liver failure. It is the most common reason for lever transplant.

The side effects of pain killers have been a common concern of both physicians and patients. This has gotten a new actuality recently when death from overdose of opioid has increased profoundly.

Overdosage of opioids can cause respiratory arrest. Recent statistics for the USA shows that during the year 2016, more than 64,000 died from drug overdosage, 33,000 people died from opioid overdose, approximately half of these involved prescription opioids.

The need for more effective treatments of pain was stated in a recent article in Science Daily by a group of known world experts [748].

Drugs with no effect on acute pain

Drugs that have little or no analgesic effect on acute (physiological pain) have found use in the treatment of chronic neuropathic pain either alone or together with other drugs. Benzodiazepines (such as diazepam) may have an indirect effect in the management of pain that is caused by muscle contractions (spasm) because they are GABA$_A$ agonists and therefore increase inhibition in neurons that either generate or facilitate muscle activity.

GABAergic inhibition also affects descending neural activity from the PAG, which normally suppress pain by its effect on neurons in the dorsal horn (the RVM pathway).

This means that enhancement of GABAergic inhibition from the administration of benzodiazepines may, in fact, decrease the (natural) inhibitory influence on the transmission of pain signals, intensifying the pain experience.

Other examples of drugs that do not affect acute pain but may have a beneficial effect on chronic neuropathic pain are the antidepressants such as imipramine, amitriptyline, nortriptyline and some sodium channel blockers [635].

Gabapentin (Neurontin) and pregabalin (Lyrica) are in extensive use for treating various forms of neuropathic pain conditions without it is known in detail how these drugs have their effects.

Studies of the effectiveness of antidepressants have indicated that the serotonin system is involved in chronic neuropathic pain, but the fact the SSRIs are less effective than non-specific drugs such as imipramine and nortriptyline [635] may set that assumption in question and indicate a more complex relationship between chronic neuropathic pain and the serotonin system.

Comparison of the efficacy of different drugs to relieve chronic neuropathic pain has shown that sodium channel blockers such as carbamazepine and Mexilitine were some of the least effective of these drugs. Sodium channel blockers are effective in the treatment of some forms of neuralgia, but best known for treatment of trigeminal neuralgia.

Treatment of itch

Opioids can have a beneficial effect on itch, but itch can also be a side effect of opioids. Whichever one of these opposite effects is greatest will dominate, but the analgesic and antipruritic effect of tends to dominate. This balance between beneficial and harmful effects may be shifted for unknown reasons and the condition so some patients may be worsened under certain circumstances. In those instances, the effect of the treatment may appear confusing to both patient and physician.

Treatment with non-pharmacological substances

Recently, several non-pharmacological drugs have been shown to be effective in relieving chronic neuropathic pain. Somewhat surprisingly, it has been shown recently that administration of omega 3 fatty acids can relieve pain [388]. Omega 3 fatty acids are usually regarded as food supplements and with no known side effects. Substances derived from Omega 3, such as lipoxins and D and E-series resolving [640] can prevent excessive inflammation [609] and promote removal of microbes and apoptotic cells. These substances are classified as specialized pro-resolving lipid mediators (SPM) and are candidates for becoming new and efficient pain relievers in the future.

There is some evidence that particularly a lowering of the ratio of omega 6 and omega 3 have a beneficial effect on plasticity disorders such as chronic neuropathic pain. α-linolenic acid (ALA) is a plant-based essential omega 3 polyunsaturated fatty acid that has anti-inflammatory effects, pleiotropic effects in neuroprotection, vasodilation of brain arteries, and neuroplasticity.

Administration of omega 3 and in particular decreasing the ratio between omega 6 and omega 3 increases the brain-derived neurotrophic factor (BDNF), a widely-expressed protein in the brain that plays critical roles in neuronal maintenance, and in learning and memory. BDNF also increases from physical exercise [63].

Omega-3 fatty acids are required for normal health, especially for the brain development and function. A study of Greenland Eskimos has shown that a seafood-rich diet is associated with low rates of coronary heart disease and autoimmune disorders. These effects have been ascribed to the intake of eicosapentaenoic acid (EPA) and docosahexaenoic acid (DHA) [630].

It has been shown in many studies that some of the active substances of cannabis such as delta-9-tetrahydrocannabinol (THC) and cannabidiol (CBD) can have beneficial effects in neurological disorders such as some forms of epilepsy, and many forms of pain [8, 551] and tinnitus [638]. THC is responsible for causing most of the euphoria associated with smoking cannabis, but CBD does not have such effects. Nabiximols, (Sativex) a cannabis-based formulation [325] has been licensed in the UK and Canada since 2010.

Nabiximols is an extract from selectively cloned cannabis plants that especially rich in CBD. Nabiximols contains a 1:1 ratio of THC and CBD and it is recommended as the second or third line in treatment of chronic neuropathic pain [523].

Wilsey and colleagues (2012) suggested that inhalation of vaporized cannabis even had a considerable therapeutic effect on people with drug-resistant neuropathic pain [723] (see also [461]). The important property of nabiximols for the relief of pain is that it has a high CBD content. This study showed that some plants tend to have vastly more CBD than THC [258].

The pharmacology of the active substances of the cannabis plants has been studied extensively [554], and our understanding of how the administration of these substances can provide pain relief has increased rapidly.

Treatment with electrical stimulation and lesioning

The recent development of methods that aim at affecting specific parts of the central nervous system has brought new ways of treating previously difficult to treat forms of neurological diseases. Electrical stimulation is in many ways attractive; it aims at specific structures, and it is not destructive. This is why electrical stimulation has replaced some old methods that used lesioning in the brain.

Stimulation of peripheral nerves (TENS)

Transcutaneous electrical stimulation of (peripheral) nerves (TENS) [718] has been used for many years in the treatment of pain. The underlying mechanisms for immediate pain reduction using TENS are most likely related to activation of large (Aβ) nerve fibers that inhibit pain neurons in the dorsal horn.

Electrical stimulation of peripheral nerves or dermatomes with impulses of a sufficiently high frequency is used [697]. This may, in turn, suppress neural activity in pain circuits at several segments above or below the targeted root due to the inhibitory effect of Aβ fibers. TENS may also promote expression of neuroplasticity in the spinal cord and supraspinal structures (such as the trigeminal nucleus).

This may be the cause of the long-term effect of TENS on chronic neuropathic pain but the exact mechanisms for this action are poorly understood.

Stimulation of the dorsal column

The theory behind dorsal column stimulation relates to the Melzack-Wall gating hypothesis [410]: the assumption that antidromic stimulation of dorsal column fibers influences cells in the dorsal horn, although the wide dynamic response (WDR) neurons are most likely involved also. Orthodromic activation of dorsal column fibers is assumed to exert suppressive actions through descending pathways [419] but ascending activity may also have a beneficial effect by inducing plastic changes in supraspinal structures.

The main targets of physiological (nociceptive) pain information are parts of the insular cortex, secondary somatosensory cortex, and several cortical areas in the cingulate sulcus. Many of these structures may also be activated in chronic neuropathic pain, but little is known about the extent of brain involvement in these kinds of pain.

Thalamic stimulation

There is increasing evidence that the thalamus is involved in different forms of pain, which has intensified attempts to treat some forms of pain through electrical stimulation of specific thalamic nuclei with implanted electrodes (deep brain stimulation, DBS) [357].

Stimulation of premotor cortical areas

The use of electrical stimulation of the motor cortex or the prefrontal cortex to control neuropathic pain that is resistant to other treatments has recently been studied by many investigators [98, 310, 418]. Electrical stimulation of premotor areas (PMA) and supplementary motor areas (SMA) [680] has been shown to reduce pain, suggesting an involvement of motor areas in pain perception.

Stimulation of the prefrontal cortex

The exact mechanism through which such stimulation works is unknown, but there is much that is known. Connections from the prefrontal motor cortex to the amygdala and other limbic structures could be responsible for the beneficial effect of electrical stimulation in pain, though other connections to limbic structures could mediate the beneficial effect. Connections from the prefrontal motor cortex could activate the descending PAG pathways.

The fact that stimulation of the prefrontal cortex has a beneficial effect on some forms of pain has likewise increased our knowledge regarding the pathophysiology of neuropathic pain. The beneficial effect of motor cortex stimulation [98] decreases with time of use, as is the case for many other treatments of neuropathic pain.

Use of TMS for pain control

Studies have shown that some forms of pain such as deafferentation pain can be influenced by transcranial magnetic stimulation (TMS) of the brain. TMS uses strong magnetic impulses to induce electrical currents in brain tissue. In that way, TMS activates or inactivates underlying brain tissue depending on the stimulation parameters.

TMS has been shown to have the ability to suppress the effects of deafferentation. Subsequent implantation of electrodes in the brain for permanent stimulation (deep brain stimulation, DBS) of the structures in the brain that have been found to reduce the pain when activated by TMS provides a constant relief of many neurological symptoms such as some of those created by maladaptive neuroplasticity.

How does DBS work?

DBS has now replaced many of the destructive lesioning procedures previously used for the treatment of severe pain. DBS is also utilized for the treatment of movement disorders. The development of these techniques, besides providing a much-needed therapeutic tool, has brought forth new knowledge regarding the pathophysiology of some forms of neuropathic pain. Animal experiments have shown indications that high-frequency electrical stimulation can block sodium and L-and T-type calcium current, which could conceivably be the cause of the observed inhibition (inactivation of neurons) [57, 568]

It has also been suggested that high-frequency stimulation may re-synchronize abnormal impulse patterns that are associated with pathologic functions such as pain [568] and it has also been hypothesized that electrical stimulation works by inactivating brain tissue by constantly depolarizing nerve cells. This would be expected to cause a similar effect as that of ablations but reversible.

Deep brain stimulation (DBS) may also activate structures beyond the location of the electrodes, possibly activating anatomically distant regions of the central nervous system in abnormal and unanticipated ways. While electrical stimulation may constantly hyperpolarize many nerve cells, the stimulation is also likely to activate many nerve fibers in adjacent fiber tracts.

Such activation is abnormal and may cause temporally coherent high-frequency firings of many fibers (rates of stimulation of 120-180 pps is commonly used).

Lesions as treatment for chronic neuropathic pain

Lesions have been made in almost all structures, including fiber tracts and nuclei, along with the neuroaxis of pain pathways connecting the spinal cord or trigeminal nucleus to the cerebral cortex. Lesioning is a form of treatment that is not reversible. This is a severe disadvantage, and there are many examples of treatment where lesioning has been replaced by other forms of treatment such as electrical stimulation.

Lesions of dorsal roots

Some forms of chronic pain have been treated surgically by a destruction of the dorsal root entry zone (DREZ) that is, the selective destruction of the layers that are dominated by C-fiber entrances (Lissauer's tract) [632]. The DREZ procedure has been largely abandoned, except for cases of brachial plexopathy.

Lesions of CNS structures

Many, or perhaps most, of these methods were introduced without knowledge about their mode of action. Only later, if at all, has it become understood how these methods produced their beneficial effects on the various forms of pain they were aimed at treating. The implementation of these methods and the evaluation of their prognoses have brought forth a new understanding of the pathophysiology of many different pain conditions. Studies even go as far as considering the effects of thalamotomy [744] and cingulotomy [248, 520].

Many structures of the brain have been the target for lesions for the treatment of chronic neuropathic pain. Many, or perhaps most, of these methods were introduced without knowledge about their mode of action. Only later, if at all, has it become understood how these methods produced their beneficial effects on the various forms of pain they were aimed at treating.

The implementation of these methods and the evaluation of their prognoses have brought forth a much new understanding of the pathophysiology of many different pain conditions.

Lesions in the sympathetic nervous system

While sympathectomy often produces good short-term effects on different forms of pain, the long-term effects are poor according to two studies [562, 669] and post-sympathectomy pain is an obstacle in that form of treatment. The effect of a sympathectomy may wane with time. Chemical sympathectomy using α-blocking agents such as phentolamine or phenoxybenzamine may be successful at treating pain. α-adrenergic blockade cause side effects such as orthostatic reactions, observable when an individual attempt to rise from a prone position. Treatment with β-adrenergic blocker such as those commonly used medication for heart ailments was found ineffective in treating pain in one study [583].

Lesion of limbic structures

Lesioning the cingulate gyrus has been used with some success to treat severe chronic pain [248, 520]. Although lesions in other limbic structures are effective in treating psychiatric disorders, their efficacy in treating pain has not been established [232]. DBS has now replaced many of the destructive lesioning procedures previously used for the treatment of severe pain.

The vagus nerve

Matters regarding the vagus nerve was discussed in Chapter 2. Here we will discuss specifically its relationship to chronic neuropathic pain.

Electrical stimulation of the vagus nerve

Vagus nerve stimulation can suppress acute pain, but it does not appear to produce an analgesic effect on chronic neuropathic pain [320, 479].

The finding that electrical stimulation of the vagus nerve is beneficial in the treatment of pain [89, 320] was met with astonishment when first publicized. It was discovered in connection with the use of electrical vagus nerve stimulation to control epileptic seizures.

While the mechanisms for its effect on pain are still incompletely understood, it is apparent that the vagus nerve plays a major role in endogenous pain [206].

Studies in animals have shown that electrical stimulation of the vagus nerve attenuates the response of dorsal horn neurons to many different type types stimuli, both noxious and innocuous [108]. Vagal nerve activity elicited by endocrine stimulation from the adrenal medullae has a similar effect [284]. The effect seems to be related to anatomical connections between the vagus nerve and the dorsal horn neurons that mediate pain [206] [284].

Other studies have shown that stimulation of the vagus nerve reduces the pain from controlled stimulation of nociceptors and it reduces the temporal integration of pain elicited by consecutive impulses ("wind-up") and pain from tonic pressure [320]. The same study, however, did not show an effect on pain associated with single impulses of heat [320]. This indicates that activity in the vagus nerve mainly affects the central processing of pain (central inhibition). Other studies have indicated that the effect of vagal activity on pain is mediated through the NA-serotonin descending system [668].

The vagus nerve seems to be involved in the opioid-induced analgesia as studies in rats have shown that vagotomy decreases the analgesic effect of intravenously administered morphine [206]. A functional vagus nerve is thus necessary to appreciate the analgesic effect of morphine.

The involvement of the vagus nerve in sexual functions, particularly those of women, has been the focus of a few studies that indicate that the vagus nerve bypasses the spinal cord to supply sensory input to the brain [327, 709]. There are indications that the vagus nerve transmits sensory input from the genitalia to the brain and that such activation of the vagus nerve may decrease pain perception.

Placebo effect

It is well known that placebo treatment can have a positive effect on pain, and placebo treatment has been recognized as an effective form of treatment for pain [226, 361].

Patients who are given inactive medication, but told that they are receiving real pain medication, improve and experience a decrease in their pain symptoms.

The placebo effect could be caused by endogenous opioids that were produced due to the expectation that the pain would be relieved by the medication that was assumed to be active.

One study of postoperative patients supported that hypothesis and showed that those people, who responded positively to placebo, responded to subsequent administration of naloxone with increased pain. Those who did not respond to the first administration of placebo did not respond to naloxone either [361].

Administration of naloxone instantly eliminates the effect of opioids. (Naloxone is a drug that blocks opioid rectors.) Considering the complexity of pain perception and its interplay with emotional factors in many forms of pain, it is understandable that additional mechanisms may be involved in the observed effect of placebo treatment for pain [226]. The limbic structures and descending pathways from the prefrontal cortex are most likely involved.

Experimental new treatments

Intravenous guanethidine that reduces norepinephrine in adrenergic neurons and blocks re-uptake is effective in the treatment of some persons with CRPS I, but some persons have experienced the brief increase of pain following days or weeks of improvement. There are some indications that treatment with oxytocin may reduce pain [220]. (See Chapter 4 for a detailed description of oxytocin).

It has been suggested that treatment with α-adrenergic blockade would be beneficial but studies have shown side effects such as orthostatic reactions, observable when an individual attempt to rise from a prone position. Treatment with α adrenergic blocker such as those commonly used medication for heart ailments is ineffective in treating pain [583].

Chapter 7

Tinnitus

Abstract

1. Subjective tinnitus and auditory hallucinations are the phantom sensations of the auditory system.

2. Subjective tinnitus is the perception of meaningless sounds that occur without any physical sounds activating the ear.

3. Hallucinations are the perception of speech, music and other meaningful sounds.

4. Objective tinnitus is caused by a (physical) sound that is generated in the body that reaches the ear by transmission in bones and other tissue.

5. Chronic subjective tinnitus has many similarities with chronic neuropathic pain.

6. Subjective tinnitus often has two components, one that is a sensation of sound the other is an effect on a person that can be best described as suffering.

7. The suffering is not directly related to the loudness of the tinnitus sound.

8. The most common way of evaluating the severity of tinnitus is from an analog scale from 1 to 10.

9. Tinnitus is often accompanied by such abnormalities as hyperacusis (lowered tolerance level for sound) and sound distortion.

10. Chronic tinnitus may be initiated by events in the ear or exposure to loud sounds but can persist through neuroplastic changes after these initial events have ceased.

11. Stress and mood related disorders can make a person's tinnitus worse.

12. The sympathetic nervous system is involved in some forms of tinnitus.

13. Studies have shown signs that some forms of tinnitus may involve the non-classical auditory pathways.

This may explain the observed cross-modal interaction that some persons with tinnitus experience.

Introduction

There are two kinds of tinnitus, subjective and objective tinnitus. Objective tinnitus is sounds generated in the body and conducted to the ear. Subjective tinnitus is hearing of meaningless sounds such as noise-like sounds, tones, or other continuous or transient sounds. It is not caused by a physical sound but generated in the ear or the brain. Subjective tinnitus is therefore a phantom sensation as are hallucinations. An observer can hear objective tinnitus, but only the person who has subjective tinnitus can hear the tinnitus sound.

Tinnitus is meaningless sounds while auditory hallucinations are meaningful sounds such as music or speech. Of those two kinds of phantom sounds, tinnitus is by far the most common.

Subjective tinnitus is another of the common diseases where maladaptive plasticity plays a major role in the creation of the symptom (perception of sound without physical stimulation). Subjective tinnitus and chronic neuropathic pain, discussed in the previous chapter have many similarities [444, 451].

The sounds of subjective tinnitus may be different from normal (physical) sounds that reach the ear. In addition to the sound component, subjective tinnitus has a component that can best be described as suffering (or distress).

Tinnitus may start from insults to the ear such as loud sounds, and it can be maintained without further external input. Plastic changes in the brain are involved in the generation and maintaining most forms of severe chronic subjective tinnitus.

This chapter mainly discuss subjective tinnitus because objective tinnitus and hallucinations are not directly linked to activation of neuroplasticity.

Objective tinnitus

Objective tinnitus [598] is often caused by blood flow in arteries close to the cochlea. Blood flow through narrow passages creates noisy turbulence. The sound may be transmitted to the cochlea via bone conduction. Tinnitus that is caused by blood flow is pulsatile and is synchronous with the heartbeat which makes it easy to identify. Contractions of muscles in the head may produce clicking sounds. Spontaneous contractions of the middle ear muscles or palatal myoclonus are examples of phenomena that may generate other kinds of audible sounds and appear as clicking noises [28, 598]. Objective tinnitus is usually of low intensity, and when a person becomes aware of its etiology, it becomes easier to ignore.

Subjective tinnitus

Subjective tinnitus is a common disorder that can have many forms [456]. Subjective tinnitus is mainly a disorder of the central nervous system (including the auditory nerve); only in a few instances can it be caused by diseases of the ear. Together with neuropathic pain, subjective tinnitus is one of the most frequent and most debilitating forms of phantom sensations [451, 456].

The loudness and the nature of the sounds that a person with tinnitus perceives varies widely, from being barely noticeable in a quiet environment to being so loud that it disturbs work and sleep [453]. The intensity and character of the tinnitus often depend on factors such as stress and physical work, but for many people, tinnitus does not seem to be related to any discernable factors.

Eye movements (changing gaze) or neck movements can often change the loudness and the frequency (pitch) of a person's tinnitus [453].

Signs accompanying tinnitus

Some forms of severe tinnitus are accompanied by changes in the processing of sounds such as causing hypersensitivity, hyperacusis (lowered tolerance of sounds) or distortion of sounds; tinnitus may be accompanied by impaired speech discrimination [456].

Some people with tinnitus may experience affective (mood-related) symptoms and of disorders such as depression are more frequent in people with tinnitus [348].

Lack of objective signs of severe tinnitus

Subjective tinnitus has no objective signs and classification of the severity of subjective tinnitus must, therefore, be based solely on the patients' assessment of the severity of the tinnitus. When evaluating the severity of tinnitus, it is most often the level of the sound (loudness) that is evaluated, but it is for most persons with tinnitus the other sign of the disease, namely what is best described as suffering that is the most bothersome. That part of the disease is more difficult to evaluate and often ignored in the assessment of a person's tinnitus.

Subjective tinnitus cannot be evaluated through the use of known clinical tests, and only the patient's description can be used to characterize the strength and character of the tinnitus from which an individual suffers. Tests such as loudness matching and masking tend to produce very low estimates of loudness of tinnitus, even when the tinnitus causes severe annoyance to the patient [221, 687].

In one study [687] 75 % of the persons with tinnitus on one side (one ear) matched the loudness of their tinnitus to a (physical) sound that was presented to the other ear at only 10-20-dB sensation level (SL). (Sensation level (SL) is the sound level (in dB) above a person's threshold of hearing). Such matches can therefore not be used to as estimates of the severity of tinnitus [187, 550]. Sounds of these relatively quiet loudness levels ought not to produce the degrees of annoyance that the person with tinnitus experience.

Physiological signs of tinnitus

The search for physiologically verifiable abnormalities in the auditory nervous system in people with subjective tinnitus has been disappointing. Short latency auditory evoked potentials do not show the degree of abnormalities expected for a person with severe tinnitus [437].

Middle latency responses (MLR) obtained in persons with severe tinnitus (defined as "problem tinnitus") show some abnormalities that may be related to the tinnitus. Gerken 2001 [213] has reported that persons with tinnitus have an abnormally large amplitude in their MLR in as many as 56% of the people with tinnitus who were tested.

Similar abnormalities, but smaller, were found in elderly persons who did not have tinnitus [213]. Studies in animals have shown similar changes in auditory evoked responses after noise exposure [661, 663].

Classification of tinnitus

A commonly used classification based on a person's self-evaluation of his/her tinnitus [550] defines three degrees of severity: "slight," "moderate," or "severe." "Slight" describes intermittent tinnitus that only bothers the person in a quiet environment; "moderate" describes tinnitus that is constant and more intense, disturbs sleep and bothering the person when trying to concentrate.

The classification "severe" is reserved for tinnitus that is a constant annoyance and interferes greatly with the ability to concentrate and inhibits sleep. People with "severe" tinnitus are often incapacitated, and some people with that degree of tinnitus resign from work due to a disability caused by the tinnitus. Others commit suicide. The response to severe tinnitus is more severe if the tinnitus is regarded to be inescapable.

Tinnitus has similarities with chronic neuropathic pain

Tinnitus has many similarities to pain, and in particular, chronic neuropathic pain [451]. Both diseases lack visible signs of illness, and these diseases are not life-threatening but can affect a person's quality of life severely. Both diseases can cause severe suffering, and they often have emotional components in the form of affective (mood-related) diseases such as depression [348]. People with these conditions do not get much sympathy from relatives and friends, and the attention that people with tinnitus get from their physicians is minimal.

A few audiologists specialize in the treatment of tinnitus. Both tinnitus and pain can lead to suicide.

Causes of tinnitus

Activation of neuroplasticity plays an important role in creating subjective tinnitus and maintaining it. Most forms of subjective tinnitus are caused by activation of neuroplasticity [454].

Subjective tinnitus may occur after exposure to loud sounds, especially impulsive or high-frequency sounds. The duration of the tinnitus may be brief, abating gradually after the end of the exposure, over minutes, hours or days. Tinnitus may also start without any distinct cause can be identified. This is often the case for tinnitus that occurs at old age.

There is a considerable individual variation in the contraction of tinnitus from sound exposure. In some persons, however, the tinnitus that occurs after exposure to a loud sound may last a lifetime. Some persons may even experience severe and lasting tinnitus from a single exposure to loud noise such as from a fire alarm.

Intake of large dosages of pharmacological agents such as aspirin (acetylsalicylate), aminoglycoside antibiotics, loop diuretics (furosemide, ethacrynic acid), quinine, indomethacin, cisplatin, and other cytostatics used in cancer treatment can cause tinnitus and hearing loss [606]. Carbamazepine, tetracycline, antipsychotic drugs, lithium, tricyclic antidepressants, monoamine oxidase inhibitors, antihistamines, β-adrenergic receptor blockers, local anesthetics, and steroids (to name only a few) can also induce tinnitus, but rarely hearing loss. Caffeine and alcohol can also cause tinnitus.

Tinnitus caused by pharmacological agents usually disappears after cessation of administration of the agent that caused the tinnitus, but in some persons, the tinnitus becomes permanent. This is, in particular, the case for tinnitus caused by cytostatics and aminoglycoside antibiotics [557].

Some specific disorders are associated with tinnitus and abnormal sound processing. Williams-Beuren (WBS) syndrome, (infantile hypocalcemia) has a high comorbidity with hyperacusis [75].

Tinnitus is usually the first symptom of vestibular schwannoma (acoustic tumors), but vestibular schwannoma is a rare etiology for tinnitus. Tinnitus is one of the three symptoms that characterize Ménière's disease

Various forms of disorders that have been assumed to affect the cochlea have been associated with tinnitus [535]. For example, exposure to loud noise, or the administration of ototoxic drugs that cause morphological changes in the sensory epithelium in the cochlea, promoting disorders accompanied by tinnitus. However, recent studies show that these relationships are complex and insufficiently known [507].

Tinnitus often occurs together with high-frequency hearing loss. It is not known why only a few people with high-frequency hearing loss experience severe tinnitus.

While people with tinnitus usually have some form of hearing loss, persons with hearing loss do not always have tinnitus. The hearing loss that occurs together with tinnitus may not be caused by the same morphological changes in the cochlea as those causing the tinnitus, and the anatomical location of the anomalies that cause the tinnitus may not be the same as those associated with common forms of hearing loss. Like other pathologies, some yet unknown factors seem to be necessary for the development of tinnitus in addition to hearing loss.

Overexposure to sound as a cause of tinnitus

Animal experiments have shown that overexposure to sound, similar to that which is known to cause tinnitus in humans, also causes signs of hyperactivity in the cochlear nucleus [307] and alters temporal integration in the inferior colliculus (IC) [666]. Other animal studies have shown that injury to the peripheral auditory system can cause these central auditory structures to become hyperactive [211]. The observed changes in function are most likely induced by expression of neuroplasticity, either as a result of the overstimulation, or, more likely, as a result of deprivation that was caused by the noise-induced hearing loss (NIHL) from the sound stimulation that was used in these experiments.

Deprivation of sound as a cause of tinnitus

The effect of reduced high-frequency input on the auditory system in people with the cochlear type of high-frequency hearing loss may be similar to the pain that is caused by a reduced sensory input to dorsal horn nerve cells.

The fact that it has been reported that 40% of people with otosclerosis also have tinnitus and that such persons obtain relief from successful stapedectomy [215] might indicate that the cause of the tinnitus was located in the conductive apparatus of the ear. A more plausible explanation would be that the sound deprivation due to the (conductive) hearing loss that had activated neuroplasticity.

That some forms of tinnitus can be caused by deprivation of high-frequency input from the cochlea is supported by the finding that cochlear implants set to generate high-frequency stimulation of the cochlea (4,800pps) are beneficial to some people with tinnitus [572].

Auditory nerve injuries as a cause of tinnitus

Tinnitus often occurs after acute injury to the intracranial portion of the auditory nerve, such as may occur from surgical manipulation or in connection with the surgical removal of tumors in the vicinity of the auditory portion of the eighth cranial nerve (mostly vestibular schwannoma) [92, 425, 435]. The fact that tinnitus often occurs immediately after operations in the cerebellopontine angle (such as microvascular decompression, MVD, operations to treat hemifacial spasm or trigeminal neuralgia) where the intracranial portion of the auditory nerve has been manipulated surgically is strong evidence that injury to the auditory nerve can cause tinnitus [425, 435].

These observations, however, must not be taken to indicate that the anatomical location of the physiological abnormalities that cause the tinnitus is the auditory nerve. Rather, there are several indications that the forms of tinnitus that are caused by injury to the auditory nerve are caused by changes in the function of central nervous system structures.

Some rare forms of tinnitus can be relieved by moving a blood vessel off the root of the auditory nerve (MVD operations) [466] which may indicate a similarity between some forms of tinnitus and diseases such as hemifacial spasm and trigeminal neuralgia.

Bilateral tinnitus is different from unilateral tinnitus, and MVD of the auditory nerve has a lower success rate for treatment of the bilateral form compared with the unilateral form of tinnitus [686].

Pathology of subjective tinnitus

The pathophysiology of subjective tinnitus is poorly understood, and since there are so many forms of tinnitus, a single mechanism cannot explain the pathophysiology for all its various forms, and some of these different pathologies affect different parts of the auditory system.

Difficulties differentiating between different forms of tinnitus have hampered efforts to find effective treatment [453].

Since tinnitus is perceived as a sound, it is intuitively but erroneously considered to be a phenomenon of the ear. The early models assumed the anatomic location of the pathophysiology of subjective tinnitus was within the ear. These models had to be revised when it became evident that some forms of subjective tinnitus occurred in deaf individuals, and that tinnitus could occur after that auditory nerve was severed [460]. These observations belie the assertion that tinnitus was due to a pathology within the ear and provided strong evidence for the concept that many forms of tinnitus are due to functional abnormalities in the brain.

The complexity of the pathophysiology of tinnitus even in selected populations is evident from the results of a study of 72 patients [466] who underwent microvascular decompression (MVD) of the auditory nerve for severe tinnitus, had a success rate of 54.8 % in males, but only 29.3% in women.

There are several possible causes of this difference. It is possible that the gender-specific reproductive hormones contribute differently towards the condition of tinnitus. Alternatively, the causes of the tinnitus may have differed between the groups.

Those people with less favorable outcome had had tinnitus for a longer period than those with better outcome [466, 595].

The higher level of testosterone in males likely plays a role, but the higher incidence of noise exposure in men than in women may also have contributed to this observed difference in treatment results.

The difference in treatment results of other MVD disorders (hemifacial spasm, HFS) and trigeminal neuralgia (TGN)) for men and women are small, and success rates (80-90%) are higher than it is in patients with tinnitus [44, 45, 466].

The prevalence of tinnitus increases with age. This can have many causes. Changes in the GABA system that normally occur with age [101] may be one such cause of some of the observed changes in the processing of sensory information including tinnitus.

Altered functional connectivity

More recently studies of connectivity in the brain have led to new understanding of the pathological changes that cause phantom sensations such as tinnitus. Thus several studies of conductivity have indicated that changes in the strength of the connections between different structures in the brain might be involved in creating tinnitus [139, 594].

There is now considerable evidence that the functional connections in several parts of the brain are different in people with tinnitus compared with people who do not have tinnitus. Several recent models that describe the pathology of chronic tinnitus [139, 593, 594] indicate that changes in the connections between several structures in the brain may be involved in the creation of tinnitus.

Maladaptive neuroplasticity as a cause of severe tinnitus

There is now evidence that activation of maladaptive neuroplasticity plays an important role in many forms of tinnitus [163]. However, studies of such phenomena are demanding, and so far, only a few studies have been published that relate neural synchrony and neural coherence to symptoms and signs of disease.

Studies in animals have shown that deprivation of input to the auditory system can cause hypersensitivity [211]. Altered temporal integration such as may occur after overstimulation of the auditory system [666] or deprivation of input [212] are examples of altered processing of sensory information. These physiological changes may be due to an altered balance between inhibition and excitation.

Neuroplastic changes in the processing of sensory information may be triggered by deprivation of input, overexposure, exposure to chemical agents, or from morphological changes such as from injuries, tumors or age-related changes. Reduced input from sensory receptors is a common trigger of functional changes and causes abnormal processing of sensory information and often increased sensitivity. The functional changes that are related to abnormal sensory input) may involve changes in synaptic efficacy or the elimination of synapses and axons.

The theory that tinnitus may be caused by a compensatory mechanism for loss of sensitivity that has overreached and caused "self-oscillation" is supported by many studies [592]. The fact that tinnitus can be affected by psychological means (such as the tinnitus retraining program [293]) supports that hypothesis.

Re-routing of information in the brain

Information may be re-routed in the central nervous system as a result of expression of neuroplasticity. Such re-routing can also occur through morphological changes such as sprouting of axons and dendrites, and through the formation of new synapses. Changes in the function of synapses can unmask dormant synapses that are normally not conducting, [697]), opening new routes for information to take in the central nervous system. Changes in discharge patterns, such as from continuous firing to burst firing, can also unmask dormant synapses.

Reorganization of the central nervous system

Expression of neuroplasticity by deprivation of input may cause reorganization of the auditory cerebral cortex but is the reorganization a contributing factor for generating tinnitus? We do not know.

The parahippocampus is involved in multiple networks that are active in different forms of expression of tinnitus. The electrical activity generated by the parahippocampus is oscillations with several frequencies and the connectivity in the brain is related to distress network activity. One hub can be involved in multiple overlapping networks that generate oscillations with different frequencies.

A few studies have shown indications that reorganization of the auditory cortex is involved in some forms of tinnitus [478]. However, more recent studies have set that in doubt [347]. Other studies have shown that reorganization of the cerebral cortex may occur because of deprivation of input [559, 600] in a similar way as has been shown for other sensory cortices [548]. Some studies [292] indicate that the prefrontal cortex is a potential location for abnormalities that result in or contribute to tinnitus.

Structures that may be involved in tinnitus are many as is seen in Figure 7.1.

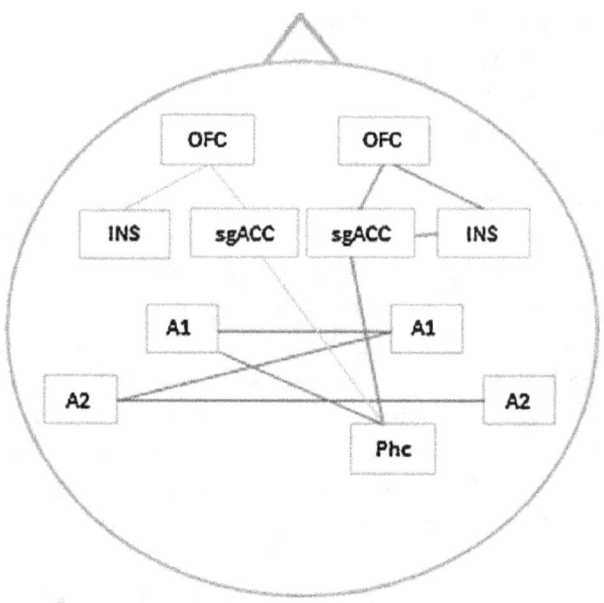

Figure 7.1 Connections between structures in the brain that may be involved in tinnitus. From: [140].

Functional connections in the brain are different for people who have had tinnitus for a short period compared with people who have had tinnitus for a long time (Figure 7.2).

short duration

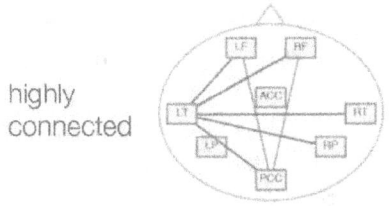

highly
connected

long duration

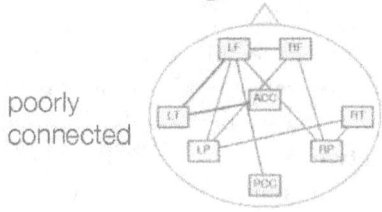

poorly
connected

Figure 7.2 Functional connections in the brain of people who have had tinnitus for a short time and a long time. Short time: Strong connections concentrated to the temporal part. Long time: Widespread strong connections. LF = Left Frontal, RF = Right Frontal, LT = Left Temporal = Right Temporal, LP = Left Parietal, RP = Right Parietal, ACC = Anterior Cingulate Cortex, PCC = Posterior Cingulate Cortex. (Adapted from [593]).

Abnormal cross-modal interaction

The abnormal cross-modal interaction between the somatosensory and auditory systems that occurs in some people with tinnitus has been interpreted to indicate an abnormal involvement of the non-classical (extralemniscal) auditory pathways [438, 446]. Such interaction is not found in healthy adults who do not have tinnitus.

A presence of subcortical cross-modal sensory interaction between sensory inputs in adults [368, 438] has been interpreted as a sign of abnormal involvement of non-classical sensory pathways.

The cross-modal interaction between the auditory and the somatosensory system [10, 438, 664] is also an example of re-routing of information that is caused by expression of neuroplasticity. Animal experiments have located some cross-modal interaction between the auditory and the somatosensory systems in neurons of the external nucleus, the dorsal cortex of the IC [10, 11, 662, 664], and in the cochlear nucleus [282, 620].

The direct subcortical route to the lateral nucleus of the amygdala nuclei from the thalamus may explain why chronic neuropathic pain and severe tinnitus often are accompanied by affective disorders such as fear and depression [349].

Activation of the non-classical auditory pathways that use nuclei in the dorsal and medial thalamus [353, 446] may explain the affective symptoms that are parts of the symptoms of plasticity disorder such as tinnitus and chronic neuropathic pain. It is also noteworthy in this connection that tinnitus and pain involve many perceptual networks, the subgenual anterior cingulate cortex (sgACC), the dorsal anterior (dACC) and posterior cingulate cortex (PCC).

The cross-modal sensory interaction between somatosensory and auditory systems that exist during childhood [446] is an indication of the activation of the non-classical auditory system. These signs decrease with age and are absent in most adult individuals indicating changes in the routing of auditory information. Similar cross-modal interaction can occur later in life in connection with tinnitus as indicated by the reoccurrence of the abnormal cross-modal interaction between the auditory system and the somatosensory system [95, 438].

The subcortical connections in the non-classical pathways may explain why some persons with severe tinnitus experience fear from sounds (phonophobia) and as well as the high incidence of depression in individuals with severe tinnitus [348].

The studies that have demonstrated the presence of cross-modal interaction between the auditory and somatosensory systems, therefore, support the hypothesis that the non-classical auditory pathways are involved in some forms of tinnitus. Imaging studies have shown a greater involvement of limbic structures in some persons with tinnitus [368], indicating abnormal participation of the non-classical auditory pathways.

The interaction between the auditory, somatosensory and visual systems has been reported in animal studies in which it was shown that sound-evoked activity in neurons in the thalamus could be modulated by visual or somatosensory stimulation [267].

The specific effect of visual input on tinnitus is unknown. However, sound can evoke phosphenes in some individuals with optic nerve disorders [360, 505].

The role of cross-modal interaction in tinnitus

Electrical stimulation of the skin can initiate, decrease or exacerbate existing tinnitus in some people [438]. The fact that electrical stimulation of the skin can have different effects on tinnitus may be explained by the diversity in the pathophysiology of tinnitus, and it may explain why, for instance, temporomandibular joint (TMJ) disorders are often associated with tinnitus [472, 473]. TMJ disorders are likely to cause abnormally increased neural activity in the trigeminal sensory system.

Some observations indicate that stimulation of receptors of one sensory modality may be perceived as a different modality in people with tinnitus. This is most apparent in people who experience tinnitus after injuries of their auditory nerve close to the brainstem; they report to perceive sounds from specific tactile stimulation. Møller and Møller (unpublished observation, 1982) noted one patient who reported that rubbing his back with a towel gave rise to a sensation of sound.

The fact that some persons with tinnitus can change their tinnitus by voluntary muscle contractions (such as eye muscles and jaw muscles) [93, 94, 114] is another sign of an abnormal cross-modal interaction.

Some persons report that they can alter their tinnitus by pressing on their check, mastoid, or any other spot in head-neck region [362].

The importance of temporal coherence

Temporal coherence in the activity of nerve cells seems to play an important role in many basic neurological functions. (Temporal coherence is a form of phase-locking of neural activity, or it can be interpreted as a correlation between the occurrences of nerve impulses in different cells in a population of many nerve cells).

It is becoming evident that correlation between the firing of many cells in a population of neurons is more important than the discharge rates of individual cells. Sensory thresholds seem to be related to the degree of temporal correlations of the discharges of many nerve cells.

When no sound is present, the time pattern of the spontaneous neural activity in the axons of the auditory nerve is normally uncorrelated.

When a stimulus such as a sound elicits neural activity that is phase-locked to the waveform of the sound, the neural discharges in individual axons consequently also become correlated (phase-locked) to each other. It is now believed that it is the degree of correlation that signal the presence of a stimulus and thereby eventually elicit an awareness of a sensory stimulus.

We lack suitable tools to determine the degree of temporal correlation of the discharges of cells in a population of nerve cells such as it occurs in a nucleus with hundreds of thousands of nerves cells.

There are many factors that can alter the correlation between the firing of cells in populations of nerve cells. Damage of various kinds can degrade the coherence of neural activity. Age-related degradation of the auditory nerve can cause impairment of temporal coherence. It has been suggested that tinnitus may be related to abnormal temporal correlations between the neural activity in individual auditory nerve fibers [164, 425].

Impairment of temporal coherence of the neural activity in the auditory nerve contributes to poor speech discrimination. Reorganization of the auditory nervous system that is caused by expression of neuroplasticity may also contribute to the poor speech discrimination that accompanies high-frequency hearing loss in some individuals.

Understanding coherence in brain networks is important for understanding the normal function of neural systems as well as the pathophysiology of brain injuries and harmful neuroplasticity.

The role of the sympathetic nervous system

There are several signs that the sympathetic nervous system is involved in subjective tinnitus. Studies conducted as early as the 1950s and 1960s have shown that stellate ganglion blockade was effective in treating the tinnitus in some patients with Ménière's disease [5]. It is not known exactly how the sympathetic nervous system is involved in generating the tinnitus, but sympathetic activation does affect the blood flow to the cochlea [350], which may affect the function of the cochlea.

Sympathetic fibers are located close to the hair cells of the cochlea [147], and noradrenaline secreted from these adrenergic fibers, may similarly sensitize cochlear hair cells as that of the adrenergic fibers proximal to the mechanoreceptors of the skin.

Reduction of noradrenaline secretion through sympathectomy and the subsequent reduction of the sensitization of hair cells could then explain the beneficial effects of sympathectomy on tinnitus.

Treatment of subjective tinnitus

Many forms of treatment have been tried for tinnitus, but the diversity of the pathophysiology and etiology of tinnitus makes it unlikely that a single treatment will have a beneficial effect on all forms of tinnitus. The focus on treatment has moved from the ear and the periphery of the nervous system to more central parts of the nervous system. This means that the treatment of tinnitus was directed towards correcting the functional changes in the nervous system either by reversing the plastic changes that caused the pathologic signs and symptoms or by correcting the balance between inhibition and excitation with the appropriate medications.

Studies from in the 1950s and 1960s have shown that stellate ganglion blockade was effective in treating the tinnitus in some people with Ménière's disease [5, 510, 704]. Beneficial effect (56% relief) were obtained in these persons, while persons with other causes of tinnitus had less benefit (27% relief) from that procedure [510, 704].

Some people experience relief of their tinnitus from the administration of benzodiazepines (that are GABAA agonists) such as Alprazolam [275, 301, 688] or Clonazepam [631], a clear sign that the anatomical location of the physiological abnormality is the central nervous system.

Baclofen, a GABAB agonist, has been found ineffective, as has gabapentin even though theoretically these two drugs should enhance GABAergic inhibition. In animal experiments, the (-)-isomer of baclofen is more effective than benzodiazepines [665] in reducing signs of hyperactivity in the IC (induced by sound stimulation).

Intravenous administration of lidocaine [409] can relieve tinnitus in some persons [355], but the effect of the oral forms of the drug (tocainide) [355] on tinnitus have been disappointing. This drug is associated with serious side effects even when given in therapeutic dosages. Another sodium channel blocker, Mexiletine, has been tried [400] but the beneficial effect has been difficult to establish. The active substances of cannabis have been used in the treatment of subjective tinnitus with some success [638].

In general, pharmacological treatment of tinnitus has been disappointing, and when drugs that have benefited individual patients have been tested in double-blind studies, they are not much better than placebos. Again, one reason for the poor results in population studies may be that persons with tinnitus makes up a heterogeneous group. Any single treatment, would most likely only be effective in a small subgroup of the population that is studied.

Some people experience tinnitus relief after moving a blood vessel of the auditory nerve (microvascular decompression, MVD) [137, 329, 443, 466]. Clinical studies show that MVD of the auditory portion of the CN VIII is effective in alleviating tinnitus in a selected population of tinnitus patients [377, 466] [462]. This has been taken to indicate that tinnitus in these patients was caused by the close contact between a blood vessel and the auditory nerve.

Electrical stimulation through electrodes placed on the cochlea [31, 104], or behind the ear [622] has been used with some success. Anatomical connections between the somatosensory system and the auditory system [457, 621, 750] may explain how stimulation of the skin may affect tinnitus. It may also explain why electrical stimulation from electrodes placed on the surface of the cochlear capsule can suppress the tinnitus some people have; the mucosa in the middle ear cavity is innervated by sensory nerve fibers that terminate on cells in the second segment of the spinal cord. Even stimulation of the fingers [540] has been shown to decrease tinnitus, probably through this connection.

The Tinnitus Retraining Therapy (TRT) developed by Pawel Jastreboff makes use of sound stimulation, psychological counseling, and education about the cause of the tinnitus and the function and anatomy of the auditory system [294]. The TRT is based on a neurophysiological model of tinnitus [292]. Other forms of training and different counseling methods have been described [558, 601].

Transcranial magnetic stimulation of the auditory cerebral cortex has been successful in eliminating tinnitus in some individuals [134, 323, 522]. Electrical stimulation of the cortex using permanently implanted electrodes has also been effective for some groups of patients [134].

When interpreting the effect of electrical or magnetic stimulation, it is important to consider how electrical stimulation acts on neural activity. High-frequency electrical stimulation can inactivate cells by constantly depolarizing the cells, which is normally the anticipated effect of electrical stimulation, but electrical stimulation is likely to also activate fiber tracts. Even the electrical current elicited by extracranial magnetic stimulation with single impulses can deactivate cells in the visual cortex [24]. This means that the same electrical stimulation may activate some parts of the nervous systems while inactivating other parts.

The beneficial effect of cortical stimulation is based on the assumption that the auditory cortex has re-organized in patients with tinnitus [478], and that electrical stimulation reverses these changes.

Other investigators find beneficial effects of electrical stimulation of the auditory cortex in specifically selected persons [136].

The beneficial effect that some tinnitus patients experience through stimulation of the auditory cortex might instead be caused by activation of thalamic cells through the descending cortico-thalamic tracts, rather than from reorganization of the primary auditory cortex.

A model of phantom sensations involves abnormalities in the thalamus causing arrhythmias in the cortico-thalamic loop [367, 700].

Other evidence points to the thalamus as being involved in tinnitus (perhaps through non-classical pathways). Whether electrodes placed on the surface of the cerebral cortex, in fact, stimulate neurons in the thalamus is irrelevant for treatment, and it is technically easier to place electrodes on the cortex rather than on the auditory thalamus.

Since stimulation of the nucleus of Meynert or stimulation of the vagus nerve can promote activation of neuroplasticity, electrical stimulation of the vagus nerve would be expected to facilitate reversing maladaptive neuroplasticity when paired with an appropriate sound stimulus. Such "pairing" of stimuli described in studies in animals [316] and later developed for clinical use in treating severe tinnitus [141]. Stimulation of the vagus nerve [168, 169, 492] has an advantage in that it requires a less invasive surgical procedure than deep brain stimulation.

Chapter 8

Movement Disorders

Abstract

1. Expression of neuroplasticity contributes to the signs of many movement disorders.

2. Activation of maladaptive neuroplasticity is involved in creation of the symptoms of spasticity and some forms of muscle spasm such as hemifacial spasm.

3. Spasticity is a common sequel to the spinal cord and cerebral injuries. It often includes increased muscle tone, hyperactive spinal reflexes, more for extensor reflexes than flexor reflexes.

4. Synkinesis that follows interruption of axons (axonotmesis) and inflammation of motor nerves may be caused by the reorganization of the respective motoneuron pools through expression of maladaptive neuroplasticity.

5. The role of neuroplasticity in movement disorders has not been recognized to the same extent as it has been for the sensory and nociceptive systems.

Introduction

The role of neuroplasticity is probably best recognized in the sensory and pain systems, but it can also affect the neural circuits that are involved in motor function in major ways [153, 233, 525].

There is evidence that expression of neuroplasticity may contribute to movement disorders such as spasms, spasticity and other forms of dystonia. Also, some forms of synkinesis may be caused by activation of neuroplasticity.

Expression of neuroplasticity often occurs in connection with injuries or various disorders of the motor system. It has been shown in many studies that functional re-organization of the motor system can contribute to the symptoms and signs of injuries to motor nerves, brain, and spinal cord [153, 525].

Extensive neural reorganization occurs after spinal cord injuries (SCI), and such re-organization may have beneficial as well as harmful effects, causing beneficial restoration of function and symptoms of plasticity disorders such as spasticity and spasms.

The motor systems are plastic and, as discussed in Section II, neuroplasticity related to motor systems is involved in many forms of beneficial changes of motor functions such as learning of new skills and restoration of function after injuries. Maladaptive neuroplasticity contributes to the development of several plasticity disorders that involve motor systems such as different kinds of spasm and spasticity and some forms of synkinesis.

We owe much of our understanding of motor system functioning in humans to a few scientists who used the neurosurgical operating room as their laboratory to study the function of the normal, as well as the pathologic human motor system. One of the first to use this opportunity was Wilder Penfield [513]. Currently, contributions to our understanding of motor system functioning and neuroplasticity come from studies using recent technological developments in imaging.

In this chapter, we will first describe disorders of the motor system where plastic changes play a major role. We will discuss how activation of maladaptive neuroplasticity may be involved in initiating and maintaining the symptoms and signs of spasticity and spasm. After that, we will discuss some diseases where recent research has shown indications that activation of neuroplasticity may play a major role in creating and maintain the symptoms and signs.

Pathophysiology of movement disorders

There are many causes of movement disorders; one important cause is functional changes initiated by activation of maladaptive neuroplasticity.

The role of neuroplasticity is probably best recognized in the sensory and pain systems, and it was discussed extensively in earlier chapters in this book. Its role in movement disorders has not received the same attention.

There is considerable evidence that similar reorganization can occur in the spinal cord and brain circuits that are involved in motor functions [233] [525], although not as well-known as neuroplasticity in sensory systems. Expression of neuroplasticity often occurs in connection with injuries disorders of the motor system, and it has been shown in many studies that functional reorganization of the motor system occurs following injuries to motor nerves, to the brain or the spinal cord. Extensive reorganization of the spinal cord and brain circuits occurs after spinal cord injuries (SCI).

It is well-known that expression of neuroplasticity occurs in response to pathologies such as reduced sensory input, but neuroplasticity is also activated by injuries to the motors system including reduced motor utilization.

Damage to motor nerves affects the function of the cells in the associated motonucleus [336] and that activate neuroplasticity resulting in compensatory functions such as spasticity. There is evidence that some of the symptoms of hemifacial spasm are caused by plastic changes in the facial motonucleus [424]. The function of motor systems in the brain and the spinal cord can change widely as a result of activation of neuroplasticity causing many forms of functional changes.

Neuroplasticity may be induced artificially by electrical stimulation of specific neural structures, or by exercise and training, to alleviate symptoms and signs of neurologic disorders such as pain, and to restore movements in movement disorders or to reduce spasm and synkinesis.

For example it has been known for many years that reflexes are plastic as are the interneuron in the descending motor pathways that leads to the α motoneurons [286, 525]. Other motor systems also show varying degrees of neuroplasticity.

Spasticity and spasm

Spasticity and spasm are the most common plasticity disorders of the motor system. Disorders and injuries affecting the spinal cord can cause spasticity.

The term spasticity is used to describe increased resistance against rapid stretching of muscles and increased stretch reflexes. The resistance against slow, passive stretching of muscles is less affected in people with spasticity.

Spasticity usually occurs several months after the occurrence of injuries to the spinal cord. During the first 4-6-month period after the injury, flexor and extensor spasms may alternate; after 6-12 months symptoms are predominantly affecting extensor muscles. The extensor reflexes may be abnormally affected by input from cutaneous receptors while innocuous (non-nociceptive) stimulation of specific skin areas may also provoke extensor reflexes. Stimulation of skin receptors in people who have had SCI may cause autonomic responses such as changes in blood pressure.

The signs of spasticity have been explained by abnormalities of spinal reflexes, mainly affecting the stretch reflex [86]. The flexor spasm that is typical for spasticity may be regarded as an exaggerated withdrawal reflex that is uncontrolled due to insufficient supraspinal input to the reflex circuit. Delwaide and Oliver showed indications that the tendon reflex (Ib inhibition) is reduced or not active in spasticity [145].

Pathophysiology of spasticity and spasm

The pathophysiology of spasticity is complex and poorly understood. The anatomical location of the physiological abnormalities that cause spasticity may be local circuits at the segmental level of the spinal cord that innervates the affected muscles. The abnormality may also be located in supraspinal structures. It is more likely, however, that the symptoms are caused by a complex interplay of physiological and morphological abnormalities, involving structures at several different anatomical locations.

The increased excitability and hyperactivity of the monosynaptic stretch reflex [86, 602], characteristic of spasticity may be caused by activation of neuroplasticity that causes increased excitatory input or decreased inhibitory input to α motoneurons, either directly or by presynaptic modulation. The loss of function or the trauma itself may initiate compensatory changes in the spinal cord through neuroplasticity. These plastic changes may then cause overcompensation in the form of hyperactivity to the extent of spasticity.

Since the neural circuits in the spinal cord gray matter are not "hard-wired," their connections and functions are task-dependent and can be modified in response to new conditions by expressions of neuroplasticity causing maladaptive changes in synaptic efficacy.

Many of the signs of spasticity that develop after spinal cord injuries or supraspinal disorders (e.g., cerebral palsy), may be regarded as a natural compensatory response to restore normal excitability of α motoneurons by increasing the gain of spinal reflexes. The symptoms of spasticity may be explained by an overcompensation to loss of function.

Expression of maladaptive neuroplasticity in spasticity may be caused by the deprivation of supraspinal input, or from changes within one or a few spinal segments. The decreased supraspinal input may cause hyperactivity of neurons at the segmental level. Increased excitability can also be caused by a decreased inhibitory input from local (segmental) or from supraspinal sources, or it may be due to an increased synaptic efficacy of the motor neurons themselves.

Understanding the regulation of α motoneurons and spinal reflexes excitability is, therefore, important for understanding the pathophysiological signs of spasticity (see Appendix B). As was discussed above, the excitability of the monosynaptic stretch reflex can be modulated by both supraspinal and segmental levels. The axo-axonic synapses are GABAergic, which may explain why GABA agonists such as benzodiazepines affect the excitability of the stretch reflex and are effective in the treatment of spasticity.

While it has been assumed that the excitability of α motoneurons is altered in spasticity, there is little direct evidence for this [602].

Changes in the recurrent (Renshaw) inhibition provides a short loop feedback to α motoneurons that is inhibitory, could offer an explanation to some of the signs of spasticity. This reflex is normally modulated by input from supraspinal structures [525]. If this modulation is altered because of SCI or strokes, that would affect motor functions.

Hyperactivity of the gamma system causing increased fusimotor activity [574] could cause abnormalities in the stretch reflex and exaggerated tendon reflexes. It was earlier assumed that increased gamma motor activity caused the increased excitability that is typical for spasticity, but more recent studies have not shown an increased firing frequency of Ia neurons. This means that the pathophysiology of spasticity is still incompletely understood.

Treatment of spasticity

We will here review some of the treatments used to alleviate the symptoms of spasticity. Many of these treatments have been found effective, although the physiological basis for their effectiveness was not completely known at the time they were introduced, and the basis for many of the different kinds of treatments that are in current use are still not completely understood.

Surgical treatment

One form of therapy for spasticity consists of severing fascicles of dorsal roots, thus decreasing proprioceptive input [634]. Surgical severance of dorsal roots of the spinal cord to treat spasticity was inspired by animal studies of decerebrate rigidity. Sherrington demonstrated in 1898 that the rigidity in a decerebrated animal could be abolished by sectioning of dorsal spinal roots. This observation was taken as a sign that sensory input to the spinal cord facilitates the monosynaptic stretch reflex as well as the polysynaptic withdrawal reflex.

Surgical operations using severance of dorsal roots to correct spasticity were performed by Foerster in 1908 [634]. Such operations are now reserved for patients in whom less severe treatments have failed. Dorsal root partial rhizotomies have had good effects in children with cerebral palsy [634].

Selective dorsal root rhizotomy (SDR) [2] was introduced in the USA by Peacock for cerebral palsy spasticity [512] and based on the work by Fasano, 1988 [177]. DeCandia [142] had demonstrated in animal experiments that, in the normal spinal cord, electrical stimulation of the dorsal roots promoted adaptation in such a way that the second of a train of impulses elicited a smaller response than the first if the rate of stimulation was higher than 15 pps. This depression did not occur in upper motoneuron injury.

Fasano, 1988 [177] applied this information to children with spasticity and found that sensory root fibers behaved differently. Some behaved normally and showed adaptation, but others did not even respond when stimulated at rates of 30-50 pps. Spasticity was reduced when the abnormally responding rootlets were severed.

Peacock and others [2, 512, 634] improved the safety of this procedure, while Deletis [144] developed an intraoperative mapping technique that could identify rootlets that were involved in micturition and should be spared. The response to dorsal root stimulation was studied by recording compound muscle action potentials (CMAP), and the ratio between the first and second response was used as a measure of the excitability of a particular fascicle of a dorsal root.

Treatment using administrations medications

Administration of GABAA agonists (benzodiazepines/valium) and GABAB receptor agonists (baclofen/Lioresal) enhance GABAergic inhibition and are effective in alleviating some of the symptoms of spasticity which supports the hypothesis that inhibition of circuits in the central nervous system is reduced in people with spasticity.

Local application of baclofen on the spinal cord (by intrathecal infusion using implantable pumps) has also been found effective in treating spasticity such that resulting spinal cord injury or cerebral palsy, where the supraspinal input is diminished, altered or absent. Other agents such as tizanidine (Zanaflex), a α-2 agonist, have had positive effects. It is a sign of the complexity of the phenomenon of spasticity that agents such as dantrolene, which inhibits calcium influx in peripheral muscles, and botulinum toxin, which works at the neuromuscular junction, is also effective in treating spasticity. These drugs have no known effect on the central nervous system, and their efficiency in alleviating symptoms of spasticity may be related to effects of neuroplasticity that was evoked by reduced muscle activity.

The Cannabis-derived substances THC (delta-9-tetrahydro cannabidiol) and CBD (cannabidiol) have also demonstrated efficacy in the treatment of spasticity and bladder dysfunction [523].

Electrical stimulation

Electrical stimulation of the rectum can induce ejaculation in men or orgasm in women with SCI and is effective in reducing the hyperexcitability of the monosynaptic reflex characteristic of spasticity [236, 636] with effects lasting many hours after cessation of the stimulation [235, 650].

This procedure may have directly stimulated the pudendal nerve itself or produced the positive effects on spasticity through the complex processes associated with orgasm or ejaculation. The anal canal is also innervated by visceral afferents, which are also stimulated by the electrical stimulation used in these studies and could also contribute to the observed effect.

In a study of the effect of anal stimulation, all six males and three females with SCI [236] experienced a decrease in spasticity lasting an average of 4-10 hours after each treatment. This study also showed that rectal stimulation in itself caused long-lasting relief without ejaculation and that this treatment was more effective than antispasticity medication. All subjects experienced an increase in spasticity during the stimulation, which consisted of one-second-long stimulation presented over 5-10 minutes [236].

Treatment of synkinesis

It is a common clinical experience that damage to the facial nerve can cause synkinesis when muscle function recovers. Synkinesis was earlier ascribed to a misdirected outgrowth of axons of the facial nerve, but this has been discounted.

It has recently been shown that facial synkinesis after trauma to the facial nerve can be alleviated by exercise [77]. Functional training of mimic facial muscles can speed up the recovery and reduce the synkinesis that often is experienced by people who have had moderate and severe facial nerve injury [96, 685]. This finding indicates that the synkinesis is instead caused by changes in synaptic efficacy on the facial motonucleus that were induced by activation of neuroplasticity.

There are anatomical connections between motoneurons in the facial motonucleus that serve different groups of muscles and the synapses that connect these motoneurons are normally dormant.

However, activation of neuroplasticity by injuries to the motor nerve is obviously able to unmask such synapses, creating synkinesis.

The role of neuroplasticity in rehabilitation of motor disorders

Physical therapy is the most commonly used means to facilitate activation of neuroplasticity. The mechanisms behind such promotion of expression of neuroplasticity for recovery (or replacement) of functions in brain injuries such as from strokes have been studied in animal (rat [304] and monkey) models. An example is the treatment of synkinesis [77].

Electrical stimulation of the cerebral cortex using implanted electrodes has been developed for that purpose in animal experiments (rats [4] and monkeys [521]). The technique has been tried in a few studies on humans, with good results [84]. Individual differences in the organization of the motor cortex are considerable, and it may, therefore, be necessary to map the motor cortex of individual stroke victims to instigate effective treatment [124].

Effects of deprivation of motor functions

A few studies have shown that deprivation of motor function such as may occur after severance of motor nerves can cause cortical reorganization [157]. Such reorganization of motor areas most likely occurs after amputation of limbs, and because motor functions are closely linked to perception, this form of post-injury reorganization may contribute to abnormal sensations that are experienced after limb amputation. Cortical representation can also be induced by changes in utilization of specific muscles [314].

Creation of proprioceptive brain maps

Proprioceptive brain maps, encompassing the brain's awareness of its body are dynamic, constantly updated based on input from the senses, particularly the touch and sight. Many brain structures have maps of the body, not only the cerebral sensory cortex. Mapping of the body on structures of the brain may be involved in creating the feeling of "self." Errors in cortical maps may cause symptoms of disease Activation of neuroplasticity can remap the cerebral cortex.

Section 4

Common Disorders
of
Nerves, Sensory and Motor Systems

This section provides a brief description of some common disorders of peripheral nerves, sensory and motor systems in which activation of neuroplasticity may play a role in creating the symptoms and signs. Also included are brief anatomical and physiological descriptions of these systems. For a more detailed discussion of the neuroscience of sensory system, please see [460], the biology of pain is described in a book [461].

The pathophysiology of most disorders of the central nervous system structures is poorly understood. The symptoms of inflammation of sensory nerves strokes or tumors are not only related to the morphological changes but also to a great extent to functional changes that occur as a result of activation of neuroplasticity.

Many of these changes in the central sensory nervous systems are induced by disorders of peripheral structures through the expression of neuroplasticity.

Studies of connectivity have brought new and important information regarding both normal and pathological functions of sensory and motor systems. For example, it has been shown that functional connections are more extensive than earlier believed and that connections may change rapidly. It is also evident from recent studies that altered functional connectivity contributes to symptoms of neurological diseases and age-related disorders. Activation of neuroplasticity is an important factor in these changes of functional connectivity.

Chapter 9

Nerves and their Common Disorders

Abstract

1. There are three main categories of trauma to peripheral nerves: Neurapraxia (no structural damage) axonotmesis (interruption of axons with preservation of the support structures of the nerve) and neurotmesis (interruption of axons and damage to their support structures).

2. A more detailed classification includes three grades of neurotmesis (Sunderland).

3. The term neuropathy is used by neurologists for diseases involving peripheral and cranial nerves.

4. Interruption of axons causes degeneration of the stump that is distal to the cell body of the axon (Wallerian degeneration) and subsequent sprouting of the proximal end of the axons. If the support structure is preserved, the axons will regrow towards their original targets and make contact with these targets.

5. A slight injury causes the conduction velocity of nerves to decrease resulting in increased conduction time.

6. This decrease in conduction velocity varies between individual nerve fibers within an injured nerve which can cause reduced temporal coherence as the nerve impulses arrive at their targets.

7. The axons of injured nerves have an increased refractory period, and abnormal firing such as burst firing may occur.

8. Abnormal firing such as burst firing can alter function of nerves and induce expressions of neuroplasticity.

9. Slightly injured or inflamed nerves become sensitive to mechanical compression. Normal nerves are little affected by mechanical manipulations or compression.

10. The functions of large diameter axons are more affected by mechanical compression than are those of small diameter myelinated fibers or unmyelinated fibers.

11. Inflammation (neuritis) from diabetes or alcohol intake (deficits of vitamin B_1) are common causes of conduction deficits of nerves as are age-related neuropathies.

12. Alcohol neuropathy is mainly caused by a vitamin B_1 deficiency.

13. Nerves may become impulse generators when injured causing ectopic activity. Other abnormalities include a reflection of neural activity from the point of injury.

14. It has been hypothesized that a direct (ephaptic) transmission may occur between bare (denuded) axons such as may be found in injured nerves. Evidence that this phenomenon occurs, however, is sparse except for short periods in connection with acute injuries of nerves.

Introduction

Symptoms and signs of diseases of peripheral nerves can result directly from changes in the function of the axons or indirectly through subsequent neuroplastic changes in information processing occurring in more central structures of the nervous system. Disorders of nerves can, therefore, present many different and often complex symptoms. Neuropathy of sensory nerves can produce pain, paresthesia and other abnormal sensations as well as induce neuroplastic reorganization of central nervous system structures. Neuropathy of motor nerves can cause paresis, paralysis and abnormal muscle activity. Pathologies of nerve have a strong influence on the function of neural circuits in the spinal cord and the brain through activation of neuroplasticity. The resulting changes are normally harmful thus examples of the dark sides of neuroplasticity.

Pathologies of motor nerves, the neuromuscular junctions (muscle endplates) or muscles themselves mostly resulting in reduced or loss of function (paresis or paralysis).

Disorders of muscles and motor nerves can also induce reorganization of neural circuits in the central nervous system including the motor cortex.

Most peripheral nerves are mixed nerves consisting of both large and small diameter myelinated fibers and unmyelinated fibers. Interruption of mixed nerves can indirectly influence motor function when the proprioceptive input to the spinal cord or cranial nerve motor circuits changes.

Nerve disorders can initiate changes in the function of central nervous system structures through the expression of neuroplasticity; these changes develop gradually and may persist even after healing of an injury to a peripheral nerve. The resulting central nervous system changes may be permanent or reversible with or without intervention. There are many similarities between signs and symptoms of disorders affecting spinal nerves and cranial nerves though the latter displays slightly more variance.

Nerves have often been regarded as entities separate from their nuclei and from the structures to which their nuclei communicate in the central nervous system. The extensive interaction between pathologies of nerves and processing of information in related central nervous system structures makes it more appropriate to regard nerves, their nuclei and the subsequent targets of the nuclei as an integrated system in which the different components interact closely with each other in both healthy and in pathological conditions.

Symptoms and signs of disorders of nerves

The symptoms of nervous disorders depend on whether sensory, pain or motor fibers are involved and the nature of the pathology. Below is a brief taxonomy of nervous system pathologies according to the symptoms and signs each produces (Figure 9.1). Some of the symptoms and signs originate directly from the pathological function of the nerve in question whereas other symptoms arise from subsequent changes in the function of central nervous system structures brought about by expression of neuroplasticity.

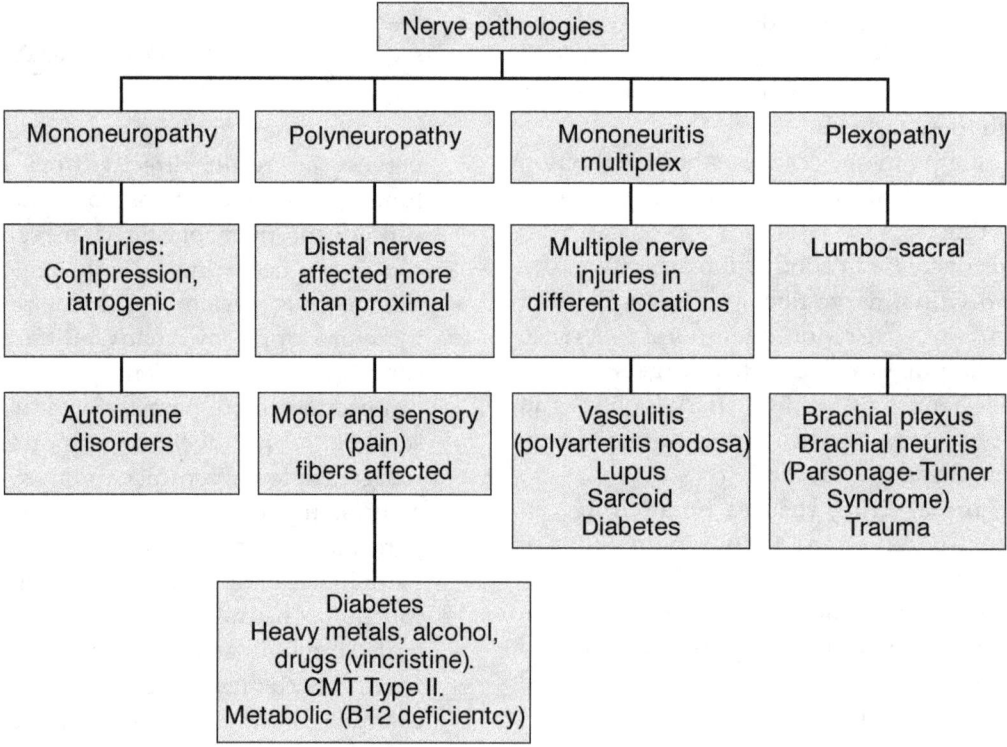

Figure 9.1. Pathologies of nerves.

Severely damage to nerves can cause total interruption of neural conduction causing paresis, paralysis or loss of sensory functions. Nerves damaged to a lesser extent may still retain some imperfect conductivity through the normal impulse pattern may be transformed [127, 584] or the nerve may inappropriately generate neural activity on its own [127]. Disorders of motor nerves the neuromuscular junction muscles and α motoneurons normally cause paresis or paralysis. Loss of function in sensory nerves can in addition to sensory deficit cause expression of neuroplasticity and produce cause complex symptoms such as paresthesia [707] and other phantom sensations such as tinnitus [92].

Injuries to motor nerves can also cause expression of neuroplasticity that causes changes in the function of motonuclei [336] and spinal cord structures [671]. Regeneration of motor nerves is often associated with synkinesis perhaps caused by a failure of the regenerating axons to make contact with their correct target. This occurs, especially in neurotmesis. Synkinesis that occurs in connection with axonotmesis, however, is more likely to be caused by altered central processing in the motonucleus brought about by expression of neuroplasticity [77, 570].

Neurotmesis of motor nerves is also likely to cause expression of neuroplasticity with subsequent changes in the function of central nervous system structures. Various forms of irritations of a nerve especially of its root may create symptoms and signs such as spasm [439] or pain and these symptoms are mostly caused by the expression of neuroplasticity [195, 369]. Injuries to mixed nerves can cause complex motor symptoms because proprioceptive fibers are affected. This kind of synkinesis can often be treated successfully by training.

Disorders caused by pathology of nerves

Neurologists usually restrict the use of the general term neuropathy to disorders of nerves but distinguish between mononeuropathies [394] affecting a single peripheral nerve and polyneuropathies affecting multiple nerves [587].

The terms mono- and polyneuropathy are used to describe the symptoms but are not related to the causes of the pain. Mononeuropathy may be caused by trauma to a single peripheral nerve. Polyneuropathy frequently occurs in association with diabetes and age-related changes [538]. Pain from nerves can also be caused by inflammation or entrapment of nerves or nerve roots, but in many cases the cause is unknown.

Viral infections such as those caused by strains of the herpes virus can cause painful conditions specifically in a radiating pattern from a single or multiple nerves (shingles, Ramsey-Hunt syndromes etc.). Neuropathology such as those associated with inflammation or ischemia can cause chronic neuropathic pain through an expression of neuroplasticity induced by altered function of the injured nerves. The secondary neuropathic pain often compounds with that caused directly by initial pathologies.

Pathologies of peripheral nerves often have more than one cause. That means that in addition to viral infections other factors often contribute to the symptoms. For example, deficiency of vitamin B is may be present and intake of vitamin B as a supplement often has beneficial effects.

Diabetes is often accompanied by disorders of peripheral nerves (peripheral nerve neuropathy). Age-related changes in peripheral nerves are common. Some drugs used in the treatment of cancer can cause peripheral nerve neuropathy causing pain.

Young people have considerable reserves, which makes it possible for peripheral nerves to withstand some damage without causing any symptoms. When the reserves are used up slight damage will result in symptoms. People who have undergone chemotherapy for cancer are typically more sensitive to neuropathies of various kinds to some extents because of their loss of reserves caused by the destruction from chemotherapy. The symptoms of peripheral nerve neuropathy first manifest at the distal part of nerves because of the long distance to the cell bodies which supplies nutrition to the axons.

Effects of mechanical irritation (compression)

There are two ways that mechanical irritation (compression) of peripheral and cranial nerves can cause pain: through the stimulation of nociceptors in the *nervi nervorum* and the transformation of the nerve into mechanoreceptive impulse generators.

This may occur either spontaneously or in response to mechanical stimulation.

Peripheral nerves under normal conditions have a low degree of sensitivity to mechanical stimulation (negative Tinel's sign), but injuries and other pathologies may change the membranes of axons so that they become mechanosensitive to stretching compression and other deformation similar to what normally occurs in Pacinian corpuscles.

Entrapment of normal sensory nerves causes tingling but rarely pain (compression does not affect small myelinated fibers or unmyelinated fibers). Only in injured or inflamed nerves does entrapment or compression cause pain.

Many studies have shown that nerve injury promote neuroma formation and nerve fiber degeneration can cause spontaneous discharges in nerve fibers proximal to the injury level [698]. Such pathologies may cause pain because the generated neural activity is interpreted in the same way as an activity that is caused by stimulation of nociceptors.

The specific perception that is caused by abnormal neural activity or activity from mechanical stimulation of slightly injured nerves depends on the kind of fiber that is affected. Injury of large diameter myelinated somatosensory fibers (Aβ fibers) typically causes paresthesia described as tingling or "pins and needles" sensations. Mechanical stimulation of slightly injured (or inflamed) nerves can cause pain when C fibers or Aδ fibers are activated. The nature of the pain depends on the kind of fibers that are activated. Activating C fibers is more likely to cause a burning sensation that is diffusely localized while activating Aδ fibers is more likely to cause stinging and well-localized pain.

Various insults to nerves or the myelin sheaths covering them can produce symptoms and signs of disorders. Inflammation and age-related changes could also cause deficits and other symptoms and signs of disorders. Inflammation in conjunction with compression of peripheral nerves can cause pain.

Mixed nerves

Stretching or compression of a mixed nerve affects axoplasmatic flow. Temporary obstruction of axoplasmatic flow or ischemia may cause signs of neurapraxia with large diameter fibers being affected more than small fibers. This may explain why sensation can be lost from compression of a nerve while maintaining pain sensation.

Unmyelinated fibers and small myelinated fibers (i.e., pain fibers) are more susceptible to local anesthetics than large fibers but less affected by compression or stretching of a nerve.

Focal injuries

Focal injuries affect a limited portion of a (single) nerve while general injuries affect an entire nerve. Mononeuropathy describes injuries that affect a single nerve. Injuries to more than one nerve are known as polyneuropathy.

Morphological changes in nerves from injuries have been classified into three main types namely neurapraxia axonotmesis and neurotmesis or in 5 groups according to Sunderland [655] (Figures 9.2 A&B).

Neurapraxia

The mildest form of focal lesions of a nerve is neurapraxia (Sunderland grade 1 (Figure 9.2) in which the morphologic structure of a nerve is preserved, but neural conduction is blocked partially or totally. Neural conduction in a nerve can recover totally from neurapraxia without any intervention.

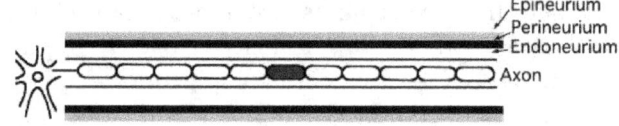

Figure 9.2. Illustration of a nerve with a conduction block without morphological changes (neurapraxia, Sunderland grade 1 [655]).

Axonotmesis

Axonotmesis (Sunderland grade 2, Figure 9.3) involves interruption of axons of a nerve without damage to its supporting structures. Axonotmesis may be caused by crushing pinching or vigorous compression or stretching of a nerve.

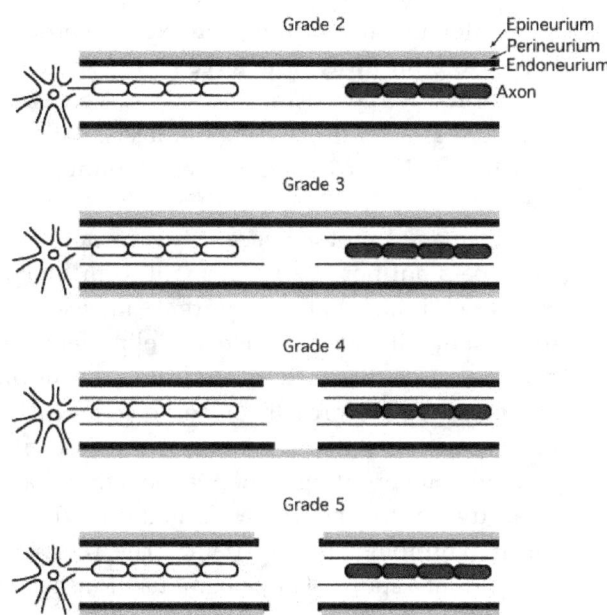

Figure 9.3. Different types of nerve injuries (Sunderland grades 2,3,4 and 5)

When lesions occur distally to the location of the cell body the parts of axons that are distal to the location of the lesion begin to degenerate immediately after the lesion. This degeneration is categorized as Wallerian degeneration in which degenerative changes to the distal segment of a nerve fiber occur when continuity with its cell body is interrupted.

Though the distal portion may conduct nerve impulses for 24-72 hours after an injury, it is usually effectively disconnected from the proximal portion within 48-72 hours after the injury. Regeneration of a peripheral nerve progresses at a rate of approximately 1 millimeter per day. Nerve fibers in the central nervous system do not regenerate.

Neurotmesis

Neurotmesis (Sunderland grade 3 4 and 5 [655]) involves interruption of not only axons but also injury to the support structure. Grade 3 is a mixture of axon damage (axonotmesis) and damage to the support structure (loss of Schwann cells, the basal lamina and the endoneurial integrity).

Partial regeneration and restoration of function can occur without intervention. Grade 4 describes injuries that are more severe and involve scar formations spanning the entire cross-section of the nerve, preserving the physical continuity of the nerve. Functional regeneration, however, is blocked by the scar tissue.

A grade 5 injury represents a total transection of a nerve and is often referred to as neurotmesis. It requires surgical intervention (grafting) to regain function.

Symptoms and signs of focal nerve injuries

Nerve injuries often produce a mixture of pathologies. Some axons may have total blockage of conduction while other axons conduct nerve impulses but abnormally. The degree of injury varies among the different axons in a nerve bundle. Naturally, complete interruption of a nerve abolishes the function of that nerve be it a sensory or a motor nerve.

Some symptoms from focal injury to nerves are directly related to the altered function of the injured nerves. Other secondary symptoms are caused by abnormalities in the central nervous system resulting from activation of neuroplasticity in responses to the altered function brought about by the initial injury. Impairment of conduction in sensory nerves primarily causes loss of sensory function, and in motor nerves, it causes weakness or paralysis of the muscles that are innervated by the nerve in question. Impaired conduction in proprioceptive fibers can affect motor functions in different complex ways.

Severe damage to nerves can cause total interruption of neural conduction causing paresis, paralysis or loss of sensory functions. Nerves that are damaged to a lesser extent may still retain some imperfect conductivity although the normal impulse pattern may be transformed.

Normal nerves carry nerve impulses without changing their pattern or generate additional activity. An injured nerve may modify the impulse pattern for example to burst pattern, or an injured nerve may generate neural activity on its own (ectopic activity).

Secondary to the initial injury impaired conduction of nerves can cause neuroplastic reorganization of central nervous system structures.

It is often difficult to distinguish between the symptoms of initial and secondary effects because the symptoms of both are often referred to the site of original injury despite the anatomical location of the physiological abnormality in the secondary pathology being the central nervous system.

Changes in the function of central nervous system structures may persist after healing of nerve injuries.

Activity in large sensory fibers can modulate activity in the target neurons of smaller fibers (pain and temperature) in the dorsal horn. Injury to only the large fibers within a mixed somatic peripheral sensory nerve may also change the modulation of information that is carried in the intact small fibers. Injury to large fibers may, therefore, promote pain without stimulation of the specific pain receptors.

The axons of an injured nerve may transmit nerve impulses abnormally, and slightly injured nerves can create many different pathological conditions. Slightly injured nerves can cause many different severe and intractable symptoms the cause of which is mostly unknown. Partial conduction block in sensory nerves causes a decrease in the input to target cells. A partial block in motor nerves can result in paresis and reduced muscle strength.

Loss of function in sensory nerves can in addition to the sensory deficit cause expression of neuroplasticity and it may cause complex symptoms such as paresthesia [707] or phantom sensations such as tinnitus. Pathological impulse pattern in nerve fibers may also affect the target cells in one or another way.

Injuries to motor nerves can also cause expression of neuroplasticity that causes changes in the function of motonuclei and spinal cord structures.

Regeneration of motor nerves is often associated with synkinesis perhaps caused by the failure of the regenerating axons to make contact with their correct target.

Synkinesis that occurs in connection with axonotmesis, however, is more likely to be caused by altered central processing in the motonucleus brought about by expression of neuroplasticity.

Neurotmesis of motor nerves is also likely to cause expression of neuroplasticity with subsequent changes in the function of central nervous system structures.

Regeneration of injured nerves

After an interruption of an axon, it sprouts and begins to grow away from its cell body and towards its normal target using the preserved support structure as a conduit. In axonotmesis, the support structure is intact and serves as a conduit for the sprouts.

Damaged motor nerves may sprout multiple fine fibers but not every fiber will form functional motor endplates at the target muscle. These redundant filaments must be eliminated [239] because they may form neuroma (a normally benign excessive growth of nerve tissue) that are pain sensitive. Although natural repair of nerves depends on sprouting of new axons, this is also an opportunity for neuroma formation which can cause symptoms such as pain. The regeneration proceeds at a speed of approximately 1 mm per day.

If the interruption of a bipolar axon occurs at a location that is proximal to the cell body the axon will grow centrally. The distance that a nerve can grow is limited and that limits recovery of function after axonotmesis. Recovery of function after lesions of axons of a motor nerve that has suffered axonotmesis depends on the formation of new motor endplates or sensory receptors when the outgrowing axons of a sensory nerve reach their target.

Axons will also regenerate after neurotmesis but whether newly sprouted axons will successfully reach their target depends on the condition of the support structure of the injured nerve. An intact support structure may allow for regrowth sufficient for satisfactory recovery of function. If the lesion is extensive such as in Grade four or five grafting either end-to-end or with another nerve must be done to provide the support structures that can act as conduits for the regenerating axons. Scar tissue that may form after injuries is an obstacle to regeneration.

Reflection of neural activity

Demyelination of a segment of a nerve may cause reflection of neural activity that reaches that segment. Such abnormalities have been implicated in chronic pain [269, 499].

Slightly injured nerves

A typical nerve transmits nerve impulses initiated at the dendrites unchanged to a target which may be a nerve cell or a muscle. Slightly injured nerves, however, may not be able to transmit nerve impulses without distorting the discharge pattern. The temporal pattern of the discharges that reaches a target neuron may thus also be distorted.

Slightly injured nerves may have a longer refractory period than normal nerve fibers [319] increasing the shortest interval within which an axon can fire thus limiting the maximum firing frequency.

Such a cap on firing rate can prevent sensory nerves from activating a target cell that responds only to high-frequency impulses. For motor nerves limitation of firing rate reduces the maximal strength of a muscle.

Injury to a nerve could also increase the firing pattern from a steady to a bursting discharge. The change from a continuous firing pattern to a pattern of firing in bursts can change the central processing even when the average number of nerve impulses remains unchanged. The firing of target neurons in which the excitatory postsynaptic potential (EPSP) decays rapidly can only occur when the interval between incoming impulses is sufficiently short to allow temporal integration. This means that a target cell that infrequently responds to a continuous train of impulses will be activated frequently by the new bursting input. This change in the firing pattern may thereby unmask synapses that are normally closed. This is one mechanism through which new connections in the central nervous system are opened causing re-routing of information.

Effect of difference in conduction velocity

The temporal coherence of the nerve impulses that arrives from a peripheral nerve to its target cell is important for the ability of the cell to become activated. Several factors affect this coherence.

The conduction velocity of the different nerve fibers in a nerve varies causing the arrival time of nerve impulses at the target to be different for different nerve fibers. The difference in arrival time causes a dispersion of the nerve impulses at the target cell that is larger for a long nerve than a short nerve and it increases when a nerve is injured because different nerves fibers are affected differently.

The effect of injury on a nerve typically manifests as a decrease in conduction velocity. This may have little effect on the functions of sensory and motor systems if it affects all nerve fibers equally. However, most pathologies that cause decreased conduction velocity in axons affect different axons differently increasing the temporal dispersion of the neural activity (Figure 9.4).

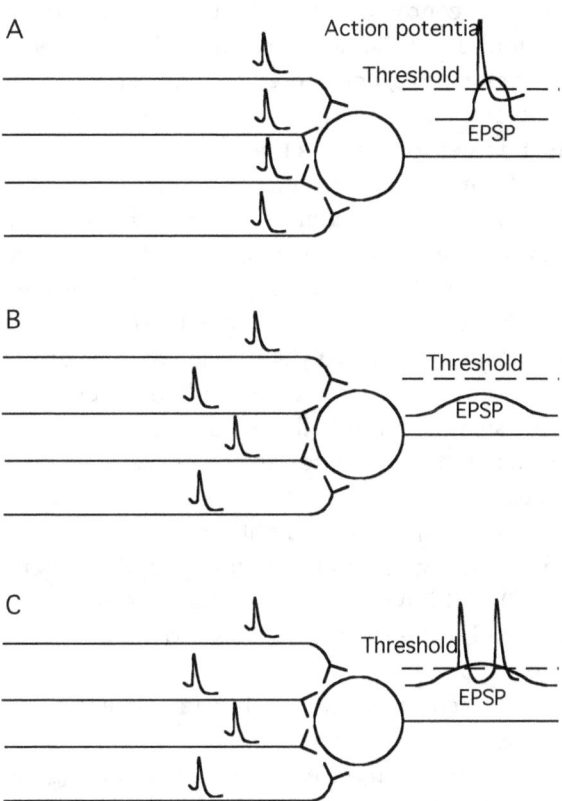

Figure 9.4. Hypothetical illustration of the effect of spatial integration by a cell on which many axons converge.

A: Little spatial dispersion. The EPSP has a short duration allowing only one nerve impulse to be delivered in the axon from the cell.

B: Increased spatial dispersion but the high threshold of the neuron prevents it from firing.

C. A large degree of spatial dispersion and a low threshold of the neuron. The prolonged EPSP makes the neuron fire twice.

Injuries to nerves often include damage to the myelin sheath which causes decreased conduction velocity and abnormal firing patterns within nerve fibers. If the conduction velocities of different fibers within a bundle are not affected uniformly the temporal dispersion of the nerve activity will increase and signal processing will be encumbered.

Temporal dispersion in the auditory nerve will cause reduced speech discrimination. In motor nerves, it may result in weakened muscle contractions.

Temporal dispersion in uninjured nerves is a function of the normal variation in the conduction velocities of the comprising fibers, and it depends on the length of the nerve.

The axon diameter and myelin coverage will affect the conduction velocity of a given fiber. The distribution of diameters of nerve fibers differs for different nerves, and thereby the dispersion differs. For example, the variation in conduction velocity is much larger for C fibers than for myelinated fibers.

A target cell on which many axons converge integrates neural activity not only in each nerve fiber over time, but it also integrates the input from all the axons that converge onto the cell. This means that both temporal and spatial coherence are important factors that determine whether or not a target cell will fire. If the nerve fibers that converge upon such a nerve cell are stimulated by a brief impulse which activates all the nerve fibers at the same time the target neuron in question will receive the nerve impulses at slightly different times and the resulting excitatory postsynaptic potential (EPSP) will have a lower amplitude than it would have had if the nerve impulses arrived at the same time (Figure 9.4).

The activity elicited at the same time in a group of fibers with different conduction velocities will arrive at their target cell with a certain degree of temporal dispersion. The effect of that can determine whether the membrane potential in the target cell reaches the threshold for delivering an action potential in its axon (Figure 9.4).

If the dispersion is small a neuron may only fire once because the amplitude of the generated EPSP decays below that of the neuron's threshold before the end of the neuron's refractory period thus preventing the neuron from firing again (Figure 9.4A) even when the amplitude of the EPSP exceeds the threshold of the neuron by a large amount.

If the temporal or spatial dispersion is large, the activity impinged on the neuron spreads out longer over time (is diluted) and therefore may not produce an EPSP of sufficient amplitude to exceed the threshold of the target cell (Figure 9.4B).

If the target cell functions according to the "integrate and fire" model of neurons it will only fire if the interval between nerve impulses in the fibers that converge on it is sufficiently small.

Temporal dispersion decreases the probability of this event which affects the ability of the input to excite the target neuron. If, however, the cell has a low threshold and the input from each fiber is sufficient to trigger an action potential by its strength the temporal dispersion can increase the activity of the neuron.

The prolonged EPSP could exceed the refractory period of the neuron, and it may fire more than once from a single input. If the threshold of the neuron is sufficiently low the neuron will fire and if the duration of the prolonged EPSP exceeds the refractory period of the neuron it may fire more than once (Figure 9.4C).

A large degree of temporal and spatial dispersion of the input to a neuron may, therefore, be more efficient in exciting a neuron than the same number of nerve impulses that occur with little dispersion provided that the threshold of firing is sufficiently low.

The same excitation at the distal end of a nerve may thus cause the target cell fire either once (Figure 9.4A) not at all (Figure 9.4B) or multiple times (Figure 9.4C) depending on the temporal dispersion and threshold of the target neuron. This means that temporal or the spatial dispersion of the input to a neuron may determine whether an injured nerve may cause less, the same, or more excitation of its target cell.

To summarize: Increased temporal dispersion (decreased temporal coherence) in nerves may have widely different effects on target neurons.

Temporal dispersion is greater for long nerves than it is for short nerves even with the same proportion of damage about the length. This may explain some of the differences between the symptoms of disorders that affect the distal and proximal portions of a nerve.

Disorders of sensory nerves that alter temporal or spatial dispersion of the input to a nerve cell in the central nervous system can, therefore, affect processing of information in the central nervous system and increased temporal dispersion can have different effects.

Electrophysiological signs of nerve injuries

Measurement of nerve conduction velocity is an important tool for diagnosis of disorders of nerves. The principles are to stimulate a nerve electrically and record the response from the same nerve at a distance from where it is being stimulated.

Clinical nerve conduction studies are often performed by recordings the responses from muscles (electromyography EMG) in response to electrical stimulation of a mixed nerve.

Examination of EMG responses from muscles to electrical stimulation of a nerve provides quantitative information about abnormalities in the function of motor nerves including abnormal neural conduction velocity.

Recording of nerve action potentials (compound action potentials CAP) from nerves can be used for determining the neural conduction velocity in all large fibers in a mixed nerve and thereby provide a quantitative assessment of demyelination and axonal injuries. A subnormal amplitude of the recorded CAP and EMG response with relative preservation of conduction velocity is a sign that some axons are not conducting.

Broadening of the CAP is a sign of temporal dispersion because the decrease in conduction velocity differs among axons. One has to remember, however, that measurement of neural conduction using these methods only reflect neural conduction in large diameter fibers and feasible clinical tools are not yet available for measurement of neural conduction in the smaller diameter Aδ and C fibers.

People with small fiber neuropathies (often seen in in people with pain) will thus have normal measurements because only their healthy large fibers are surveyed. The backfiring of motoneurons causes an F-response which can be used effectively to measure conduction velocity of the proximal part of motor nerves.

The test is performed in a similar way as recordings of the H-response: by stimulating mixed nerves electrically and recording from muscles that are innervated by the nerve that is stimulated [25]). These tests are important for the diagnosis of disorders where conduction is normal in distal nerves but abnormal in their proximal parts such as occurs in people with HMSN-I (Hereditary motor-sensory neuropathies. Charcot-Marie-Tooth syndrome).

Causes of disorders of nerves

Injuries to nerves resulting from insults such as physical trauma (compression stretching or wounding) can cause focal damage to a nerve. Gunshot wounds accidents and surgery (iatrogenic incidents) are common causes of permanent damage to peripheral nerves. Heat as experienced during accidental burns or clinical electrocoagulation may cause transient or permanent nerve injury. Other forms of focal nerve damage may be caused by entrapment such as from scar formation and surgical manipulations

General (global) injuries may be caused by chemical and metabolic factors such as those that occur with poisoning, diabetes, vitamin deficits, uremia and hepatic dysfunction or by inflammation (neuritis) of various kinds (Figure 9.5).

Such disorders that affect motor nerves are commonly studied clinically using electromyography [25]. In some nerve disorders, it is not possible to find a cause (idiopathic).

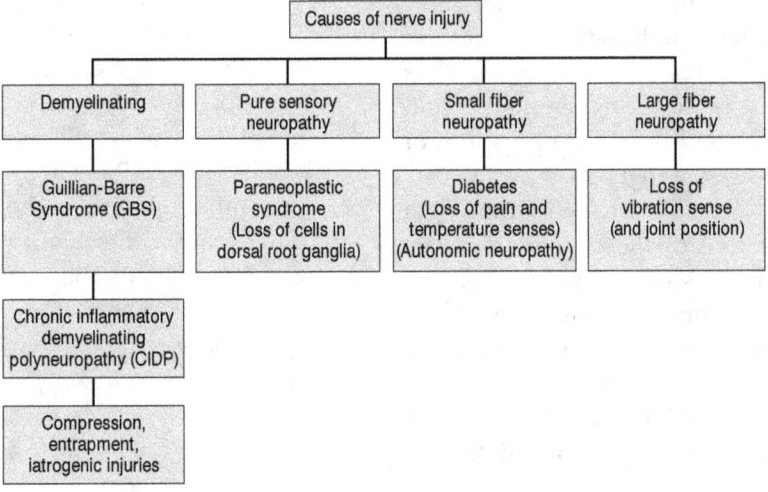

Figure 9.5. Causes of nerve injuries

Trauma

Trauma may affect all parts of a nerve, but the central portions are more sensitive to mechanical insults than the peripheral portions of nerves. The absence of the undulation of the central portion of nerves that in peripheral portions allow stretching without causing injury adds to the vulnerability of the central portion of nerves.

Before peripheral nerves enter the central nervous system (spinal cord and brain), the myelin changes from Schwann cell generated myelin to oligodendrocyte generated myelin. The transition between the peripheral portion of a nerve and the central portion is known as the root exit or entry zones or the Obersteiner-Redlich zone. Trauma to the central portion of nerves produces similar kinds of injuries like that to the peripheral portion, but the central portion of nerves is more sensitive to mechanical insults because it has fewer support structures.

Despite the central portions of nerves are insulated from insults inside the spinal canal or cranium, they are at risk of injury during surgery. The introduction of microneurosurgery and the use of intraoperative neurophysiologic monitoring, however, have dramatically decreased this risk of surgical trauma.

Nerve compression and entrapment

Nerve compression has been a common explanation for many disorders. Compression of the trigeminal and of the glossopharyngeal nerve roots has often been associated with their classical neuralgias. These hypotheses have recently been challenged, and more complex explanations have been sought. The challenge of these hypotheses has come from several sources of evidence such as clinical observations animal experiments and understanding of the effect of compression of peripheral nerves and nerve roots.

TGN can be treated successfully by moving a blood vessel off the root of the trigeminal nerve (microvascular decompression operation) or the root of the ninth cranial nerve for glossopharyngeal neuralgia. All these three (or four) different treatments have approximately the same success rate, approximately 85% [45]. We will discuss these disorders and their pathology more detail in Chapter 12.

Chronic compression of nerves may be asymptomatic, and pain that has sometimes been associated with nerve compression can occur in its absence. For example, common symptoms of "carpal tunnel syndrome" are often assumed to be caused by compression of a nerve at the wrist, but the cause may be more complex. Compression of nerves such as from entrapment may cause pain only when the nerves in question are inflamed or injured.

Scar formation after trauma or surgery can cause nerve compression or entrapment. Nerves or nerve roots may also be compressed when foramina through which they pass shrink as often happen with age (e.g. spinal stenosis).

Some forms of common lower back pain are assumed to be caused by mechanical compression of the roots of spinal nerves, yet similar morphological changes occur commonly without noticeable symptoms.

Knowledge about the effect of (mechanical) compression of a normal nerve may explain why compression of a normal nerve does not cause pain. The reason is that mechanical compression of an abnormal nerve or nerve root mainly affects the large myelinated nerve fibers such as $A\beta$ sensory fibers and $A\alpha$ motor fibers but not the smaller $A\delta$ and C fibers that are involved in pain. Compression of motor nerves can cause muscle contractions (twitches) [338, 339].

The reason may be found in the fact that normal pain nerve fibers are not sensitive to compression unless they are inflamed or injured. The symptoms of compression of large diameter nerve fibers are tingling and muscle weakness.

Deformation of peripheral nerves (mechanical stimulation) preferentially causes tingling without pain because it mainly affects large diameter myelinated nerve fibers ($A\alpha$ and $A\beta$) but not the smaller nerve fibers involved with pain.

Inflammation, however, changes this paradigm and mechanical compression or irritation can then activate these smaller caliber nerve fibers. This means that treatment of the inflammation of spinal nerves in people with the common back pain is effective in relieving the pain.

The role of neuroplasticity

Compression or irritation of spinal nerve roots may activate neuroplasticity causing changes in the central nervous system which in turn causes changes in neural function thus generating the sensation of pain.

The pathophysiology of these disorders, however, is more complex than just conduction block in nerves [369]. The subsequent involvement of central nervous system structures through the expression of neuroplasticity plays a major role in generating the symptoms and signs of many forms of nerve compression and injuries – which may explain some of the poor correlation between symptoms and morphological signs of nerve entrapment.

Periformis sciatica

A peculiar form of back pain is periformis sciatica. It causes pain and tingling in the leg and is caused by compression (or irritation) of the sciatic nerve as it travels by the periformis muscle. In some people, the nerve passes through the muscle. It is usually treated effectively with a specific exercise.

The carpal tunnel syndrome

The carpal tunnel syndrome is a common nerve entrapment disorder which is the second most common industrial injury in the U.S.A.; it has been believed to be caused by entrapment of the median nerve or pressure on the nerve. However, the carpal tunnel syndrome may occur without any detectable signs of nerve entrapment or any other morphological abnormality.

Splinting, cortisone injections massage or immersion of the hand in water can relieve carpal tunnel symptoms, and none of these remedies involve decompression of the nerve. Resting the limb or a change of activities can also relieve the symptoms. As in other pain conditions, the pain from carpal tunnel syndrome is worsened by psychosocial factors such as boredom stress job dissatisfaction monotonous routines and insecurity.

Ulnar nerve entrapment is the second most common entrapment neuropathy (with symptoms of numbness and tingling in the distribution of the ulnar nerve, the fifth finger and the lateral aspect of the fourth.

Other peripheral nerves such as the sciatic and common peroneal nerves are subject to similar entrapment.

Painful muscle contractions

Back pain is often associated with painful muscle spasms. The muscle contractions in these disorders are usually tonic and not easily observed. In clinical experience, back pain often can be treated successfully by benzodiazepines which support the hypothesis that the pain is caused by muscle contractions or has a supraspinal origin. The general lack of objective signs of back pain has suggested that the cause of some instances may be psychiatric (a not uncommon conclusion when detectable abnormalities are absent.

Diabetes and other causes of neuropathy

Neuropathy is a common complication of diabetes. Diabetes affects the microvasculature supplying the smallest nerve fibers altering their behavior. Pain and changes in temperature sensation are typical symptoms. Deficiency of vitamins B_1 B_2 and B_{12} can cause neuropathy of various kinds, including diabetes and alcohol related neuropathy. Administration of B vitamins can often relieve these symptoms.

Tamoxifen used in the treatment of some kinds of cancer often causes burning feet- a sign of peripheral nerve neuropathy. Administration of B vitamins can likewise often relieve these symptoms.

The abnormal firing brought about by these conditions can promote activation of neuroplasticity in the target nuclei of an injured nerve by abnormal firing of nerve impulses or caused by the deprivation of input from sensory nerves causing changes in synaptic efficacy, formation or elimination of synapses, sprouting of dendrites and axons and change in protein synthesis [623]. This may cause chronic neuropathic pain. Similar neuropathic changes in may occur in motonuclei after an injury to motor nerves [336] causing muscle spasm.

Nerves as impulse generators

Pathologies of nerves may cause the affected nerve to act as an impulse generator [127]. Though compression of a nerve may involve little physical damage, it can cause nerve impulses generation at the location of the compression. Such ectopic impulses can propagate both in the distal and central directions from the injured segment of a nerve and interact with the normally generated nerve impulses and elicit trains of impulses.

An injured or ischemic area of a peripheral nerve can thus act as a "trigger zone" for ectopic activity. Generation of such abnormal activity is exacerbated by hyperventilation because of hypocalcemia.

Slightly injured nerves may begin to express adrenoceptors activated by circulating catecholamines such as epinephrine and norepinephrine. Sympathetic axons then sprout and project toward dorsal root ganglia after injuries to the nerve in question. This is another way in which catecholamines can stimulate afferent pain fibers and cause sympathetically maintained pain. After-discharges also occur frequently in injured segments of nerves in response to a further input.

Ephaptic transmission

It is hypothesized that axons that have lost their myelin insulation may communicate with each other through ephaptic transmission. Ephaptic transmission is the direct transfer of impulse activity from one denuded axon to another. The word "ephaptic" is an artificial word constructed from the word synapse partly backward. It has also been hypothesized that such ephaptic transmission is involved in creating the symptoms of several nerve disorders.

Signs of ephaptic transmission in injured nerves were first described by Granit and colleagues (1944) who showed that direct transmission between injured (cut) nerve fibers could occur for a short period after the injury to a nerve [223]. The hypothesis that neural transmission may occur directly between barred (denuded) axons has been further tested experimentally by Howe and colleagues [268] who used chromic sutures to create focal demyelination of the trigeminal nerve. These investigators found evidence that introducing a single spike into injured zone could set up a reverberation generating abnormal high-frequency neural spike trains. Later similar findings were made in dorsal roots of the spinal cord [547].

Brief periods of signs of ephaptic transmission in a surgically injured central portion of the facial nerve were demonstrated in studies of the abnormal muscle contraction in a patient undergoing an MVD operation for hemifacial spasm [431] [424]. (Ephaptic transmission is also discussed in connection with hemifacial spasm in Chapter 12).

However, it is doubtful if ephaptic transmission play any noticeable roles explaining symptoms from injured nerves.

Viral inflammation

Inflammation of nerves (neuritis) is a frequent cause of symptoms and signs. Though some forms of neuritis are caused by unknown viral agents (idiopathic polyneuritis) various strains of the Herpes virus are often involved in neuritis. Varicella-zoster the herpes virus behind chicken pox causes neuropathies associated with shingles and Ramsey-Hunt syndrome. Herpes simplex is a related strain known for causing disorders of the central nervous system especially in children including encephalitis. It can also cause neuropathy of single nerves.

The herpes zoster virus resides in the sensory ganglia of most individuals without producing any symptoms, but occasionally it may cause pain and eruption of vesicles on the skin over portions of or multiple dermatomes. The pain is severe and may persist for a long time after the vesicular rash fades. Immediate treatment with antiviral agents such as Acyclovir or Famvir helps reduce the duration of the rash and the incidence of subsequent chronic pain. Herpes zoster oticus involves the eighth cranial nerve and is known as the Ramsey-Hunt syndrome. Medications such as gabapentin (or pregabalin) or tricyclic antidepressants may be helpful for persistent pain. Administration of vitamin B_{12} may also be beneficial.

Herpes simplex is the cause of blisters and sores most common to occur around the mouth, nose and genitals.

Polyneuropathies

Polyneuropathies are disorders that involve more than one peripheral nerve. They are typically divided into two groups axonal polyneuropathies in which the main pathology is a loss of axons and demyelinating polyneuropathies and in which the primary pathology is a loss of myelin. The most common causes of axonal polyneuropathies are metabolic as is the case for diabetic neuropathy.

Vitamin B_1 B_2 or B_{12} deficiency, solvents, heavy metals, autoimmune processes (lupus) and many drugs including chemotherapeutic agents such as vincristine and cis-platinum can cause polyneuropathy sometimes producing pain.

The pain is typically symmetrical across the midline affecting mainly sensory nerve fiber of small diameters and burning in nature. Distal fibers are most often affected more severely than proximal fibers. This means that pain first occurs in the hands and feet.

It is important to note that the main clinical techniques used to determine the presence of neuropathy are EMG techniques. EMG studies can provide information about neural conduction velocity but only for large fibers and hence do not reflect injury to the small fibers conducting pain impulses.

The role of neuroplasticity

Interruption of neural conduction and abnormal firing of sensory nerves may provide abnormal input to the central nervous system or induce neuroplasticity of function. Total blockage of neural conduction in sensory nerves causes not only sensory deficits but the deprivation of input may also result in a reorganization of central structures through an expression of neuroplasticity. Deprivation of input may in that way cause phantom symptoms such as paresthesia and pain for somatic nerves and tinnitus for the auditory nerve.

Demyelinating disorders

One of the most prominent signs of genetic inherited abnormalities of myelin occurs in the hereditary motor sensory neuropathy (HMSN-I) also known as the Charcot-Marie-Tooth disease (CMT-I). While Guillain-Barre (GBS) is an acquired multifocal demyelination that causes conduction block over affected segments of the nerve, HMSN-I is a hereditary disorder that causes demyelination that begins at the root entry (or exit) zone and progresses to more distal segments of nerves.

Symptoms and signs of central involvement

The symptoms and signs of these secondary effects are different from those of primary effects and often involve hyperactivity and reorganization of central structures. It can be difficult, however, to discern whether a symptom is the result of a primary effect or caused by a secondary effect.

The secondary effects through activation of neuroplasticity that involve the central nervous system, however, can have more severe consequences than the primary effects of nerve injuries. Additionally, a secondary effect will persist even after the initial trauma has healed but a primary effect may heal. The symptoms from either cause are almost always referred to the anatomical location of the injured nerves in question even after that the symptoms exclusively come from central nervous system structures.

Interventions such as training are highly beneficial for recovery of function after grafting of cut motor or sensory nerves, and it is normally necessary to retrain motor skills by inducing neuroplastic reorganization of central nervous structures to generate motor commands that compensate for the misdirection of motor nerve fibers. Training can make a recovery faster and more complete.

While the naturally occurring expression of neuroplasticity and that induced by training are aimed at restoring normal function, it may also be misdirected causing abnormal movements or abnormal sensory perception (paresthesia) and pain may result.

Deprivation of sensory input such as that results from conduction block (or severance) of a nerve is a strong promoter of reorganization of central nervous system circuits [695, 697]. Change in the discharge pattern of the peripheral or central portions of nerves or nerve roots can also cause reorganization and change of the function of specific central structures. Alteration or absence of input can cause re-routing of information and altered processing of information from sensory organs.

Changes in the function of central structures may occur to compensate for changes in the function of nerves. The hyperactivity that often results from decreased input to the central nervous system may have been invoked to make up for a decreased input by increasing the gain, but if the changes in the function of central nervous system structures are too large, hyperactivity may produce unwanted effects such as tinnitus. Injuries to motor nerves and muscles can also cause expression of neuroplasticity.

Chapter 10

Sensory Systems and their Common Disorders

Abstract

1. Sensory organs contain sensory receptors and structures that conduct the physical stimulus to the receptors, and which ultimately provide conscious awareness of physical stimuli.

2. Sensory receptors convert a physical stimulus into a code of nerve impulses in the fibers of the afferent nerve that innervate the sensory cells.

3. The axons from sensory receptors in the auditory, somatosensory, visual and taste senses form the beginning of the ascending sensory pathways.

4. These axons make synaptic contact with the cells of a nucleus (dorsal column nuclei, cochlear nuclei, and nucleus of the solitary tract) that is located on the same side of the body as the receptors. The axons of these cells cross the midline.

5. Two parallel pathways are known as the classical (lemniscal or specific), and non-classical (extralemniscal or non-specific) pathways convey information from somatosensory, auditory, visual and taste receptors to higher central nervous system centers.

6. Cells in the classical sensory systems respond distinctly to different qualities of sensory stimuli.

7. The thalamus is the first common pathway for the sensory modalities of hearing, vision, somesthesia, and taste.

8. The classical ascending pathways of the somatosensory, auditory, visual and taste senses project to modality-specific nuclei in the ventral parts of the thalamus.

9. Cells in the ventral thalamic nuclei project to the respective primary sensory cortices where the cells are modality specific.

10. Cells in the primary cerebral sensory cortices relay information to other secondary and association cortices and subcortical structures.

11. The non-classical pathways target cells in nuclei in the dorsomedial parts of the thalamus. These cells respond to stimuli of more than one sensory modality.

12. Cells in the dorsal-medial thalamic nuclei bypasses the primary sensory cortices and project to the respective secondary and association sensory cortices and to subcortical structures such as the lateral nucleus of the amygdala.

13. The olfactory system is different from the other senses in that it has no thalamic representation and the main target of olfactory information is the central nucleus of the amygdala.

14. Disorders of sensory systems are characterized by decreased or absent function or hyperactivity.

15. Disorders of sensory systems include trauma to respective nerves, viral infections, and tumors (schwannoma).

16. Symptoms of pathologies affecting the sensory nervous system can occur from an expression of neuroplasticity that can cause reorganization that changes the function of central nervous system systems.

17. Causes of sensory deficits from pathologies located to the brain include tissue damage from ischemia (stroke, trauma, etc.), tumors, viral infections (encephalopathies) age-related changes.

Introduction

Sensory disorders can affect the conductive apparatus of sensory organs, the sensory receptors, the sensory nerve and the central nervous system. Disorders that affect one of these four main steps of sensory processing have distinctive symptoms and signs. Disorders that affect the sensory nervous systems are complex, and the symptoms may be referred to locations anatomically distinct from those where the abnormal neural activity is generated. Activation of neuroplasticity can affect and contribute to the symptoms of diseases and it can be the primary cause of the symptoms as discussed in other places in this book.

The symptoms of many disorders of the sensory systems are caused by morphological changes of the sensory cells, but some are due to functional changes in the central nervous system induced by the expression of neuroplasticity.

Decreased sensory sensitivity (elevated threshold) has earlier been thought to be closely related to impairments in the function of the parts of the sensory organs that conduct the stimulus to the receptors together with pathologies of the receptors. It has become evident, however, that the sensitivity of a given sensory system is affected by complex factors not limited to the conductive apparatus and receptors and including factors such as activation of neuroplasticity that cannot be detected with available clinical testing methods.

The most common disorders of sensory systems involving neuroplasticity are subjective tinnitus and chronic neuropathic pain which was discussed in separate chapters in this book. We called these disorders plasticity disorders because of the prominent role of neuroplasticity.

Other examples of complexity include the finding that an enriched environment of sensory stimulation can affect the progression of age-related sensory deficits both in the somatosensory system [256] and the auditory system (augmented acoustic environment [721]). The visual system is subjected pathological changes in the conductive apparatus of the eye and in the sensory cells. The somatosensory system is subjected to disorders of sensory nerves and their receptors causing tingling and other sensations.

Age-related changes are perhaps the most common causes of sensory deficits [720]. In general, the sensitivity and the acuity of sensory functions decrease with age. Age-related changes in sensory function affect sensory receptor cells, sensory nerves and central nervous system structures. Activation of neuroplasticity affects the changes that occur in sensory functions with age.

The increased understanding of how neuroplasticity can alter the function of the nervous system has had an additional impact on the understanding of disorders of sensory systems, again most pronounced for the auditory system.

The division of sensory systems into the four categories discussed earlier though helpful for explaining the anatomy is not beneficial for the understanding of the complex physiology and pathophysiology of the sensory system. One should instead consider how all these components act together as a single integrated system. This means that for example disorders of the conductive apparatus and sensory receptors not only affect the function of these components but also the function of the nervous system as a whole.

The sensory systems provide much of the bases for creation of "self" and for mapping of the brain structures with the body and its movements and that of the surrounding.

In this chapter, we will first discuss disorders that are related to the structures that conduct sensory stimuli to the receptors and after that discuss disorders that are specifically related to sensory receptors. That is followed by deeper discussions of changes in the function of the central nervous system that cause hyperactive symptoms and phantom sensations and changes in the processing of sensory information.

For a more detailed description of the anatomy and physiology of sensory systems see Møller, 2014 [460].

The sensory organs and their diseases

The conductive apparatuses of the sense organs have different complexities, those of the ear and the eye being the most complex.

The anatomy and the functions sensory organs of the five senses have many interesting similarities and differences and they have different complexities.

The auditory system

In the following, we will discuss hearing in some detail because that is the sense that has been studied most extensively. The ear is also a more complex organ than that of the other senses. We will discuss the role of neuroplasticity in developing normal sensory functions, and the role of maladaptive plasticity in diseases of the sensory systems.

The conductive apparatus of the ear

The outer ear consists of the pinna and the ear canal. Cerumen (wax) can build up in the ear canal and if it obstructs the ear canal, it causes hearing loss. Disorders of the middle ear (and obstruction of the ear canal) impair sound transmission to the cochlea and cause elevated hearing thresholds [458]. Conduction of sound through the middle ear is impaired when the air pressure in the middle ear differs from the ambient pressure because of changes in the mechanical properties of the middle ear. The air pressure in the middle ear cavity decreases without proper ventilation because of resorption of oxygen by the mucosa that lines the middle ear cavity. This occurs when the Eustachian tube does not open to equalize the pressure. The inability of the Eustachian tube to open often accompanies the common cold due to swelling of the mucosa in the pharynx.

Inflammatory processes of the middle ear may cause the middle ear cavity to become filled with fluid (otitis media with effusion [64]) which will impair the transmission of sound to the cochlea if the fluid covers the backside of the tympanic membrane [458]. Such disorders are common in childhood but if not remedied may cause a deprivation of input to the ear that can hamper the normal development of the auditory nervous system [333].

Perforation of the tympanic membrane is another cause of conductive hearing loss. A hole in the tympanic membrane lets sounds into the middle ear cavity making the difference between the sound pressure on the two sides of the tympanic membrane to become less than it is normal and consequently the vibration of the tympanic membrane is reduced, and less sound is conducted to the cochlea.

A small hole in the tympanic membrane acts as a low-pass filter that lets low frequencies pass into the middle ear cavity; it affects low-frequency hearing more than hearing at high frequencies [458].

Disease processes such as otosclerosis involve the growth of bone around the stapes footplate which impairs its normal motion [78] causing hearing loss.

The Cochlea

The outer hair cells of the cochlea amplify the physical stimulus (sound). The outer hair cells act as "motors" that provide energy to the motion of the basilar membrane of the cochlea. Impairment of outer hair cells may, therefore, be regarded as a (complex) form of conductive hearing impairment.

Outer hair cells may thus be regarded to be a part of the conductive apparatus of the ear, but in contrast to the middle ear, the action of the outer hair cells is non-linear [458].

Because of this nonlinear action loss of function of outer hair cells impairs the frequency selectivity of the cochlea which can impair discrimination of complex sounds such as speech sounds. Impairment of the function of outer hair cells decreases the dynamic range over which the ear can function [458]. The active function of outer hair cells normally causes a compression of the intensity range of sounds that activate inner hair cells and thereby increases the ear's dynamic range.

Injuries to outer hair cells in addition to elevating the hearing threshold cause frequency-specific changes in the cochlear processing of sound. These changes in the function of the cochlea explain some forms of hyperacusis that often accompany a hearing loss of cochlear origin. Other causes of hyperacusis are functional changes in the auditory nervous system. There are indications that activation of neuroplasticity plays a role in these processes.

Noise-induced hearing loss

The term "noise" refers to "undesired or unwanted" sounds but is also normally used for sounds that can cause hearing loss such as industrial noise. Music and other "desired and wanted" sounds can cause hearing loss equally well if sufficiently loud though such sounds are not normally referred to as noise.

The adverse effect of exposure to high-intensity noise on the ear can be a temporary increase in the hearing threshold (temporary threshold shift TTS).

If the sound exposure is above a certain level and of a certain duration increase in the threshold will not revert completely, and some hearing loss will be permanent. The component of hearing that does not recover (or is present a long time after the end of the exposure) is known as permanent threshold shift (PTS) [87, 131]. The degree of the hearing loss depends on the intensity of the sound that reaches the ear and its duration.

Outer hair cells are most vulnerable to overexposure, but outer hair cells do not act as sensory cells regarding converting sound into a neural code. Damage to outer hair cells impairs the cochlear amplifier which is most effective at low sound intensities. As mentioned above outer hair cells may rather be regarded as a part of the sound conducting apparatus. That means that noise-induced hearing loss (NIHL) may be regarded as being caused by a complex impairment of sound conduction in the cochlea.

Outer hair cells in the basal (high frequency) part of the cochlea are normally damaged to a greater extent than hair cells in more apical (lower frequency) parts of the cochlea [423, 647] [458].

Damage to outer hair cells, therefore, affects the hearing threshold and the perception of soft sounds but it has less effect on sounds at physiological levels such as speech sounds in normal conversation speech. The nonlinear properties of the cochlea thus make the pure tone audiogram a poor indicator of a person's hearing status.

The outer hair cells normally provide amplification of approximately 50 dB and destruction of outer hair cells can consequently cause a hearing loss of up to 50 dB [423] [458]. Detectable injury to inner hair cells which perform the neural transduction of the vibration of the basilar membrane is rare.

Through their non-linear function, the outer hair cells provide amplitude compression and injuries to the outer hair cells, therefore, affect the ability of the cochlea to compress the amplitude of sounds that reach the ear.

Amplitude compression in the cochlea shrinks the range of volumes to which the inner hair cells must respond. This is important because the discharge pattern in most auditory nerve fibers is not able to code the entire range of sounds that the auditory system can process. Reduced amplitude compression affects processing of sounds especially complex sounds such as speech sounds.

Impairment of the function of outer hair cells not only reduces the sensitivity of the ear but it also affects the function of the cochlear frequency analyzer. Since the outer hair cells sharpen the frequency selectivity of the basilar membrane for low sound intensities impaired function of the outer hair cells affects the ability of the cochlea to discriminate sounds according to their frequencies.

The acquired elevation of the hearing threshold (TTS and PTS) from noise exposure depends on the immission level a construct describing the level and duration of the exposure and to some extent the physical characteristics of the sound [87]. The term immission level is used to describe the average noise level in dB plus ten times the logarithm of the duration of the exposure in months.

The hearing loss that individual persons acquire as a result of exposure to loud sounds varies widely even under similar exposure conditions [87, 237] (Figure 10.1).

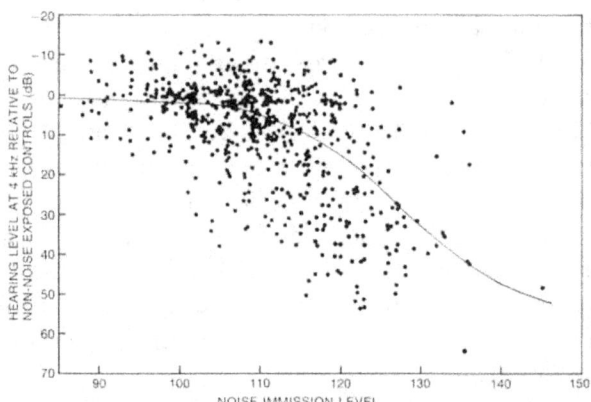

Figure 10.1. Hearing loss at 4,000 Hz as a function of immission level. (Data from Burns and Robertson 1970 [87]).

NIHL usually affects hearing in the frequency range around 4 kHz more than at any other frequency (Figure 10.2). The reason for this is the amplifying effect of the ear canal (see [458]).

The nonlinearity of the cochlea makes the location of the maximal vibration of the basilar membrane of the cochlea to shift towards the base of the cochlea when the sound intensity is increased.

This means that the shift in the hearing threshold will occur at a slightly higher frequency than that of the highest sound exposure (see below).

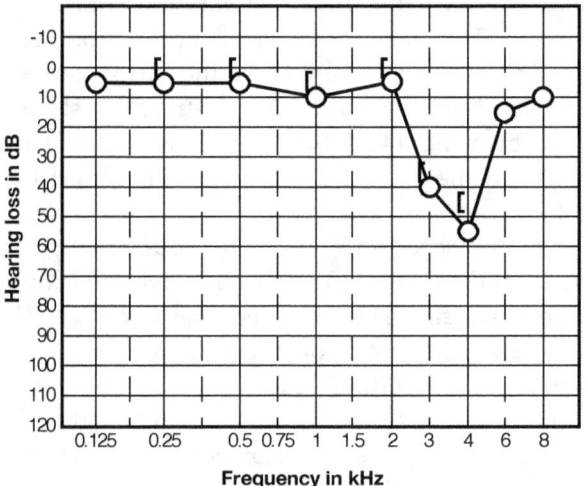

Figure 10.2. Typical audiogram of a person who has suffered NIHL. (Data from Lidén 1985 [364]).

Pathophysiology of noise-induced hearing loss

The pathophysiology of hearing loss from overstimulation (NIHL) is complex [560] and poorly understood. It seems to consist of at least two components:

One is morphological change to hair cells in the cochlea, and the other component is (morphological or functional) changes in the nervous system.

That damage to hair cells can cause a change in the central nervous system structures was shown in a study of the cochlear nucleus in animals exposed to loud noise [470, 471]. Other studies have shown evidence that functional changes occur in parts of the central nervous system in connection with NIHL [211, 212, 423, 719] [458]. These changes are signs of activation of neuroplasticity.

This difference in susceptibility to noise exposure is another sign of the complexity of NIHL [87] (Figure 10.1). Genetic factors are undoubtedly a risk factor for NIHL, but there are many other factors that may influence the risk of getting NIHL.

Studies in animals have shown that the variability in NIHL is less in the same strain of animals [743] than in humans but still considerable (Figure 10.3A). This is probably because laboratory animals have less genetic variation. The fact that exposure conditions are better controlled in laboratory studies than they are in the field of human study contribute to the observed smaller individual variation in NIHL in laboratory tests.

When the genetic variation is further decreased using heavily inbred animals, the variability in NIHL decreases further (Figure 10.3B) but even then, such genetically identical animals suffer different degrees of NIHL when exposed to the same sounds under controlled laboratory conditions.

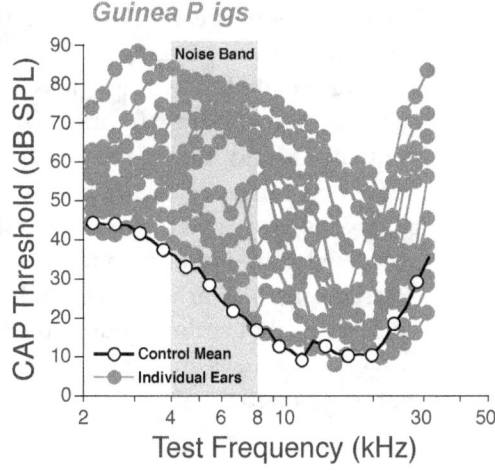
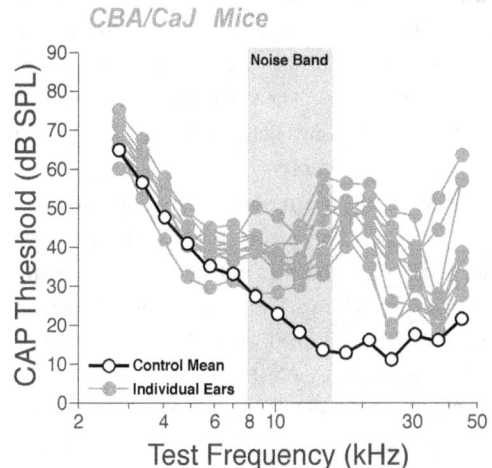

Figure 10.3. NIHL in animals of various degrees of genetic variations. Left hand graph: Data obtained in male guinea pigs (400 -500 g). The exposure was a 2-4 kHz octave band of noise at 109 dB SPL for 4 hrs with a 1-week survival. The mean peak PTS was 35.1 dB at 7.6 kHz (SD of 21.33 dB) [378]. Right hand graph: Data obtained inbred mice males (23-29 g) exposed to octave-band noise (8-16 kHz) at 100 dB for 2 hrs with a 1-week survival. The mean peak PTS was 38 dB at 17.5 kHz (SD of 4.06 dB) [743]. (Courtesy Charles Liberman).

Although these studies show clearly that the genetic makeup is important there seem to be other reasons for the variability in NIHL. One such factor may be imprinting which can silence or activate a specific gene. This would mean that NIHL is affected both epigenetically and genetically.

The implication of these findings is that the effect of noise exposure on hearing (NIHL) can only be predicted to a certain degree even in genetically identical animals under ideal (laboratory) conditions. Perhaps there are also purely stochastic components involved in the cause of biological events such as NIHL.

Further evidence of a genetic effect on NIHL comes from a study of the effect of lifetime noise exposure in two strains of rats the Sprague-Dawley strain and the Wistar Okamoto strain. The Sprague Dawley rats had normal development of blood pressure with age (normotensive) while the Wistar rats were genetically disposed for developing hypertension with age (spontaneously hypertensive) [70]. Rats that had a predisposition for acquiring hypertension ("spontaneous hypertensive rats") also acquired a greater degree of NIHL than normotensive rats [71] under the same circumstances.

After three months of exposure to 105 dB SPL noise, young (3 months), normotensive rats had acquired a mean hearing loss at 6 and 12 kHz of 38.5 dB while spontaneous hypertensive rats had an average hearing loss of 56 dB under the same conditions. (The noise consisted of a 1640 Hz wide band of noise sweeping from a center frequency of 3 kHz to 30 kHz every 2 seconds and with a duty-cycle of 1 second on and 1 second off at 100 dB Leq) for 10 hours daily). The normotensive rats had less loss of hair cells and less hearing loss than spontaneously hypertensive rats [71].

In a different study, normotensive young rats that were exposed to loud noise for one month had no detectable morphological changes in their cochleae while spontaneous hypertensive rats had considerable losses of hair cells under the same conditions. This is a further indication of the complexity of NIHL.

The fact that experimentally induced hypertension (induced by ligating a renal artery) did not make (normotensive) rats more susceptible to NIHL [72] indicates that the greater NIHL in spontaneously hypertensive rats is caused by genetic differences between these two strains of rats rather than hypertension as such.

In these studies, spontaneously hypertensive rats that were not exposed to noise also had a slightly larger hearing loss with age than normotensive rats.

That the mechanism of NIHL is complex is further evidenced by studies in animals that have shown that the amount of acquired NIHL can be reduced by exposing the ear to moderately loud sounds before exposure to the very loud noise that causes NIHL (augmented acoustic environment) [420, 681]. This "toughening" of the ear concerning acquiring NIHL was first demonstrated in studies in cats by Miller [420], but later many studies have confirmed the existence of this peculiar effect [99, 742].

The mechanisms of such toughening are poorly understood, but it may involve the central nervous system. The increased resistance to NIHL may be a result of expression of neuroplasticity involving descending auditory pathways that terminate on outer hair cells. The term "toughening of the ear" may therefore be misleading in that it in fact most likely is the function of the nervous system that is being "toughened".

Age-related changes in sensory functions

It is known that the auditory system undergoes age-related changes that primarily manifest as an elevation of the hearing threshold. Changes in the function of the auditory nerve may explain some of the decreases in speech discrimination that typically occurs as a result of aging.

Age-related hearing loss or presbycusis normally affects high frequencies more than low frequencies, and it increases gradually with age the frequency range of hearing loss expands (Figure 10.4). The degree of age-related hearing loss in people who are not known to have been exposed to excessive noise varies considerably (Figure 10.5). This means that endogenous and perhaps unknown exogenous causes may influence the hearing loss that occurs with age.

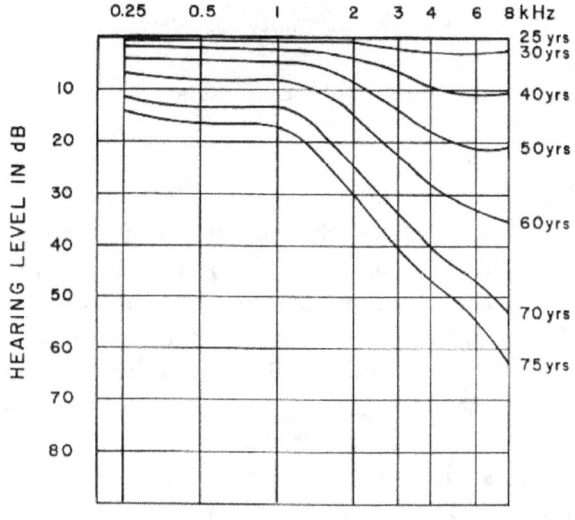

Figure 10.4. The average hearing threshold for men in different age groups. Combined results from eight studies based on examining results from a total of 7617 ears. Adapted from Spoor 1967 [649].

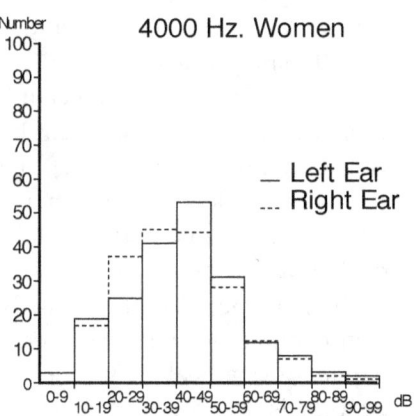

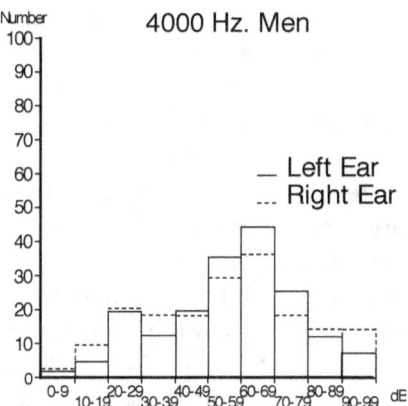

Figure 10.5. Variation in hearing threshold at 4000Hz in a cross-sectional population study of non-selected individuals age 70 years. (Data from Møller MB, 1981).

Studies of the pathophysiology of age-related hearing loss have mainly focused on the cochlea where loss of hair cells has been assumed to be the cause of age-related hearing loss [302]. The typical changes in the cochlea consist of loss of outer hair cells most prominent in the basal parts of the cochlea. These morphological changes have been associated with age-related hearing threshold elevations. Oxidative stress is likely to play a role in developing presbycusis in a way similar to how NIHL is affected by the content of melanin in the stria vascularis [46]. This may confirm the role of melanin as a free radical scavenger.

These morphological changes in the cochlea cannot, however, explain all aspects of presbycusis. In some persons, the loss of the ability to understand speech is greater than what is expected from their pure tone threshold shift which implies impairment more extensive than what would be caused by damage to the outer hair cells. Age-related hearing impairment is therefore not restricted to the loss of sensitivity of the ear caused by loss of outer hair cells rather is influenced by changes in the function of the central nervous system and auditory nerve [719, 722].

The gender difference in the age-related hearing loss has often been attributed to the fact that men are often more exposed to loud noise and that one's hormonal profile may also play a role in presbycusis. Genetic factors beyond gender are also involved in age-related hearing loss [205].

The variation of diameters of auditory nerve fibers increases with age [648], and this can be expected to impair the temporal coherence of nerve impulses that arrive at the cochlear nucleus.

Since the time pattern of the neural code of speech sounds is important for speech intelligibility these changes in the auditory nerve may contribute to the decrease in the ability to understand speech especially in a noisy environment or when more than one person is talking at the same time.

Altered GABAergic inhibition may explain some change in auditory function and perhaps also changes that occur in other sensory systems with advancing age. Some of the first studies that showed that the GABA systems change systematically with age were those of Caspary (1990) [101]. Caspary and colleagues found evidence of an age-related decrease in the production of GABA in the inferior colliculus (IC) in experiments in rats [101-103]. Other investigators have shown that age-related changes occur in the GABA systems such as the vestibular system [214].

It has been demonstrated that the sensitivity of GABA$_A$ receptors increases with age and GABA$_A$ receptor sites proliferate. From studies of GABA$_A$ receptors in the IC in rats, it has been hypothesized that the age-related changes in the composition of the GABA$_A$ receptor units are a result of a compensatory change in response to lowered presynaptic GABA release [103]. The increased sensitivity to benzodiazepines with age may be a manifestation of such a compensatory change in the sensitivity of GABA$_A$. Indications of abnormally strong GABAergic tone during aging do not necessarily contradict the observation of reduced production of GABA with age [101].

The involvement of GABA as a promoter of age-related changes has been supported by studies that show that administration of flumazenil a benzodiazepine antagonist can extend the lifespan of rats and decrease age-related deterioration of memory [385] indicate that a benzodiazepine antagonist can both increase lifetime and protect against the loss of cognitive abilities.

The extensive efferent innervation of outer hair cells [646, 702, 703] may be involved in these aging related changes because this innervation makes it possible to control the function of outer hair cells by descending neural activity.

This means that information generated in or modulated by the central nervous system can affect events that occur at the receptor level and possibly influence the presentation of deficits after injuries to the sensory cells.

Ototoxic antibiotics

It is well known that pharmacological agents such as aspirin (acetylsalicylate) and aminoglycoside antibiotics can cause hearing loss and tinnitus in some persons if given at large dosages (for a review see Forge and Schacht 2000 [186]. Other drugs such as loop diuretics, furosemide, ethacrynic acid, quinine indomethacin and cytostatics such as cisplatin can also cause tinnitus and hearing loss [606, 631]. Ototoxic aminoglycosides are also affecting the vestibular system, and the same substances that are ototoxic are often nephrotoxic.

The molecular mechanisms behind the ototoxic action of ototoxic antibiotics are beginning to be better understood [733]. It is believed that they involve a block of calcium channels [518, 732] and it has been proposed that the ototoxic action depends on the ability of aminoglycosides to form chelates with iron [530]. The redox-active aminoglycoside-iron complex activates oxygen and reduces it to a superoxide radical [733]. The electron donor in this process is assumed to be a polyunsaturated fatty acid. These discoveries have opened up the possibility to reduce the ototoxic effect by administration of iron chelation therapy [118, 641].

It has been suggested that melanin plays a role in the loss of hair cells from ototoxic antibiotics showing that the degree of skin pigmentation plays a role in acquiring hair cell loss from ototoxic antibiotics and thus suggesting an effect of melanin on the status of antioxidants in the cochlea [732]. Melanin allows ototoxic drugs to accumulate. Eye pigment correlates with ear melanin. It was mentioned above that melatonin plays a role in NIHL.

Neonatal jaundice

Neonatal jaundice that is associated with high levels of unconjugated bilirubin which causes sensorineural hearing loss specifically because of lesions of auditory brainstem nuclei (the cochlear nucleus). Studies in humans indicate that lesions in the basal ganglia may also occur [389].

Hyperbilirubinemia occurs because of the immaturity of a hepatic enzyme uridine diphosphate glucuronosyltransferase which converts unconjugated bilirubin to conjugated bilirubin [59]. The neurotoxic effect may be caused by altered expression of calcium-binding proteins [645].

Studies of the mechanisms of neural damage from hyperbilirubinemia have been done mainly in the Gunn rat [645], which is a rat that has a genetic deficiency in the glucuronosyltransferase enzyme.

Ménière's disease

Ménière's disease [208, 510, 704, 726] is defined as a triad of symptoms consisting of episodic vertigo fluctuating hearing loss. It is a progressive disorder that affects both the auditory and the vestibular systems.

The hearing loss during attacks of Ménière's disease is greatest for low frequencies (Figure 10.6), and tinnitus occurs at the same time. In the early stages of the disease hearing reverts to normal or near normal thresholds between attacks and tinnitus is absent, but the reversion to normalcy decreases over time as does the frequency range of the hearing loss which widens to include higher frequencies (Figure 10.6).

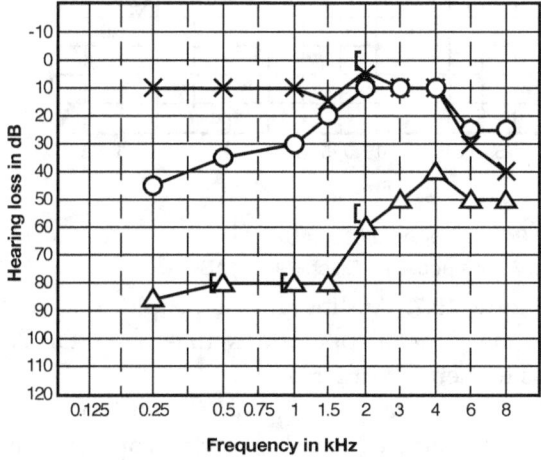

Figure 10.6. Typical audiograms from a person with Ménière's disease. Triangles: hearing loss during an attack open circles: hearing loss between attacks. Crosses show hearing loss in the unaffected (left) ear (Data from Møller, MB 1994 [468]).

It has been hypothesized that the signs of Ménière's disease are caused by an imbalance of the volume in the fluid system in the inner ear which is shared by the auditory and the vestibular systems.

More specifically it has been suggested that increased fluid volume in the endolymphatic space causes the disease [577] but the exact pathophysiology of the disorder has eluded researchers and clinicians, and it is unknown how these abnormalities in pressure (or rather in volume) are created, and their effect on the sensory cells is not completely understood.

Many different treatments are in use to alleviate the symptoms of Ménière's disease including sectioning of the vestibular nerve [216, 626], decompression of the endolymphatic sac [526, 612], destruction of vestibular sensory cells using ototoxic antibiotics through local application of gentamicin [627], diuretics, diet restrictions, etc. Some treatments aim at correcting the assumed imbalance of fluid systems in the inner ear. The relative inefficiency of such treatments indicates that the symptoms may have other causes and perhaps the imbalance in the fluid system is a result of the disease and not a cause. The high success rate of placebos supports the hypothesis that the anatomical location of the physiological abnormalities may be the central nervous system.

More recent treatments involve puffs of air to the middle ear cavity [146] varying the pressure applied to the inner ear fluid system. The success of that treatment indicates that the symptoms may be caused by expression of neuroplasticity thus indicating an involvement of the central nervous system. There are also indications that the sympathetic nervous system may be involved in generating the symptoms and signs of Ménière's disease [510, 704].

Other disorders of the auditory nervous system

Disorders of the auditory nerve can be caused by tumors (such as vestibular schwannoma) and close contact with one or more blood vessels in the subarachnoidal space [466]. Inflammatory and other processes affect the auditory and other nerves resulting in various forms of neuropathies. Auditory nerve aplasia occurs as a congenital malformation [117, 395].

Pathologies of the auditory nerve cause more complex forms of hearing loss than pathologies that affect the conductive apparatus or the cochlea and the impairment of speech discrimination from auditory nerve disorder are greater than that caused by the same degree of threshold shift from pathologies of the cochlea or the conductive apparatus.

The range of fiber diameters in auditory nerve is narrow which means that there are only small variations of the conduction velocities of the different axons of the nerve.

The temporal dispersion of the neural activity that arrives at the target cells (in the cochlear nucleus) is therefore very small. Lesions of the auditory nerve broaden the distribution of conduction velocities and increase the temporal dispersion of the neural activity that reaches the cochlear nucleus. That is assumed to be one of the reasons why auditory nerve lesions often cause greater degrees of impaired speech discrimination than do disorders restricted to the cochlea.

Hearing loss may occur as a complication to surgical manipulation that involved the auditory nerve. Surgical procedures in the cerebellopontine angle represented a significant risk of serious postoperative deficits before the introduction of microneurosurgery and intraoperative neurophysiologic monitoring [440].

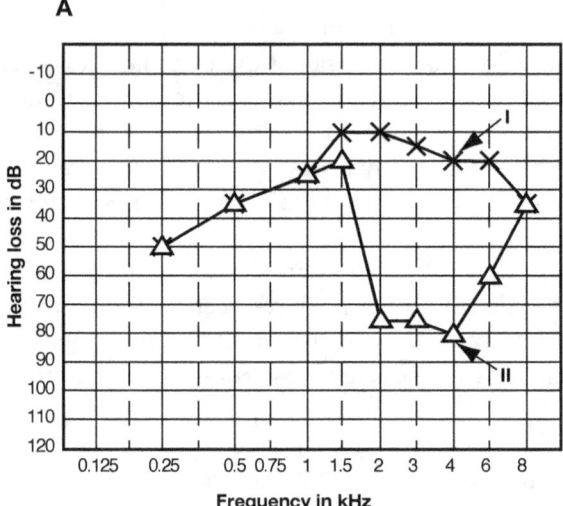

I: Pre-op Discr.=96% AS
II: 5 days post-op Discr.=0% AS

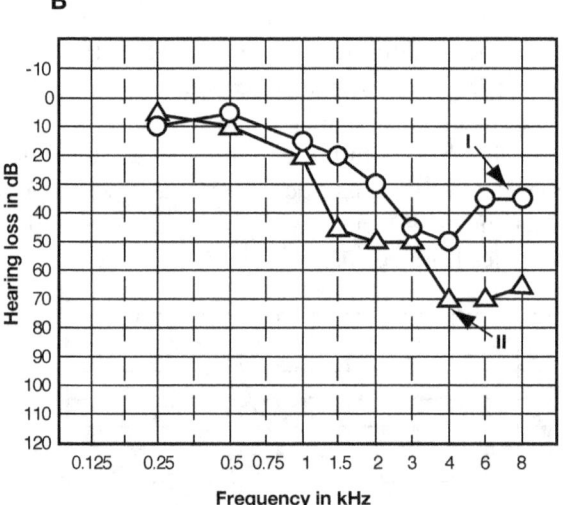

I: Pre-op Discr.=80% AS
II: 7 days post-op Discr.=30% AS

Figure 10.7. Audiogram of people who had undergone surgical operations that have caused injuries to their hearing nerve.

A: Preoperative (I) and postoperative audiograms obtained five days after an operation in the cerebellopontine angle (II). The speech discrimination decreased from 96% before the operation to 0 % after the operation.

B: Audiograms that show large changes in speech discrimination with relatively small changes in the pure tone audiogram. I: Preoperative audiogram. II Postoperative audiogram seven days after an operation in the cerebellopontine angle. The speech discrimination decreased from 80% to 30% after the operation.

Sudden deafness

A particular form of hearing loss known as the sudden hearing loss is a form of sensorineural hearing loss. It presents with a rapid onset and it occurs without any noticeable cause. It is rarely total, and it has been defined (empirically) as hearing a loss of 30 dB or more at least three contiguous frequencies [710]. The incidence of sudden hearing loss in the USA is 1.5/100,000 [272]. Other investigators have estimated that 4,000 cases of such hearing loss occur annually in the U.S.A [393].

The cause of sudden hearing loss is unknown but infectious diseases (bacterial or viral), or circulatory, immunologic, toxic and traumatic injuries have been suggested as causes. Auto-immune disease, Ménière's disease, trauma, vestibular schwannoma, multiple sclerosis, perilymphatic fistula, and vascular disorders have also been suggested as cause of sudden hearing loss [183] as has microvascular compression of the root of the auditory nerve [527, 694]. Two-thirds of the people with sudden hearing loss recover within days, and most recover within two weeks without treatment. The prognosis is worse for the most severe cases and those with downward-sloping audiograms and in addition to the hearing loss [393].

Treatments that often include steroids acyclovir and hyperbaric oxygen therapy have been tried without any noticeable effect on the natural history of the disease [344]. A recent study [298] using antioxidant (Vitamin E; d--tocopherol acetate 400 mg twice daily) in addition to other treatments showed some benefit (79 % recovered compared with 45% in the group who did not get Vitamin E).

The fact that antioxidants seem to improve recovery from sudden hearing loss indicates that oxidative processes may be involved.

Hyperacusis

A reduction of the tolerance level for sounds is known as hyperacusis [35]. Hyperacusis is common in connection with hearing disorders such as tinnitus. A parallel condition in the visual system involves low tolerance for light occurs in head injuries. The physiological basis for these phenomena is unknown. The fact that hyperacusis occurs in connection with diseases such as Williams syndrome [75] may indicate that biochemical abnormalities can cause it.

Misophonia and phonophobia

Some people experience adverse reactions to specific sounds. Misophonia is a condition in which very specific sounds such as those produced by eating cause very strong negative emotions, feelings of aversion and sometimes autonomic reactions [452]. Phonophobia is a condition where some individuals react to some specific sounds with fear [452]. While misophonia and phonophobia are adverse reactions that are elicited only by specific sounds most individuals experience unpleasant reactions to most forms of sounds above certain intensities.

Misophonia typically manifests around the age of 8-12 years. This early onset could indicate that it is related to a postnatal development that involves a blocking of the non-classical ascending auditory pathways [446] that involve the dorsal-medial thalamus.

The role of activation of neuroplasticity

Activation of neuroplasticity is important for the normal development of the auditory system. Studies of the morphological changes of the ear have dominated research in hearing loss for many years. Recent progress in the understanding of the role of functional changes in the auditory nervous system that occurs as a result of activation of neuroplasticity has directed research efforts to the auditory nervous system.

It has become evident that pathologies of the conductive apparatus can affect the function of structures in the auditory nervous system through activation of neuroplasticity. Disorders of the conductive apparatus, including the cochlea, can decrease the input to the nervous system and that can activate neuroplasticity because of deprivation of input to the nervous system.

Age-related changes in the function of sensory receptors are often followed by the compensatory actions of neuroplasticity which may give rise to symptoms more troublesome than the deficits in sensitivity. Examples are tinnitus induced by hearing loss.

Age-related decreases in sensitivity of sensory receptors occur in all sensory systems [720] perhaps most pronounced in the auditory system where it is known as presbycusis [458, 649]. Again, it is the outer hair cells that are most vulnerable and inner hair cells are rarely affected [249].

Reduction in the sensitivity of olfaction and taste with age may cause lack of appetite.

Vision

The conductive apparatus of the eye projects an image on the retina. Focusing the image from near and far objects depends on the ability of the lens to change (accommodation). Failure of accommodation affects most people around the age of forty necessitating the use of spectacles for reading and other tasks at a short distance.

The most common disorder of vision is a defect in the light conducting apparatus. Incorrect properties of the cornea and the lens cause unfocused images and nearsightedness. Many older people experience cataract's clouding of the lens.

Disorders of the retina are macular degeneration that usually occurs in older age (age-related macular degeneration AMD). Other diseases are retinitis pigmentosa, an inherited disorder consisting of degeneration of the retina [244].

Retinitis pigmentosa

Retinitis pigmentosa is an inherited disorder that causes severe impaired vision and blindness. This disease affects light receptors from the outside inward in the retina and from the center outward. It can also affect receptors in patches in the retina. The disorder is progressive and has no known cure.

Macular degeneration

Macular degeneration is a common age-related progressive disorder that causes visual deficits in the form of blurred vision. It affects the macula of the eye either by causing bleeding (wet macular degeneration) or by causing a breakdown of cones in the retina. It is associated with small bright (yellow) spots (drusen) in the retina. It is assumed to be caused by oxidative stress, but unlike similar age-related degeneration of auditory sensory cells, macular degeneration is not known to cause phantom phenomena (phosphenes).

The dry form is characterized by debris that collects between the retina and the choroid [133]. The wet form is characterized by blood vessels growing from the choroid behind the retina. Both forms can result in retinal detachment. Laser coagulation or angiogenesis inhibitors are common treatments.

Intake of dietary supplements (Lutein and zeaxanthin) can reduce the risk of age-related macular degeneration [376].

Exposure to the sun

Sensory receptors in the eye can be damaged permanently from looking into the sun without protection. A temporary reduction in sensitivity occurs from normal light exposure which is not regarded as a trauma but rather an adaptation to light. (The term adaptation is used differently in perceptual literature and physiology literature).

In the sense of vision dark adaptation means the gradual increase in sensitivity that occurs in darkness while light adaptation means a decrease in sensitivity because of exposure to light. In other sensory systems, adaptation means a decrease in sensitivity caused by exposure to stimulation. In physiology, the term adaptation is often used to describe the decrease in the firing of nerve fibers or nerve cells that occur after applying a stimulus.

The somatosensory system

Age-related loss of sensitivity also occurs in the somatosensory system where it probably has its greatest effect in connection with proprioception because a reduction of proprioception contributes to the impairment of movement. Disorders of the somatosensory system are less profound than disorders of hearing and vision. Deficits of touch vibration, or temperature sensation can progress much further without the person noticing any deficits.

The somatosensory system also includes proprioception which is involved in motor control. Proprioceptive input is important for the normal use of the motor system.

Reduced sensitivity of receptors for proprioception impairs the somatosensory feedback required for dexterous use of the hand and fingers.

Substances that often are found in common food such as organic compounds that include heavy metals can reduce the sensitivity to touch and vibration as well as that of proprioception.

Deprivation of input (such as occurs in limb amputations or severance of nerves such as the auditory nerve) to sensory and other central nervous system structures can be a strong promoter of neuroplasticity.

The somatosensory system modulates other functions such as pain. Loss of somatosensory input can, therefore, cause pain. Loss of somatosensory function in the mouth and throat (CN IX) can cause swallowing problems and result in choking.

Somatosensory input from different parts of the body is integrated to form a unified picture of our body and that contribute to the perception of a "self". For example, probing of a location of the body by one's finger not only provides information through tactile stimulation of receptors in the finger but the concomitant stimulation of receptors in the skin at the location being probed contribute to the sensation. That is normally not obvious, but it can become apparent when a part of the body is rendered without tactile sensation by local anesthesia.

Probing one's face after it has been numbed by a nerve block at a dentist's office provides a different impression of the size of parts of the face than it does without the effect of the local anesthesia. Normally a person has access to information obtained from both the face and the finger; after local anesthesia, only the finger can report its position.

Paresthesia

The term paresthesia is commonly used to describe somatosensory sensations such as tingling "pins and needles" burning etc. These phantom sensations are typically present in the extremities particularly in the lower limbs and often in the presence of diseases that affect peripheral nerves such as diabetes. Paresthesia may be transient such as that which may occur from compression of the sciatic nerve when sitting on a hard surface or more persistent such as that that may occur from nerve entrapment. It may also be caused by damage to peripheral nerves or chemical imbalance. Pain from peripheral nerve pathologies may be regarded as a form of paresthesia.

Paresthesia frequently occurs in elderly people without any other known diseases (except perhaps subclinical forms of polyneuropathy). It can be caused by a deficiency of vitamins mainly B_1 and B_{12}. Older people often have reduced absorption of vitamins and other essentials. Pathologies of the central nervous system can also cause paresthesia and paresthesia often occur together with pain and itch.

It must be emphasized that the symptoms of such injuries and insults to nerves are often accompanied if not dominated by subsequent symptoms that developed through neuroplastic changes to the central nervous system.

Gustation and olfaction

Disorders of the olfactory and gustatory systems have attracted little attention, but age-related changes occur particularly in olfaction. This sentence does not belong in this discussion of hearing.

Phantom taste (phantageusia) [252] consisting of metallic taste often occurs after section or injury of the chorda tympani. Other abnormal taste sensations may occur as a side effect of medications. Phantom smell or phantosmia [228, 252] is usually unpleasant.

Disorders of the central sensory nervous system

The symptoms of lesions of central structures of the sensory nervous system such as the cerebral cortex are less distinct than those that are caused by lesions to peripheral structures.

For example, the deficits from tumors or strokes that affect the auditory cortex are subtle, and speech discrimination is not profoundly affected (except in tests of low-redundancy speech comprehension) [65, 332]. Reports of meningioma causing deafness are usually related to cerebellopontine tumors with direct involvement of the vestibulocochlear nerve [514]. Brainstem tumors that affect nuclei in the ascending sensory pathways usually affect other systems to the degree that makes symptoms from sensory systems perceived as minor.

Phantom sensations are often accompanied by changes in the perception of sensory stimuli that activate sensory receptors in a normal way indicating changes in the way that ordinary sensory stimuli are processed.

Sensory hallucinations (meaningful sensations such as music speech and pictures) often occur in connection with psychiatric disorders such as schizophrenia as well as lesions of various kinds to the brain [81]. Auditory hallucinations may occur in conjunction with temporal lobe lesions or psychiatric disorders [81] [252].

Many of the drugs used commonly in anesthesia can cause hallucinations. Most of these hallucinations disappears after a few days but a few drugs such as those belonging to the Ketamine-family (arylcyclohexylamine, known to produce dissociation, anesthesia and hallucinogenic effects) can cause hallucinations that may last years.

Some of the disorders of sensory nervous systems are caused by trauma and other insults, but many disorders are jointly caused by expression of neuroplasticity. We have already discussed how deficits of sensory receptors can affect the function of central nervous system structures through the expression of neuroplasticity. Also, trauma and other insults to the nervous system are normally accompanied by expression of neuroplasticity some of which may be compensatory for deficits other plastic changes such as phantom sensations may be signs of disease.

Age-related changes in the nervous system may be regarded as an insult to nerves and the central nervous system but can also be regarded as a normal process. Age-related changes in sensory nervous systems have complex symptoms and some few objective signs.

Phosphenes are the term for a phantom visual sensation that does not include specific patterns or meaningful pictures. They can interfere with sleep. Phantom eye syndrome can occur after removal of an eye and is characterized by visual sensations [644]. The sensations usually take the form of phosphenes: flickering or permanent light. A few people experienced contours, objects or scenes. These sensations are mostly experienced in darkness and before falling asleep. Black patches in the visual field (scotoma) are also signs of disorders of the visual portion of the central nervous system.

Chapter 11

Movement Systems and their Common Disorders

Abstract

1. Movement disorders are characterized by decreased or absent function (paresis or paralysis) or hyperfunction such producing hypertonia, hyperreflexia, and spasm. Traumatic spinal cord and cerebral injuries account for a large part of movement disorders.

2. Strokes, various degenerative or genetic disorders are common causes of movement disorders. Movement disorders have been categorized as upper and lower motoneuron disorders. Signs of upper motor neuron disorders are spasm hypokinesia or hyperkinesia. The symptoms of lower motor neuron disorders are hypotonia and hyporeflexia.

3. The term multiple system atrophy covers a wide range of degenerative motor disorders. Deficits in gait and balance, as well as the lack of coordination (ataxia), are other features of movement disorders.

Introduction

The pathology of movement disorders may be localized to either the muscles, the motor neurons, the motor nerves or the central nervous system. The motor weakness (reduced motor activity) can be caused by disorders of motor nerves (peripheral neuropathy compression of motor nerves) or by central nervous system causes. Parkinson's disease is an example of hypokinesia.

Neuroplasticity has a central position when it comes to movement function in that it is the basis for learning motor skills. Neuroplasticity also plays central roles in creating the signs of movement disorders although the involvement is far less obvious than in the learning of motor skills.

Activation of neuroplasticity is involved in creating the spasm that occurs after healing of injuries to motor nerves. Spasticity may occur after spinal cord injuries. Spasm occurs in diseases such as spasticity, hemifacial spasm, and spasmodic torticollis.

Pathology of movement disorders

Movement disorders were earlier divided into disorders of pyramidal and extrapyramidal origin. Extrapyramidal signs were earlier assumed to be associated with disorders of the basal ganglia while pyramidal disorders were assumed to have their origin in the pyramidal tract (the corticospinal tract). The distinction between disorders with pyramidal and extrapyramidal signs lost its anatomical relevance when it became known that information from the basal ganglia could reach the motor cortices (primary motor cortices (MI) premotor cortices (PMA) and supplementary motor cortices (SMA)) and thereby reach the spinal cord through descending spinal tracts. The term extrapyramidal signs are still in clinical use for describing symptoms. Here we will distinguish between lower and upper motor neuron disorders.

Lower motoneuron deficits often cause flaccid paresis or paralysis ipsilateral to the lesion, but upper motoneuron disorders are likely to include more complex symptoms that often include spasms and spasticity contralateral to the lesion. Upper motoneuron disorders can be bilateral.

Many of the fibers in the motor tracts of the motor system terminate in synapses that do not normally conduct. The existence of such dormant connections represents a redundancy that may be activated through the expression of neuroplasticity.

Many phenomena can activate neuroplasticity in the motor system such as injuries or changes in demand (inactivity or increased use) opening connections that are normally not conducting. Spinal reflexes can change as a result of usage (training) thus showing the effect of activating neuroplasticity.

Lower motor neuron disorders

Many forms of reduced function of motor systems may be related to the α motoneurons (the "final common pathway"). Amyotrophic lateral sclerosis (ALS) causing death or impairment of the function of the α motoneuron. The death of these neurons may be caused by a combination of many factors such as increased oxidative stress, glutamate excitotoxicity or disruption of calcium homeostasis that initiate subsequent apoptosis.

Amyotrophic lateral sclerosis (ALS) is a progressive degenerative disorder closely associated with the degeneration of α motoneurons in the spinal cord or the brainstem, but it also includes the degeneration of motor fiber tracts and pyramidal cells in the motor cortex.

The disorder is progressive from the onset and from the time of diagnosis respiratory failure ensues within six months to 10 years with a mean of 2 years. No known therapy has been effective. The pathophysiology is unknown, but familiar ALS is associated with mutations in a gene that controls the synthesis of SOD (superoxide dismutase).

Upper motor neuron diseases

Upper motoneuron disorders may cause paresis, but this is usually accompanied by other symptoms and signs of movement disorders such as spasm, tremor, etc. of different muscle groups. Cerebral palsy is a common term for a group of non-progressive motor disorders that are caused by events that have occurred in utero or are acquired during birth or early in life. Ischemic strokes, bleeding, and inflammation that affect different central nervous system structures involved in motor control are also common causes of paresis and paralysis.

Traumatic injuries and ischemic insults to the central nervous system from various causes such as strokes, birth injuries, surgically induced trauma, and other common causes of movement disorders.

Spinal cord injuries (SCI), disorders of the basal ganglia and the motor cortices are the most common causes of movement disorders. Other pathologies such as multiple sclerosis (MS) and degenerative diseases such as Parkinson's disease (PD) and Huntington's disease (HD) cause various forms of movement symptoms.

It is only recently that activation of neuroplasticity has been recognized as a contributing factor in the cause of symptoms and signs of movement disorders. (In a previous chapter, we discussed diseases where activation of neuroplasticity was the primary cause of the symptoms and signs).

Age-related changes include deficits in neural transmitters from degeneration of neural tissue such as occurs in PD and HD. Age-related decrease in production of gamma-aminobutyric acid (GABA) [102] in the central nervous system results in a shift in the relationship between excitation and inhibition.

The changes that occur as a function of age occur at different rates in different individuals. Many disorders have an increasing incidence with age which indicates that age-related changes play a complex role in many movement disorders.

Demyelinating disorders such as multiple sclerosis (MS) that affect fiber tracts in the spinal cord or brain may cause paresis as well as dysfunction of the sensory systems and higher order central nervous system functions such as mood disorders etc.

Paresis and paralysis may be caused by inadequate facilitation of α motoneurons even when descending motor pathways are intact. The facilitatory and inhibitory input to the α motoneurons from spinal and supraspinal sources may be altered because of traumatic injuries to the spinal cord or strokes. The facilitatory input to α motoneurons has several sources such as the reticular formation through the reticulospinal tracts as well as through the medial descending motor tracts. These pathways are often overlooked, but a better understanding of how such facilitation occurs may aid in the development of treatments for paresis and paralysis.

Rostral structures normally supply complex input to the spinal segment that is both inhibitory and excitatory on motor neurons. Changes in the balance between inhibition and excitation can cause movement disorders.

The altered sensory input to the spinal cord also plays a role in producing symptoms of dyskinesia. It is assumed that many movement disorders are caused by inefficient utilization of input to the pattern generator (CPG) that makes it possible to perform walking movements without control from the spinal cord) defective spinal cord reflexes in the spinal cord and misdirected or incorrect compensatory processes.

All three of these components are affected by injuries or deprivation of input but malleable and correctable through activation of neuroplasticity that is evoked through training and other means such as electrical stimulation of peripheral structures (transdermal electrical nerve stimulation, TENS) or the cerebral cortex.

Other movement disorders related to supraspinal structures are congenital movement disorders like hyperkinesia syndromes which include tremor, spasm and various forms of involuntary movements (chorea). Tremor is an oscillating movement that may consist of alternating contractions of antagonist's muscles. It can be hereditary or caused by systemic diseases such as thyroid disorders, drugs or age-related changes.

Spasm and Spasticity

The term muscle spasm is usually used to describe involuntary muscle contractions that are accompanied by EMG activity. Irritation of or injury to motor nerves may cause motor abnormalities such as spasm and synkinesis by altering the processing in cranial motor nuclei such as the facial nucleus and nuclei found in the ventral horn of the spinal cord. Some forms of spasm and synkinesis are, however, often caused by more complex mechanisms including abnormal proprioceptive or other somatosensory input. The involvement of proprioception in causing signs of movement disorders is important and will be discussed below.

Examples of involuntary muscle contractions are spasmodic torticollis, trismus, stiff-man syndrome and nocturnal leg cramps, but even tension headaches belong to this group of disorders. Trismus is an involuntary closing of the jaw due to tonic spasm of the muscles of mastication. Maladaptive neuroplasticity is assumed to be either the primary cause of some forms of muscle spasm or a contributing cause.

Dyskinesia

Hypokinesia and hyperkinesia can result from injuries and other causes that result in morphological changes such as destruction of central nervous system tissue or ischemia. Traumatic injuries, tumors and side effects of surgical operations can cause interruptions of pathways and alterations of the function of gray matter regions involved in the processing of movement commands and initiation of a movement. Altered function of the motor system may also occur because of reorganization of the nervous system caused by activation of maladaptive neuroplasticity.

Chorea

The many different types of chorea (abnormal involuntary movements) are often congenital and involve both cortical and subcortical structures with diffuse morphological abnormalities. Chorea often occurs together with mental disorders. Involuntary sound production is ranging from non-verbal sounds to obscenities (coprolalia) also occurs. The etiologies of these disorders are often understood poorly, and the anatomical location of the underlying physiological abnormality may not even have been identified. Some of these disorders, however, have been associated with abnormalities of specific neurotransmitters.

Chorea is a part of the symptoms of Huntington's chorea (HC), but chorea is also a typical sign of other disorders of the basal ganglia. Chorea often occurs together with mental disorders.

Disorders of the spinal cord and the control of motor function in the brainstem

Spinal cord and brainstem disorders can be divided into two categories: those that affect the spinal cord or brainstem in general and those that only affect α motoneurons selectively. Disorders that affect structures rostral to the motoneuron normally cause more complex signs and symptoms such as hypokinesia and hyperkinesia in addition to paresis and paralysis.

Spinal cord injuries

Spinal cord injuries (SCI) subsequent inflammatory and healing processes and tumors can cause a host of complex movement disorders. SCI may cause a total or partial lack of motor function, and it may involve inadequate function such as weakness, spasticity, clonus, and spasm. The symptoms and signs depend on the nature, location, and extent of the pathology.

SCI can cause paresis and paralysis but disorders and injuries that affect the spinal cord in general usually also present with symptoms and signs of other movement disorders such as hyperkinesia and hyperkinesia.

The symptoms and signs are often the results of the initiation of a chain of events that involves many parts of the central nervous system (CNS) including the expression of neuroplasticity.

The response to the familiar "Jendrassik maneuver" is an example of modulation of motor excitability. When a person's reflexes are tested there will usually be some unconscious inhibition. The Jendrassik maneuver removes or reduces this inhibition. Using this maneuver, a person clenches his jaw and interlocks his hands but pulls them apart while his patellar reflex is elicited. This reflex response should be larger than what is observed without the Jendrassik maneuver.

Traumatic SCI that occur from automobile accidents, falls, gunshots, etc. do not usually involve total anatomical transection (approximately 33%) yet many people (approximately 50%) experienced neurologically total severance. Surgical operations, particularly tumor removals arterial-venous malformation correction and spinal procedures may also cause SCI as a complication. Operations for scoliosis was earlier a not uncommon cause of SCI, but the introduction of intraoperative neurophysiologic monitoring and improved surgical techniques have reduced the risk to a very small figure.

The symptoms and signs of people with SCI likely go through several phases after the occurrence of the injury each one being characterized by different abnormalities of the spinal reflexes. Symptoms are initially characterized by a spinal shock which transitions to weakness and flaccid paresis before progressing into hyperkinetic signs such as spasticity.

Many of the symptoms and signs of SCI may be explained by the altered relationship between excitatory or inhibitory supraspinal input to segmental spinal reflex circuits.

Basal ganglia, cerebellum and cerebral cortex

Movement disorders caused by physiological abnormalities in the basal ganglia and the cerebral cortex are more complex than those anomalies with more caudal anatomical locations. Abnormal movements (dystonia, hypokinesia, and hyperkinesia) often occur together with paresis and paralysis such as can be seen in cerebral palsy. Some of the disorders of the cortex and basal ganglia are inherited congenital disorders. Acquired disorders of these structures are from injuries (accident or iatrogenic) and strokes and intracranial bleeding.

Disorders related to the basal ganglia

The two most characteristically disorders that are associated with the basal ganglia are Parkinson's disease (PD) and Huntington's disease (HD) [61]. Both are age-related.

These two disorders are both chronic neurodegenerative disorders with certain commonalities but also characteristic differences. The basal ganglia are the primary anatomical location of degeneration of basal ganglia structure that causes the movement signs and symptoms for both PD and HD but different nuclei are affected in these two disorders. The incidence of PD increases with age while the incidence of HD is highest in the fourth decade of life.

Parkinson's disease

The typical symptoms of PD, slow movements, rigidity, and low-frequency tremor are assumed to be caused by selective degeneration of dopamine-producing cells in the substantia nigra compacta (SNc). The motor symptoms of PD also include "freezing" reactions in many people with PD.

The impairment of the function of the substantia nigra causes a re-routing of information in the basal ganglia. The cause of these signs is not completely understood, but there is evidence that multiple factors are involved such as hereditary factors oxidative stress and age which is the most significant risk factor. PD includes other typical age-related changes.

The motor symptoms and signs typical of PD are assumed to be caused by deficits in the substantia nigra's production of dopamine. The cause for the decrease in production of dopamine is not known, but there is evidence that mitochondrial defects oxidative processes, stress, degeneration of specific structures and inflammation together with age-related changes are involved [50]. Neurotoxicity by the neurotransmitter glutamate most likely contributes to the development of the disease. Activation of neuroplasticity most likely is involved in the creation of these symptoms.

Exposure to certain environmental factors may induce symptoms similar to those associated with PD. It has been suggested that some natural chemicals that are present in the environment can contribute to the development of PD.

Symptoms of PD may be induced by dopamine receptor antagonists as seen in many psychoactive drugs used to control psychotic behaviors. PD is more complicated than a mere motor symptom syndrome. The motor deficits are often accompanied by other typically age-related degenerative changes such as cognitive deficits, dementia, and depression. Though the motion symptoms have attracted most of the research interest and treatment attention, the effects on the other affected systems should not be ignored.

Abnormalities in proprioceptive function have been considered to contribute to the motor symptoms of PD. It has been suggested that at least some of the motor deficits are caused by impaired sensory function.

Research regarding the motor deficits in PD has benefited from studies of animal models involving the administration of MPTP a substance that causes degeneration of dopamine-producing neurons in the substantia nigra in monkeys. The discovery that MPTP induces neural degeneration causes similar to that which occurs in PD also suggests that environmental toxins may be implicated in the development of PD.

Studies of the pathophysiology of PD have focused on the changes in the functions that are caused by the morphological changes which mostly involve the SNc. However, the functional changes that these pathologies cause can also evoke the expression of neuroplasticity aimed at compensating for the deficits resulting from these morphological changes.

The involvement of neuroplasticity has been mostly ignored in forming hypotheses about the pathologies of PD.

The fact that training of various kinds is beneficial in reducing the symptoms and signs of PD indicates that expression of neuroplasticity is involved in creating the symptoms and signs of PD.

Treatment of Parkinson's disease (PD)

Before the advent of L-dopa for treating PD, surgical lesions were made in the basal ganglia mostly in the pallidus (pallidotomy). The feasibility of this procedure was discovered empirically by a surgeon who accidentally ligated the artery supplying the globus pallidus in a patient with PD while performing a surgical operation for a different disorder on the patient [119]. Surgical treatment of PD almost fell out of use after the introduction of L-dopa in 1967 but has recently been reintroduced because of the loss of L-dopa efficacy after prolonged continual treatment. Lesions were initially made primarily in the globus pallidus (pallidotomy), but also thalamotomy became popular for a period.

Surgical lesions have now been largely replaced through chronic electrical stimulation through implanted electrodes (deep brain stimulation, DBS). The targets for implantation of electrodes for permanent stimulation are the GPi, STN and the ventral intermediary nucleus of the thalamus (Vim). The substitution of DBS for surgical lesions was made under the assumption that DBS causes inactivation of nerve cells which is similar to that of lesions but is reversible.

Electrical stimulation of brain tissue can have two effects: it can activate nerve cells or fiber tracts or inactivate nerve cells through constantly forced depolarization. Only stimulation of a high frequency (100-250 pulses per second) has been found to be therapeutic for treating PD. It has thus been suggested that it works primarily by deactivating inhibitory neural structures by keeping the cells depolarized [747]. This effect is similar to that of depolarizing muscle relaxants such as succinylcholine.

However, electrical stimulation also stimulates fiber tracts and fibers may be able to follow the high-frequency stimulation. This means that DBS is likely to have complex effects on the function of the structures that are subjected to such stimulation. DBS being reversible and adjustable and having a relatively minute risk of morbid complications.

Some of the first stereotaxic placements of stimulating electrodes in subcortical structures for the relief of movement symptoms in PD were made in the thalamus (the Vim). Such stimulation effectively suppressed tremor in PD. Later stimulation of the STN was found effective in reducing movement signs of PD. Electrical stimulation of structures of globus pallidus followed and showed great benefit in the treatment of PD.

The observed tolerance effect is an obstacle in the use of this technique [568]. It seems likely that the tolerance that gradually made the stimulation less effective may have to do with functional changes that occur through the expression of neuroplasticity. DBS represents an abnormal stimulation of specific brain tissue, and many studies have shown that such stimulation causes the expression of neuroplasticity.

Physical therapy and exercise play critical roles in the rehabilitation of patients with PD thus another example of the importance of activating neuroplasticity in the treatment of deficits and abnormal functions of motor systems.

Huntington's disease

HD is a progressive disease that primarily affects the caudate nucleus and the putamen, but other areas of the central nervous system become affected as the disease progresses. While the SNc is the most affected nucleus in PD, the major abnormalities in patients with HD occur in the caudate nucleus and the putamen which show massive degeneration. Also, the globus pallidus is often affected in HD, and there is a neuronal loss in the cerebral cortex mainly affecting layers III V and VI.

The functional abnormalities in HD are different from those of PD. The inhibitory and excitatory input to the striatum from the SNc is unaffected in HD, but inhibition from the striatum onto the LGP is decreased while the inhibition on the STN from LGP is increased. The excitation from the STN to SNr and MGP is both decreased in HD while increased in PD.

The inhibition on the thalamus from MGP and SNr is decreased in HD while it is increased in PD. The excitation from the thalamus to the cortex which was decreased in PD is increased in HD. It is believed that this increase in thalamic excitation of the cortex is the cause of the increased and often inappropriate motor activity in HD.

Tardive dyskinesia

Tardive dyskinesia is a category of itself and is not a PD-like syndrome. Tardive dyskinesia affects mainly the facial muscles and the tongue with involuntary movements and is also known as oral, buccal dyskinesia. Tardive dyskinesia occurs as a side effect of some antipsychotic and neuroleptic drugs used primarily in treating schizophrenia. These antipsychotic and neuroleptic drugs are finding increasingly used in the treatment of other disorders including disorders in children.

Strokes

There are two kinds of stroke, ischemic stroke (80%) and hemorrhagic strokes (20%). Ischemic strokes have their effects by obstruction of blood flow in a specific cerebral vessel while hemorrhagic strokes involve bleeding from disruption of a blood vessel. Ischemic strokes cause a focal destruction of cerebral tissue with symptoms related to the structures affected. Bleeding such as from hemorrhagic strokes causes a more diffuse damage to brain tissue.

Strokes that cause damage to one of the two visual pathways in the association cortices affect processing of spatial and object information independently. Mel Goodale and colleagues have shown that visual information that guides grasping is processed within different areas of the association cortices from that where a "stream" which is involved in the perception of form is processed. Individuals with strokes in these regions may have selective deficits in either grasping or visual perception [480]. An individual with a stroke that affects the dorsal stream may lose the ability to use vision to guide motion whereas another stroke victim in whom the ventral stream is affected may be able to guide hand motion using vision while unable to recognize the form of objects.

Strokes are different from simple deficits in perfusion such as those caused by low blood pressure which causes general symptoms of ischemia typically with a loss of consciousness.

The initial phase of ischemic strokes destruct brain tissue and the following events are complex and involve activation of neuroplasticity [297] [483].

The available treatment of the acute phase of ischemic stroke have poor results, but preventive actions can reduce the risk of strokes considerably [416] [508].

Transient ischemic attacks (TIA) are short lasting strokes with full recovery from neurologic deficits, typically within a few hours.

The symptoms and signs of movement disorders are often caused by damage to motor pathways such as from ischemic strokes that affect sensory systems. Damage to sensory systems may produce signs of movement disorders because the normal proprioceptive sensory feedback is affected. Any damage to proprioception may affect the ability to control posture and control voluntary movements.

Complex central nervous system disturbances

Integration of sensory and motor systems is observed in reaching, and it has been hypothesized that the primary motor cortex is involved in somatosensory processing. A person may have the ability to discern the distance of an object and be capable of extending his arm and hand to that distance to a high level of precision when these tasks are attempted independently.

The person may be unable, however, to perform these tasks in conjunction with one another if the connection between the sensory and motor systems is impaired. In a reaching task which requires continual feedback regarding the precise location of the hand about the target, this deficit will become apparent. Visual feedback is important. Visual processing follows some of the principles of stream segregation and visual processing in the dorsal stream is the most important for control of movements such as reaching. Some of the complex effects of strokes on voluntary movements can be related to deficits of the visual system.

Other multi-symptom atrophies

Many of the disorders that are associated with a Parkinson-like syndrome are known as multi-symptom atrophies (MSA). Some like striato-nigral degeneration produce Parkinson-like symptoms but do not respond to levodopa since the pathology is in the striatum and not the substantia nigra.

Progressive supranuclear palsy also produces PD-like symptoms but is associated with prominent eye motion abnormalities and increased axial tone and also does not respond to levodopa.

Some of these syndromes are referred to as Parkinson Plus syndromes. These include the Shy-Drager syndrome in which autonomic dysfunction is prominent in addition to Parkinson symptoms.

Many related syndromes now classified as SCA (spinocerebellar atrophies—older names included olivopontocerebellar atrophy dentatepalidoluysian, Machado-Joseph Disease, etc). most prominently are characterized by abnormalities in the cerebellar systems but are also associated with parkinsonian symptoms. It is common to see some Parkinsonian symptoms even in unrelated degenerative diseases such as Alzheimer's disease.

Other forms of dystonia

There are numerous other forms of dystonia but they are rare disorders, and their pathophysiology is unknown. Many of the disorders related to the basal ganglia are congenital or hereditary, and the movement disorders are often accompanied by other central nervous system abnormalities. Many of these other forms of dystonia include hyperkinesia and display a wide spectrum of movement disorders from tremor to spasm and various forms of chorea.

Tremor can be inherited or caused by systemic diseases such as thyroid disorders drugs or age-related changes. Gilles de la Tourette Syndrome [285] is a movement disorder (dystonia) that is characterized by sudden rapid, recurrent movements that often include a production of odd sounds. It begins in childhood, and it can be either less pronounced with age or become worse. The anatomical location of the physiological abnormalities producing these symptoms are supposed to be the cortical-striatal-paleo-thalamic circuit and treatment using DBS (bilateral thalamic stimulation) has been shown to be effective in reversing these symptoms [3].

The fact that people with Tourette's syndrome have cognitive deficits supports the hypothesis that either other systems are affected or that the function of the basal ganglia is not limited to motor function.

Also, persons with these disorders benefit from physical therapy and other forms of training; again, an example of the important role of neuroplasticity in the treatment of disorders of the nervous system.

Wilson's disease is interesting because it has a motor behavioral and psychiatric signs. It is also known as hepatolenticular degeneration. It is an autosomal recessive disorder of copper metabolism associated with reduced amounts of the copper-binding protein ceruloplasmin, and the symptoms are assumed to be caused by excess accumulation of copper in the brain and the liver. It occurs in approximately 1 in 40,000 people.

In adults, these movement disorders resemble that of PD and include tremor dystonia postural instability and ataxia. In addition to hepatic dysfunction more or less pronounced psychiatric symptoms occur. Other typical findings are Kaiser-Fleischer rings in the cornea representing depositions of copper.

Common for all these disorders is that the cause is poorly understood and even the anatomical location of the physiological abnormality is incompletely known. Therapy rests on the use of agents that inhibit copper absorption (such as zinc) and agents which facilitate removal of copper by chelation.

Gait and balance disturbances

Gait and balance disturbances are common, and their incidence increases with age. Control of posture is complex, and many disorders of the motor system affect the control of posture.

Control of posture depends on the proper function of the motor system and correct proprioceptive input from the vestibular system together with input from receptors in joints tendons muscles and the skin. Visual input is important and can substitute for the loss of vestibular input.

The most obvious consequences of balance disturbance are falls. Falls are a frequent cause of injuries - including head injuries – which result in disabilities and deaths. The incidence of falls increases with age.

The pathophysiology of gait and balance disturbances is complex and poorly understood. There are many anatomical locations of abnormalities that can cause gait and balance disturbances.

Failure to control posture can be caused by motor proprioceptive or vestibular dysfunction. These two different causes of balance and posture control can be distinguished by the Romberg test which for which a positive result indicates a sensory cause. The patient stands steady with feet together first with eyes open then with eyes closed.

Ataxia

Ataxia is an inability to coordinate voluntary movements -- especially walking -- which becomes jerky. Involuntary movements are not included in the term ataxia. Ataxia is a general term that describes the lack of motor coordination. Ataxia may occur because of various lesions to the motor system (motor ataxia) or sensory deficits (sensory ataxia). Motor ataxia is often caused by disorders of the cerebellum, but disorders of other supraspinal structures can also cause motor ataxia. The most common cause of ataxia is from ingestion of alcohol and other hypnotic drugs. Such drugs also cause ataxia in animals including insects.

People with motor ataxia may or may not be unsteady in this position, but their unsteadiness is not affected by having their eyes open or closed (negative Romberg sign). Patients with sensory ataxia become unsteady with closed eyes (positive Romberg sign). Otolaryngologists often use a more difficult version of the test where the patient places his/her feet ahead of each other instead of together.

Defects in the ventral spinocerebellar tracts are often involved in motor ataxia. Sensory ataxia can be caused by faulty proprioceptive input, especially from the vestibular system. In addition to ataxia cerebellar disorders are typically associated with a tremor of various types. Ataxia can affect limbs, trunk, eyes and other bulbar structures. A gaze-evoked nystagmus is a form of ataxia.

Little is known about the involvement of neuroplasticity in these disorders. Treatment such as training and exercise has a beneficial effect on these disorders indicating that expression of neuroplasticity may be involved in generating some of the symptoms.

Resistance developing from medical treatment (tolerance) may also be caused by expression of neuroplasticity in an attempt to compensate for the changes caused by the treatment.

Disorders of the cerebral cortex

Movement disorders of the cerebral cortex can be caused by cell destruction or ischemia resulting from vascular trauma. Cerebral palsy is the most common disorder of the motor cortex which presents with symptoms of paresis paralysis and hypoactive and hyperactive movement disorders of various kinds. It is a non-progressive disorder that can be caused by many different forms of insults such as asphyxia trauma vascular events congenital abnormalities and kernictus (Jaundice associated with high levels of unconjugated bilirubin or in small premature infants with more modest degrees of bilirubinemia)

Loss of dexterity is the primary sign of corticospinal tract interruption. Injury to the corticospinal tract also causes abnormal posture abnormal reflexes (spasticity) and abnormal cutaneous reflexes [86]. More of the fibers of the corticospinal tract terminate on interneurons than on motoneurons and influence the motoneurons through their effects on reflexes that involve the interneurons on which they terminate. Changes in the function of local circuits in the spinal cord, therefore, play an important role in creating the symptoms and signs that are experienced after interruption of supraspinal input to spinal segmental circuits. For example, the cutaneous reflexes are often diminished in individuals with upper motor neuron lesions while the deep tendon reflexes are increased - yet another sign of the complexity of motor control systems.

Many factors that lead to these diffuse symptoms and signs are difficult to identify. The pathophysiology is poorly understood. Other disorders that are related to the cerebral motor cortex may be induced through the expression of neuroplasticity that can cause reorganization of the cerebral cortex.

Reorganization of motor cortices

Evidence points to the presence of reorganization of cerebral cortices the brainstem and the spinal cord at segmental levels. Deprivation of input is the strongest promoter of neuroplasticity and injuries that cause interruption of pathways may thus (immediately or later) cause changes in function that is not directly a cause of the original morphological changes.

Changes in the function of peripheral structures - including motor nerves and proprioceptive input - may promote such expression of neuroplasticity.

The changes in function are normally not accompanied by any detectable abnormality in morphology. Even changes in muscles and motor nerves may affect central nervous system structures. The symptoms from altered function of central nervous system structures may change over time. Expression of neuroplasticity may involve the unmasking of dormant synapses formation or elimination of synapses sprouting of axons and the changing of synaptic efficacy. Hyperactivity which can cause spasticity and tremor may result from increased synaptic efficacy in excitatory neural circuits or decrease in synaptic efficacy in inhibitory circuits.

Changes in the balance between inhibition and excitation are a common outcome of expression of neuroplasticity that involves altered synaptic efficacy.

The severing of a peripheral nerve in adult rats causes a reorganization of the primary motor cortices [283]. The cortical areas adjacent to those represented by the muscles innervated by the severed nerve expand into the territory of the severed nerve. This is similar to what occurs in the sensory cortex after sensory deprivation, which means that adult cortical motor maps are not as had been assumed earlier.

Within a few hours after transection of a peripheral nerve stimulation of the affected cortical area elicited contraction of muscles that normally were represented by adjacent areas of the primary motor cortex (MI). The rapid change in responsiveness indicates that existing synaptic connections have altered their efficacy rather than forming new relationships (spouting). These investigators [283] found evidence that this re-organization was caused by a release of tonic inhibition that normally exists in the cortical interconnections and was able to induce a similar re-organization by pharmacological means such as by applying bicuculline methyl bromide to the M1 region of the cerebral cortex. Bicuculline is a $GABA_A$ receptor antagonist ((-)) to cause a release of GABAergic inhibition.

It is not known how such reorganization of the motor-cortex affects control of movement, but it seems logical to assume that some of the unexplained symptoms and signs from motor nerve injuries may be related to such cortical re-organization.

Strokes that cause damage to one of the two visual pathways in the association cortices affect processing of spatial and object information independently. Mel Goodale and colleagues have shown that visual information that guides grasping is processed within different areas of the association cortices from that where a "stream" which is involved in the perception of form is processed.

Pesrons with strokes in these regions may have selective deficits in either grasping or visual perception [480]. An individual with a stroke that affects the dorsal stream may lose the ability to use vision to guide motion whereas another stroke victim in whom the ventral stream is affected may be able to guide hand motion using vision while unable to recognize the form of objects.

Disorders of the brainstem and sleep

The power of brainstem mechanisms in blocking descending motor pathways is evident from the fact that skeletal muscles are paralyzed during rapid eye movement (REM) sleep (paradoxical sleep). The observation that some people occasionally experience waking up paralyzed for a few seconds (sleep paralysis) indicates that the normal reversal of the blockage of descending activity was delayed after the end of REM sleep (waking up). A few people have an abnormal or absent blockage of descending motor activity during REM sleep [502].

This disorder is known as the "rapid eye movement sleep behavior disorder" (RBD). Individuals with RBD often make extensive body movements during sleep sometimes physically acting out their violent dreams while unconscious and sometimes injuring other people [588, 589]. The disorder occurs most often in men, and it is often associated with other neurodegenerative diseases. Individuals with RBD are at a higher risk of acquiring PD [66].

In a recent study, 57% of RBD persons had other neurological disorders all of which (except 14%) were PD dementia without parkinsonism and multiple system atrophy (MSA) [66, 502]. These investigators concluded that RBD might be the first manifestation of other disorders such as PD [502]. That administration of a benzodiazepine such as Clonazepam was effective in treating RBD [502] thus supporting the hypothesis that decreased efficacy of GABA$_A$ receptors plays a role in this disorder.

The absence of normal paralysis during REM sleep could be caused by the failure of brain neurons to block the facilitator descending activity to α motoneuron. This facilitatory input is necessary for the signals from the brainstem to activate the α motoneurons. Without this facilitation, the motoneurons cannot respond to commands from the motor cortices (M1, PMA, and SMA).

Disorders of Cranial Nerves and Neurotology

Abstract

1. Cranial motor nerve symptoms include paresis, paralysis, and hyperactivity.

2. Symptoms from sensory cranial nerve symptoms include pain, paresthesia, and reduced function.

3. Cranial nerve disorders are associated with unilateral spasm (hemifacial spasm, unilateral spasmodic torticollis) or bilateral spasm (blepharospasm, bilateral spasmodic torticollis, and spasmodic dysphonia).

4. Unilateral hyperactive disorders such as trigeminal neuralgia and hemifacial spasm can be successfully treated by microvascular decompression of the respective cranial nerve roots as can glossopharyngeal neuralgia and unilateral spasmodic torticollis.

5. Disorders such as blepharospasm, atypical face pain, bilateral spasmodic torticollis and also spasmodic dysphonia have a different pathophysiology probably involving the basal ganglia.

6. Symptoms of vestibular disorders (vertigo unsteadiness, lightheadedness, and nausea) may be caused by pathologies of the inner ear the vestibular nerve and the vestibular nervous system.

7. Neoplastic disorders affecting cranial nerves are rare except vestibular schwannoma (acoustic tumors) which are benign tumors consisting of myelin-forming Schwann cells that originate from the eight-cranial nerve most commonly the superior vestibular nerve. Similar kinds of benign tumors can occur on CN V CN VII and CN X but rarely.

8. Neuroplasticity plays an important role in the disorders of the cranial nerves.

Introduction

Disorders of cranial nerves include paresis and paralysis of motor nerves such as facial palsy, hyperactivity of motor nerves such as hemifacial spasm (HFS) and some vestibular (balance) disorders. Trigeminal and glossopharyngeal neuralgia (TGN and GPN) are disorders of the sensory systems that result in neuralgia, a severe and sharp shooting pain that is perceived in the distribution of a nerve. Disorders of cranial nerves such as HFS, TGN, and GPN are known as "vascular compression disorders" because they can be effectively cured by moving a blood vessel off the respective cranial nerve root (microvascular decompression (MVD) operations [439, 443] [424]).

The pathophysiology of HFS serves as a model of other hyperkinetic disorders. Cyclic oculomotor spasm with paresis and Bell's palsy are other examples of disorders of cranial nerves.

The vestibular system is extremely plastic. Neuroplasticity, therefore, plays an important role for the normal function of vestibular system and neuroplasticity is involved in many of its disorders.

Disorders of cranial sensory nerves

Trauma and diseases that affect cranial nerves produce similar symptoms and signs like that of spinal nerves, but the symptoms of injury from cranial nerves are often more complex than those from injury of spinal nerves.

Neuritis (nerve inflammation) of the vestibular portion of CN VIII produces violent symptoms from the vestibular system consisting of vertigo (the sensation that the world is spinning), vomiting and dizziness. Neuritis of the auditory portion of the CN VIII usually results in deafness that is sometimes accompanied by severe tinnitus.

Sensory cranial nerves can be damaged during neurosurgical operations [440]. The auditory-vestibular nerve is especially vulnerable because approximately 1 cm of this nerve (its total length is approximately 2.5 cm) has central myelin and lacks the supportive tissue found in the peripheral portion of the nerve [654, 656]. Surgically induced injuries to the CN VIII can result in vertigo, tinnitus and hearing loss. The introduction of intraoperative neurophysiologic monitoring has reduced such iatrogenic injuries, most noticeably for the auditory nerve [229, 434, 440] and to a lesser degree the vestibular nerve [604].

Some cranial nerve disorders such as trigeminal neuralgia (TGN) and disabling positional vertigo (DPV) can be treated effectively both by medicine and by surgical operations [462]. The choice between treatments often depends on the specialty to which the patient's physician belongs.

Expression of neuroplasticity is involved in some forms of spasm and synkinesis that are related to cranial motonuclei. There is evidence that expression of neuroplasticity is involved in pain conditions such as TGN glossopharyngeal neuralgia (GPN) and nervus intermedius neuralgia. Other hyperactive disorders in which neuroplasticity plays an important role include some forms of tinnitus.

Disorders of cranial nerves often affect the function of their respective nuclei. Cranial nerves and their nuclei must, therefore, be regarded as single units.

Trigeminal neuralgia

Trigeminal neuralgia (TGN) (also known as tic douloureux) is a typical mononeuropathy. It is a progressive disorder that has been studied extensively, and it is the best-known neuralgia of cranial nerves [195, 711]. TGN occurs with an incidence of 5.9 per 100,000 in women and 3.4 per 100,000 in men (in a white population in the U.S.A) [311]. It is most prevalent in older persons.

TGN seems to occur spontaneously with no known cause. Attacks of TGN involve lacerating pain that is referred to specific areas of the face most commonly to the second and third branches (ophthalmic and maxillary) of the trigeminal nerve that also innervates the mucosa inside the mouth.

TGN usually has distinct trigger points locations on the skin or in the mouth where sensory stimulation such as touch, cold or warmth can provoke an attack. The exact location of the trigger points is specific to the person. The trigger points are well-defined regions of the face or inside the mouth where sensory stimulation by touch or cold can trigger attacks of pain [196]. Eating or exposure to cold winds can often elicit pain attacks. Anesthetizing the trigger point can often relieve the pain. Severe TGN that is not effectively treated may lead to suicide.

TGN is one of only a few pain disorders that are well defined and for which several effective treatments are in use. The pathophysiology of TGN is also better understood than that of many other pain disorders [194-196].

TGN can be treated with a high degree of success with at least three different methods. Pharmacological treatment using carbamazepine, baclofen or gabapentin is highly effective [193] especially in the early phases of the disease. Surgical procedures such as microvascular decompression (MVD) operations of the intracranial portion of CN V [45, 201, 633], partial trigeminal rhizotomy [29, 660] or a glycerol injection in the trigeminal ganglion is also effective. More recently gamma radiation has been used to treat TGN [331].

MVD operations for HFS and TGN have success rates of approximately 85% [44, 45], and a partial section of the trigeminal nerve has a similar success rate. The average recurrence of the pain after these operations is approximately 15 years. Glycerol injection has a similar success rate, but the pain relief lasts a shorter time disease (for an overview of results of treatments see [436, 443]).

Although the neurosurgeon Walter Dandy reported he had seen vessels in close contact with the trigeminal nerve root, he did not develop a treatment based on this principle [443] but continued to perform partial sectioning of the root of CN V to treat TGN.

Gardner [201] was the first to suggest that vascular compression might be involved in the creation of the symptoms of TGN and he and his colleagues demonstrated the effectiveness of MVD procedures for TGN. The treatment of TGN using MVD was popularized by Jannetta [289] (see [443]).

Whether the symptoms of TGN are caused by pathologies of the nerve itself or its root or if the symptoms are caused by abnormal activity of specific populations of neurons in the central nervous system has been a matter of discussion for a long time [67, 149, 201, 202, 204].

The hypothesis that claims that pathology of the nerve root is the cause of the symptoms assumes that ectopic spikes and possibly crosstalk (ephaptic transmission) occur between fibers that have been damaged slightly through close contact with a blood vessel [202, 607].

It has been proposed that the hyperactivity is induced by the irritation of the trigeminal nerve root by a blood vessel causing increased and abnormal activity in the fibers of the sensory part of the trigeminal nerve (portio major). Other investigators have hypothesized that the anatomical location of the pathologies that cause the symptoms of TGN is the central nervous system and it has been postulated that the cause the symptoms of TGN is impaired segmental inhibition in the trigeminal nucleus causing hyperactivity in the trigeminal sensory nucleus.

The fact that TGN can be treated successfully by drugs that have a central action such as carbamazepine (a sodium channel blocker) and baclofen (agonist of the GABAв receptor) is a strong indication of central nervous system involvement in producing the pain.

The hypothesis that decreased segmental inhibition is a factor in generating the pain of TGN is supported by findings from animal studies which have shown that drugs such as carbamazepine (Tegretol) and phenytoin (Dilantin) that are effective in treating TGN affect segmental inhibition [194]. These drugs are sodium channel blockers, but they also have other actions.

The beneficial effect of baclofen is stereospecific and levo-baclofen (-)-baclofen) is at least five times more effective than racemic baclofen in treating patients with TGN [193]. Dextro-baclofen has no known effect on segmental inhibition, and it may be the cause of the side effects of racemic baclofen.

Atypical face pain

Atypical trigeminal neuralgia is a pain condition of the face that is distinctly different from TGN. Atypical face pain [222] is characterized by constant pain that is often poorly localized and without trigger points. It does not respond to the same treatments as TGN and GPN. At the time of diagnosis however atypical face pain is often mistaken to be TGN. Atypical face pain is not treatable through MVD and neuroplasticity may not be directly involved.

Neuralgias of other cranial nerves

The glossopharyngeal nerve (CN IX) is associated with neuralgia (GPN) that leads to pain similar to TGN, but the pain is located in the throat and sides of the neck. GPN is a rare disorder with an unknown incidence rate. GPN can be treated successfully by MVD of the root of CN IX and medically by carbamazepine. Earlier, a section of parts of CN IX was performed to treat the disorder, but MVD of CN IX is effective in relieving the pain [343] [553].

Nervus intermedius (Weisberg's nerve) neuralgia (also known as geniculate neuralgia) is characterized by attacks of sharp pain deep in the ear [370]. It can be successfully treated by moving a blood vessel off the nervus intermedius or by sectioning of some fascicles of the nervus intermedius intracranially (and probably by medical treatment with carbamazepine as well).

Bell's palsy

Bell's palsy usually causes total paralysis of the mimic muscles on one side of the face [561]. Bell's palsy presents with rapidly increasing facial weakness that usually turns into total paralysis within hours.

Bell's palsy has a high rate (95%) of complete or near-complete recovery with or without treatment, but the mimic muscles in some few people remain total paralyzed for the rest of their life.

The etiology of Bell's palsy is not completely known but many authors assume that it is caused by viral inflammation [6]. Other investigators have found evidence that the conduction block in the facial nerve is caused by swelling of the nerve in its bony canal (the Fallopian canal, Figure 12.1).

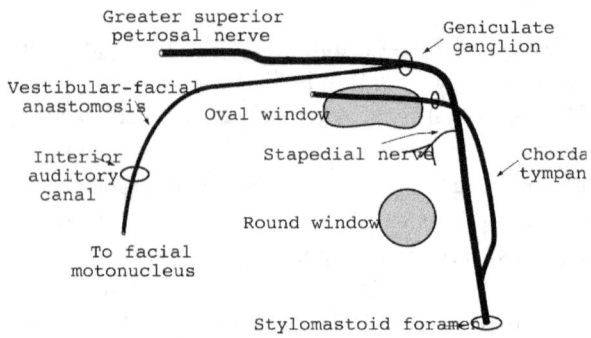

Figure 12.1 Anatomy of the facial nerve.

This hypothesis is supported by the finding that surgical decompression of the nerve is an effective treatment [533, 534]. However, the effectiveness of any treatment for Bell's palsy is difficult to prove because spontaneous recovery is high (approximately 95%). It is now generally accepted that treatment with medications such as steroids is ineffective in changing the natural history of the disease.

Recovery from facial palsy of various kinds is often accompanied by synkinesis. It has been inferred that the "Mona Lisa Smile" (Gioconda smile) may be a result of synkinesis that has developed after trauma [7]). It has been shown recently that facial synkinesis can be reduced (or relieved) by training [77, 570]. This is a strong indication that activation neuroplasticity plays an important role in the cause of the synkinesis of mimic muscles that occurs after recovery from damage to the branches of the facial nerve.

The risk of surgically induced trauma to the facial nerve in connection with surgical operations in the cerebellopontine angle is decreasing because of improved surgical methods such as microneurosurgery and the introduction of intraoperative neurophysiologic monitoring in the beginning of the 1980's [432, 440]. Earlier surgical damage to the intracranial portions of motor nerves such as the facial nerve occurred frequently in operations in the cerebellopontine angle (CPA) such as in operations for vestibular schwannoma.

Other cranial motor nerves such as CN III, IV, VI and XII may be damaged in surgical operations for other skull base tumors.

Such complications have been significantly reduced after the introduction of intraoperative neurophysiologic monitoring [432, 603] as well as by improvements in surgical techniques -- aided by the advent of technologies such as the operating microscope and microneurosurgery [545] and now more recently the use of endoscopes making minimally invasive surgery possible.

The peripheral part of the facial nerve can be injured during surgical operations. Operations on the face such as cosmetic operations (facelift) can cause paralysis because of damage to a branch of the facial nerve, often occurring to the supraorbital branch and in operations for temporomandibular joint (TMJ) disorders.

Ramsay Hunt syndrome type II is caused by Herpes zoster oticus virus. It is another disease causing facial palsy and often hearing loss [561].

Hyperkinetic disorders related to cranial motor nerves

Unilateral hyperactive motor disorders of cranial nerves are hemifacial spasm (HFS), cyclic oculomotor spasm [328] and trigeminal spasm. The treatment of these "vascular compression" disorders is similar to the treatment of TGN. Cyclic oculomotor spasm has similarities with HFS but is affecting the third cranial nerve [439].

Bilateral motor disorders that are related to cranial motor nerves (blepharospasm, spasmodic torticollis, spasmodic dysphonia) are probably disorders of central motor systems such as the basal ganglia; these disorders are discussed below.

Hemifacial Spasm

Hemifacial spasm (HFS) is a rare and progressive disorder that is characterized by periods of spasm of facial mimic muscles on one side of the face [173, 439] [424]. It has an incidence of 0.74 per 100,000 in white men and 0.81 per 100,000 in white women) [33], the onset is relatively late in life. In between attacks, the function of the facial (mimic) musculature has minimal pathological signs. Some people with HFS experience different degrees of synkinesis but only a few experiences facial muscle weakness.

The spasm often begins around one eye and over the years extends to other facial muscles on the same side of the face. After 10 to 20 years the spasm may even involve the platysma; however, the muscles above the eyes are rarely involved (perhaps related to the different innervation of the muscles of the forehead compared with other mimic muscles) [173].

HFS can be cured by moving a blood vessel off the intracranial portion of the facial nerve (MVD operations. The cure rate of such MVD operations is very high, 85-95% [44].

Pathophysiology of HFS

The great success of moving a blood vessel off the root of the facial nerve as treatment of the symptoms of HFS has naturally pointed to the root of the facial nerve as the location for the pathology responsible for the symptoms of HFS. This observation has supported the hypothesis that the symptoms of HFS were caused by ephaptic transmission between denuded facial nerve axons.

However, anatomical studies have shown that a similar location of one or more blood vessels is present in people who do not have the symptoms of HFS. In fact, anatomical studies by several investigators consistently find that similar locations of blood vessels on the root of the facial nerve is present in more than 50% of people who have not had HFS [654].

There is little doubt that the vascular contact with the root of the facial motor nerve is involved but the fact that such vascular contact is common means that another factor must be involved to cause symptoms of HFS. The hypothesis that (at least) two different factors are necessary to cause symptoms of the vascular compression disorders is supported by animal studies.

Two hypotheses about the pathophysiology of HFS have prevailed [431] [443]. One explains the typical signs of HFS namely spasm and synkinesis by assuming that ephaptic transmission occurs between demyelinated (denuded) nerve fibers at the location where a blood vessel is in contact with each other in the facial nerve root [494] [203].

Ephaptic transmission describes direct neural transmission between bare axons. It has been shown to occur for a short period in acutely injured nerves [223], but it is questionable if it plays any important role in persistent neural injuries although some studies support that hypothesis [547]).

Clinical studies of people with HFS have questioned whether ephaptic transmission could cause the symptoms and signs of HFS because it involves most of the facial muscles including the platysma as seen in persons who have had HFS for many years.

It seems unlikely that ephaptic transmission could cause such massive contractions because that would require that almost all facial nerve fibers were denuded and were in close contact with each other.

Intraoperative neurophysiological recordings in operations for HFS of the abnormal muscle contraction have demonstrated that moving such small vessels off the facial nerve causes an immediate cessation of the abnormal muscle contraction (Figure 12.2). In these studies, recordings of the abnormal muscle response were used as a sign of the pathology of HFS.

The other hypothesis of the pathology of HFS is by Ferguson [178] who postulated that the symptoms of HFS can be explained by hyperactivity of the facial motor nucleus.

The abnormal muscle response as an indicator of pathology

People with HFS have an abnormal muscle response (also known as the lateral spread. response) that can be elicited by electrical stimulation of a branch of the facial nerve while the electromyographic (EMG) response is recorded from muscles that are innervated by a different branch of the facial nerve [172, 429]. In people who do not have HFS, such stimulation does not produce any measurable EMG activity in muscles that are innervated by other branches of the facial nerve.

The latency of the initial component of the abnormal muscle response result in a person with HFS is approximately 10 msec (Figure 12.2) The abnormal muscle response is assumed to be caused by backfiring of α-motoneurons in response to antidromic stimulation of the motor nerve. It may thus be similar to the F-response, and it is, therefore, an indication that the excitability of the facial motoneurons is higher than normal.

The initial response to electrical stimulation of a peripheral branch of the facial nerve is followed by EMG potentials that may last several 100 msec. The prolonged response reflects repetitive firings of motoneurons that produce repetitive muscle contractions (spasm). The abnormal muscle response is much less affected by anesthesia than what the blink reflex is. (The abnormal muscle reflex is much less affected by anesthesia than the blink reflex).

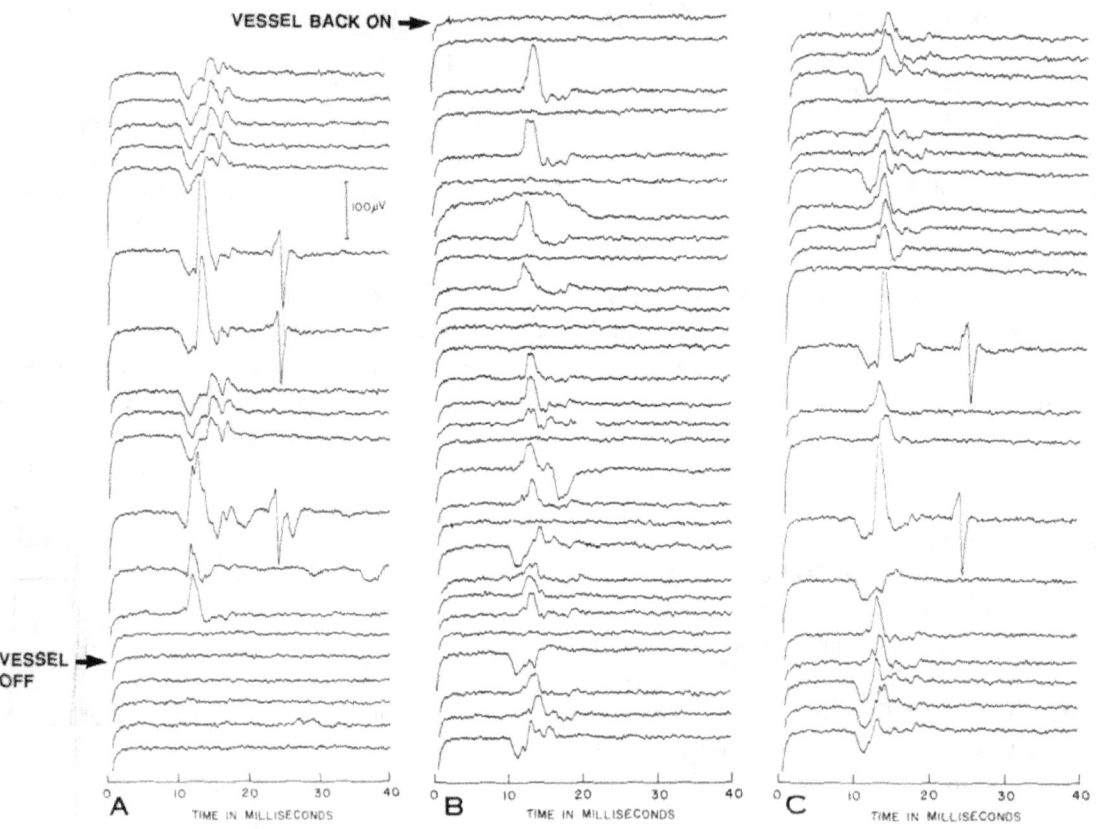

Figure 12.2 Abnormal muscle response recorded from the mentalis muscle in response to electrical stimulation of the zygomatic branch of the facial nerve in a patient undergoing an MVD operation for HFS. Consecutive recordings (beginning at the top of the left column) to stimulation at a rate of 5 pps (From: [427]).

Signs of involvement of the facial motonucleus

Results of intraoperative electrophysiological recordings in patients undergoing MVD operations for HFS have indicated that the anatomical location of the physiological abnormality that causes the crosstalk that is typical for HFS is central to the location of vascular contact [426, 427]. The same intraoperative studies, as well as animal experiments in models of HFS, have supported the hypothesis that the anatomical location of the physiological abnormality is the facial motonucleus.

Experience from MVD operations has shown that a small vessel and even a venula could cause the symptoms of HFS [290].

The fact that the symptoms and signs of HFS can be relieved permanently by moving small arteries (arterioles) or even veins off the facial nerve root (also speaks against the hypothesis that pulsatile force would cause demyelination that could enable subsequent direct communication between bare axons (ephaptic transmission) as would be a prerequisite for the ephaptic transmission.

The fact that moving very small vessels -- including veins - off the facial nerve root can cure HFS even in persons who have extensive contractions of their facial muscles during attacks indicate that the role of blood vessels is not mechanical as was assumed earlier [288].

Intraoperative studies have shown that the existence of an abnormal muscle contraction that is typical for HFS could not be explained by ephaptic transmission at the location of the vascular contact [428] [431]. Only in a single patient did such intraoperative neurophysiologic recordings show signs of the presence of ephaptic transmission.

This phenomenon lasted only a few minutes and it occurred after the facial nerve root had undergone extensive surgical manipulations and appeared to have been injured.

The signs of ephaptic transmission (shortened latency of the abnormal muscle response by approximately 2 msec) were only observed in a single operation out of many hundred operations for HFS where similar intraoperative recordings were made.

The observed of sign of ephaptic transmission between nerve fibers is in good agreement with the early descriptions of ephaptic transmission between injured myelinated nerve fibers in spinal (dorsal) roots) [223] but it cannot explain the symptoms of HFS which lasts long periods [428].

Instead, recordings from other patients showed consistent evidence that the anatomical location of the abnormality that causes the cross talk in people with HFS is central to the location of the vascular contact with the root of the CN VII [429] [441]. These studies thus supported the hypothesis that there are functional abnormalities in the facial motonucleus in people with HFS that include the establishment of connections between populations of motoneurons.

This is consistent with the hypothesis that was originally proposed by Ferguson [178]. These functional connections between neurons that innervate different groups of facial muscles may be a result of the unmasking of dormant synapses which connect motoneurons that give rise to nerve fibers of different branches of the facial nerve.

Animal studies have supported the hypotheses that the signs of HFS (spasm and synkinesis) are caused by abnormalities in the facial motonucleus.

One such animal model of HFS was created by electrical stimulation of the facial nerve according to the kindling paradigm [575, 608]. Repeated electrical stimulation of the facial nerve at the stylomastoid foramen in rats caused the development of an abnormal muscle response that is similar to that which is present in individuals with HFS [608] after approximately four weeks of daily stimulation of the facial nerve.

These findings support the hypothesis that synkinesis of facial muscles can be caused by novel stimulation of the facial nerve that is presumed to cause unmasking of dormant synapses and thereby to facilitate cross-activation of different muscle groups.

The fact that the abnormal muscle response disappears instantaneously during operations for HFS when the offending vessel is moved off the facial nerve (Figure 12.2) indicates that the abnormal activity in the facial nerve caused by the close contact with a blood vessel is necessary to sustain the abnormality in the facial motonucleus.

This suggests that some abnormal neural activity is generated in the facial nerve by the close contact with a blood vessel and that this abnormal activity is necessary to maintain the hyperactivity of the facial motor nucleus.

There is thus considerable evidence that the "vascular compression" of cranial nerves is different from the various forms of entrapment that are known to occur to peripheral nerves. Instead, the close contact between a cranial nerve root and a blood vessel is more likely to exert its effect by irritating the nerve in question and probably activate nerve fibers to produce abnormal firings which then affect the nucleus of the respective cranial nerve.

Anomalies in the blink reflex in HFS

Abnormal crosstalk (synkinesis) that is one of the signs of HFS. It can be demonstrated by recordings of the blink reflex ("lateral spread") [495] as well as from recordings of the abnormal muscle contractions that are typical for people with HFS [172, 429]. The blink reflex response is normally limited to the orbicularis oculi muscles, but in people with HFS, it also includes contractions of other face muscles -- thus a sign of synkinesis [495].

The R1 component of the blink reflex can be recorded during general anesthesia in patients with HFS on the affected side but not on the unaffected side. This indicates that the suppression of the blink reflex that is normally caused by general anesthesia is counteracted by the hyperactivity of facial motoneurons in patients with HFS thus a further indication that the facial motonucleus is hyperactive in individuals with HFS.

The latency of the blink reflex elicited on the affected side during anesthesia is slightly longer than that of the normal blink reflex [430].

(The abnormal muscle reflex is much less affected by anesthesia than the blink reflex).

The mass movements of facial muscles in very young children may also be a result of functional connections between different groups of facial motoneurons by synapses that later become dormant during normal postnatal development.

Treatment of hemifacial spasm

Treatment of HFS using MVD operations has a success rate of about 85% [44] [424]. Using the fact that the abnormal muscle response disappears instantaneously when the offending vessel is moved off the root of the facial nerve in MVD operations for HFS has made monitoring of the abnormal muscle response an important technique that improves the outcome of MVD operations for HFS. Using this technique, it is possible to achieve success rates of the MVD operation for HFS of 97% [433].

Considering the similarities in the pathophysiology of HFS and TGN one would expect that similar medical treatment as is effective in treating TGN (carbamazepine, phenytoin, and Baclofen) would also be effective in treating HFS. These drugs, however, have low if any efficacy in treating HFS [501, 578].

Other treatments of HFS have consisted of the selective severing of the branch of the facial nerve that innervates muscles around the eye [398] (summarized recently by Dobie and Fisch 1986 [156]). Surgically induced damage to the facial nerve in the middle ear has been used as a treatment of HFS [745]. These treatments, however, do not have the same efficacy as MVD and are associated with facial weakness or paresis.

More recently people with HFS have been treated with injections of Botulinum toxin (Botox) in the facial muscles that are affected by the spasm.

After being treated with injections of Botox for some time, subsequent MVD operations have a lower success rate than when done in people who have not been previously treated with botulinum toxin.

Other hyperactive cranial nerve motor disorders

Tic convulsif

Cushing [128] coined the term "tic convulsif" to describe a combination of TGN and HFS. It is a very rare disorder, and there is considerable disagreement about how this disorder should be defined and whether it exists at all. It is possible that the brief facial muscle twitches that often occur in people with TGN in connection with attacks of pain may have been misinterpreted as signs of HFS in some people and that this has been interpreted as a separate disease and named tic convulsif [515]. Some investigators [740] have defined tic convulsif as a combination of HFS and geniculate neuralgia (nervus intermedius neuralgia).

Spasmodic torticollis

Spasmodic torticollis is related to the eleventh cranial nerve and is characterized by involuntary head movements [524]. Spasmodic torticollis occurs in two forms: one that affects the neck muscles bilaterally and one that has a distinct unilateral pattern [281 1676, 576]. The bilateral form may be caused by central nervous system pathology (such as that of the basal ganglia).

Spasmodic torticollis is troublesome because a person with that disorder cannot keep his/her head steady, but most complaints are because of pain from the muscles that are constantly contracting and relaxing. Treatment with MVD has had some success but at a lower rate than the treatment of TGN and HFS [188]. MVD seems to be more successful in the unilateral form than of the bilateral form [485].

Electrophysiological studies performed during MVD operations of patients with unilateral spasmodic torticollis have shown the presence of an abnormal muscle response similar to that which is present in HFS [576] supporting the hypothesis that the unilateral spasmodic torticollis has similarities with HFS.

The bilateral form does not exhibit such abnormal muscle responses indicating that the pathophysiology of the bilateral form of the disorder may be similar to blepharospasm.

Other studies have shown that the suppression of EMG activity in the sternocleidomastoid muscle from electrical stimulation of the supraorbital nerve is lower in people with spasmodic torticollis than in people who do not have spasmodic torticollis [486]. If reduced inhibition is the cause of spasmodic torticollis, then the pathophysiology of this disorder may be similar to other forms of dystonia [54]. These investigators did not, however, differentiate between bilateral and unilateral spasmodic torticollis.

Cyclic oculomotor spasm with paresis

This disorder has similarities with HFS, and it is probably caused by hyperactivity of the third cranial nerve nucleus thus having similar pathophysiology as HFS. Close contact between a blood vessel and a portion of the third cranial nerve seems to be involved [328].

Spasm of mastication muscles

While the blood vessel that is in contact with the sensory root of CN V in people with TGN is often also in close contact with the motor portion (portio minor) of CN V (that innervate the muscles of mastication) spasm of these muscles rarely occurs. Even when the portio minor of CN V is deformed by the close contact with a blood vessel symptoms from the mastication muscles are absent. This supports the hypothesis that the close contact between a cranial nerve root and a blood vessel only creates symptoms and signs when another factor (or factors are) is present.

Bilateral cranial motor nerve disorders

Unlike hemifacial spasm which is unilateral blepharospasm is characterized by involuntary bilateral muscle contractions and is usually centered around the eyes causing forceful eye closure. It is a serious encumbrance to normal life and prevents the driving an automobile. Since it is bilateral, it is assumed to involve supranuclear structures and probably involves the basal ganglia. Blepharospasm occurs mostly in elderly persons.

Spasmodic dysphonia

Spasmodic dysphonia is caused by a dysfunction of the larynx that can affect adductor and abductor muscles or the vocal cords the former being the most common [674, 713]. Spasmodic dysphonia is related to CN X but since the vocal cords are affected bilaterally the anatomical location of the physiologic abnormalities that cause the spasm is probably central to the motonucleus of CN X. Little is known about its pathophysiology, but it likely has central cause such as dysfunction of the basal ganglia [674, 713].

Disorders of the vestibular system (balance disorders)

Some vestibular disorders are associated with vertigo and nausea initiated by head movements [40, 463] while others produce similar symptoms that occur spontaneously without body movements. Vestibular disorders especially those that are caused by disorders of the vestibular nerve may cause autonomic reactions such as vomiting. Balance disorders especially vertigo can cause falls which may result in serious trauma including head trauma and death. Vestibular disorders may, therefore, be regarded life-threatening disorders.

Vestibular disorders can have a variety of causes; anomalies in the vestibular apparatus of the inner ear, malfunctions of the vestibular portion of the CN VIII and by neuroplastic re-organization of the central nervous system. The best-known vestibular apparatus disorders are

When head movements are felt it is a sign that information from the balance organ in the inner ear has been re-directed to parts of the central nervous system other than those that normally receive such information. Symptoms from the vestibular system are related to plastic changes within the nervous system. This occurs typically as a result of intoxication such as from excessive intake of alcohol.

Loss of function of the vestibular organ in the inner ear or the vestibular nerve has a very different effect depending on how fast the changes in function occurs. Slow changes can occur without any noticeable symptoms whereas sudden changes such as occurs as a result of vestibular neuritis causes violent symptoms. Vestibular neuritis is a common cause of severe vestibular symptoms.

Most people who have lost the normal function of their vestibular system in childhood or as teenagers recover completely within a few months people in their 30s or 40s may need many months, to recover and people older than 50 years most often nerve recover completely from damage to their vestibular system and will have remaining deficits for the rest of their lives.

Even in healthy persons, excessive head movements activate the vestibular organ and subsequently the vestibular nervous system is activated and that may cause symptoms such as vertigo and vomiting. Seasickness is an example of that. The symptoms normally abate when the movements are stopped.

It is interesting to consider how vomiting in response to head movements have developed. Vomiting, nausea, and vertigo in response to abnormal head motion do not seem to be of any benefit to the organism.

Vestibular system symptoms may also be generated through incompatibility between the input from vision and body proprioceptors with that from the vestibular system. Space sickness which has achieved much attention since the beginning of space travel is another pathologic reaction to abnormal motions that generate output from the vestibular organ that is incompatible with the output of other proprioceptive and visual systems.

Abnormal eye movements (nystagmus) often present with disorders of the vestibular system either spontaneously or evoked by head movements.

Benign paroxysmal positional vertigo

The most common vestibular disorder is benign paroxysmal positional vertigo (BPPV) a non-progressive self-limiting disorder characterized by nystagmus and episodes of vertigo elicited by head movements. BPPV sometimes known as benign paroxysmal positional nystagmus (BPPN) [40] accounts for 20% of all incidences of balance symptoms. Like many other diseases of sensory organs, the incidence of BPPV increases with age [192]. In older people, however, it is the most common vestibular disorder accounting for half of the vestibular disorders. The most common cause of BPPV in people under the age of 50 is from head injury, but BPPV is also associated with a migraine [280].

Specific head movement exercise (Epley maneuver [509]) has been used successfully to treat BPPV [79].

Contemporary theories about the pathophysiology of BPPV suggest that it is caused by a mechanical disorder of the vestibular organ that stimulates the receptors in an abnormal way in response to head movements. Basophilic deposits in the posterior semicircular canal are supposed to cause the anomalies. The novel output of the vestibular organ that reaches higher central nervous system centers is assumed to cause the symptoms of BPPV. The Epley maneuver is supposed to be beneficial by the flinging of statoconia that have become stuck on the receptor in the utricle and saccule. The success of treatment that makes use of head movements (the Epley maneuver [509]) supports the hypothesis that the symptoms are caused by abnormalities in the vestibular apparatus in the inner ear.

It is possible that such abnormal activity can cause abnormal neural activity in the vestibular nerve and that this abnormality can open synapses that are normally dormant (unmasking of ineffective synapses) in the vestibular nuclei and thereby establish connections to brain regions that normally do not receive information from the vestibular organ. However, there are many vestibular disorders that are diagnosed as BPPV but which have no known cause. Some incidences of BPPV may be caused by virus, strokes and in connection with Ménière's disease.

Disabling positional vertigo

Disabling positional vertigo (DPV) is characterized by constant vertigo and nausea that are worsened by head movements [464]. DPV is a progressive and often incapacitating disorder [465, 467] [462]. People with DPV experience discomfort from any head movement and they often spend most of their time in bed because this is the body position in which they feel is the least uncomfortable [463].

The disorder can be treated successfully by MVD of the vestibular nerve root [291], and the success rate is 77% for men and 80% for women [467] thus slightly lower than that of HFS and TGN. It is believed that symptoms that can be alleviated by moving a blood vessel off the vestibular nerve root (DPV) are in fact caused by the reorganization of the central vestibular nervous system through activation of neuroplasticity.

Nystagmus

Since the vestibular system controls the position of the eyes through the vestibular ocular reflex (VOR) disturbances in vestibular function can cause abnormal involuntary movements of the eyes known as nystagmus. Nystagmus occurring spontaneously in response to head movements is an important clinical sign of vestibular disturbances.

Electronystagmography (ENG) recording of eye movements is used to test disturbances in vestibular function. Some people have spontaneous nystagmus since birth yet perfectly normal vision – again a sign of the remarkable adaptability of the nervous system.

Tumors of cranial nerves

Vestibular schwannoma are slow-growing benign tumors [49, 110]. Vestibular schwannoma were earlier known as acoustic tumors and are the most frequently occurring and best-known tumor of the cranial nerves. (The reason for the name acoustic tumor was that the most pronounced symptoms and signs arose from the auditory system).

Vestibular schwannoma have been assumed to begin to grow from the Oberstiener-Redlich zone (glial margin), but recent studies have shown that some tumors begin to grow from sites of CN VIII that are peripheral to the Oberstiener-Redlich zone (see the chapter on peripheral nerves) [734].

When it became clear that these tumors most frequently grow from the (superior) vestibular nerves and the fact that these tumors are the result of excessive growth of Schwann cells attempts were made to change the name to vestibular schwannoma. Nonetheless, adoption of the changed name has been slow.

Vestibular schwannoma that is diagnosed has been shown to occur with an incidence of approximately 1 in 100,000, but autopsies show an incidence of 2.4% (sic) [49] indicating that the occurrence of asymptomatic vestibular schwannoma is fairly common. Investigators agree that most of the small tumors that are detected by imaging methods are slow growing; many are stable, and some even regress over time [110, 625]. This information is important for treatment because it has been the routine to treat acoustic tumors surgically whenever detected. The findings that tumors, in fact, may decrease in size and many cases pose no health threat have hopefully changed the approach to treatment [263]. The risks of complications in such operations have also been re-evaluated [445, 497].

Asymmetric hearing loss, vestibular symptoms, elevated threshold, poor growth of the acoustic middle ear reflex response and abnormal auditory brainstem responses are all important signs and symptoms of a vestibular schwannoma.

The tinnitus may increase after surgical removal of vestibular schwannoma. Patients with small tumors who are operated while they still have vestibular function may experience vestibular symptoms after tumor removal because of the surgical destruction of the vestibular nerve.

APPENDIXES

Appendix A

Anatomy and Physiology of Nerves

Abstract

1. Nerves are classified in according to the diameter of their axons, in three groups of myelinated fibers: Aα Aβ, Aδ, and one group of unmyelinated fibers (C fibers): The Aα being the largest and fastest conducting fibers and the C fibers being the slowest conducting fibers.

2. The kind of myelin that covers myelinated nerves changes just before the nerves enter the central nervous system from peripheral myelin that is generated by Schwann cells, to central myelin that is generated by oligodendrocytes. The transition zone (known as the Obersteiner-Redlich zone) is located at a small distance from the central nervous system. The length of the central part varies among nerves.

3. Most nerves are mixed nerves, containing sensory (including proprioceptive and pain) fibers, and motor and autonomic fibers. In the spinal cord, sensory fibers enter the spinal cord as dorsal roots, while motor fibers exit the spinal cord as ventral roots.

Introduction

Spinal nerves originate or terminate in the spinal cord, while cranial nerves originate or terminate in the brainstem or cerebrum. Many spinal and cranial nerves are mixed nerves. Most nerves contain somatic motor fibers, sensory nerve fibers, proprioceptive fibers and pain fibers. Some nerves contain visceral and autonomic nerve fibers. Sensory and motor fibers are mostly myelinated, while some fibers that carry pain signals and those that belong to the autonomic nervous system are unmyelinated. It is common to divide myelinated fibers into three groups according to the diameter of their axons: Aα, Aβ, and Aδ. Unmyelinated fibers are C- fibers.

Nerves from the periphery enter the spinal cord as dorsal roots while nerves to the periphery exit the spinal cord as ventral roots. The ventral roots mostly consist of motor fibers, while the dorsal roots consist of fibers that innervate sensory receptors (including pain fibers and fibers that innervate proprioceptors). Some dorsal roots also contain fibers of the autonomic nervous system.

Conduction velocity in nerve fibers

The conduction velocity of myelinated nerve fibers is proportional to the axon diameters. Unmyelinated nerve fibers have a much lower conduction velocity than any myelinated fibers.

Motor nerves, primary muscle-spindle afferents (Aα) have conduction velocities ranging from 70 to 120 m/sec, and average axon diameters of 15 μm. Afferent sensory nerve fibers (Aβ) have conduction velocities from 30 to 70 m/sec and average axon diameters of 8 μm. The smallest myelinated nerve fibers (Aδ) conduct at 12-30m/sec and have average axon diameters of less than <3 μm. Pain afferents and sympathetic postganglionic fibers (Unmyelinated) have conduction velocities of 0.5-2 m/sec and diameters of approximately 1 μm.

The central portions of nerves are different from the peripheral portions in several ways. The myelin of the central portion of nerves is generated by oligodendrocytes while the myelin of the peripheral portion is generated by Schwann cells. The peripheral and the central parts of nerves differ by the type of myelination. The transition zone between the peripheral and the central part of nerves occurs near their entry to the central nervous system, where the myelin changes from Schwann cell generated myelin to oligodendrocyte cell generated myelin in the central part. This transition zone is known as the Obersteiner-Redlich zone.

The support structure of the peripheral portion of nerves is also different from that of the central portion. Each axon of the peripheral portion of nerves is covered by endoneurium to form nerve fibers. Nerve fibers are organized in fascicles (bundles) that are covered by a sheath of perineurium (Figure A.1).

The peripheral portion of nerves may consist of a single funiculus or can be composed of several funiculi (bundles) that are covered by perineurium. Epineurium covers nerve trunks.

Funiculi in the peripheral portion of nerves have an undulated course (Figure A.2) that allows the nerves to be stretched without inducing stress on the individual nerve fibers. A traction that exceeds the stretched length of a nerve will cause the typical injuries seen in traumatic nerve injuries [656].

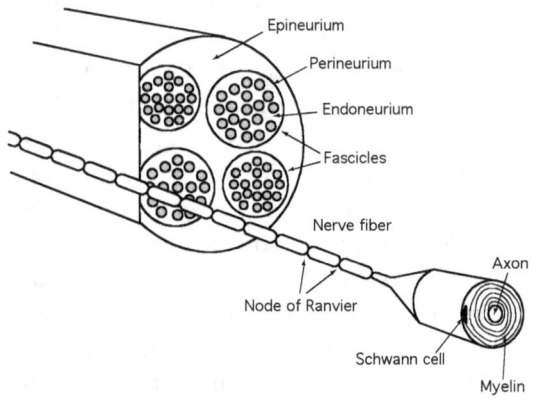

Figure A.1 Anatomy of a typical peripheral portion of a nerve [656].

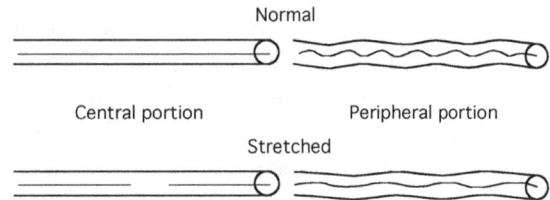

Figure A.2 Effect of traction and injury on the central and the peripheral portion of a nerve [656].

The endoneurium consists of collagen fibrils, and those in the central portion of a nerve are finer than those than in the peripheral portion.

Perineurium and epineurium are also absent in the central portion of nerves, making the central portion of nerves more vulnerable to mechanical stress.

The central part of nerves, therefore, lacks some of the protection that peripheral portions have, and as a result, the central segments of nerves are more fragile than their peripheral counterparts.

Also, the central portion of nerves lacks a funicular support structure and proceeds in parallel without the undulations of the peripheral portion of nerves (Figure A.2. This means that the central portion of nerves is more fragile with regards to stretching.

The Oberstiener-Redlich zone where the transition between the peripheral and central portions takes place is important because it is the anatomical location of pathologies such as tumors (Schwannoma). This transition zone has been studied especially about the cranial nerves where it has been shown to be sensitive to irritation from, for example, blood vessels.

Sensory nerves

Sensory fibers from the periphery are bipolar, with their cell bodies located in the dorsal root ganglia (DRG). Nerve fibers of different diameters make synaptic contact with cells in different layers of the dorsal horns. Sensory nerves from the periphery enter the dorsal horn of the spinal cord as dorsal root fibers, where they travel together with fibers that innervate pain receptors (nociceptors), proprioceptors and autonomic fibers. Low threshold cutaneous receptors are innervated by $A\beta$ fibers (6-12 μm diameter), and such fibers have conduction velocities in the range of 30-70 m/sec (Table A.1). $A\beta$ fibers terminate in lamina III-V (Rexed's classification [552]).

Proprioceptive fibers from muscle spindles and tendon organs and receptors monitoring joint movements are large ($A\alpha$) fibers. Fibers carrying pain information are small caliber myelinated fibers ($A\delta$) and unmyelinated fibers (C fibers). The $A\delta$ fibers enter laminae I, IV and V, and C fibers enter lamina II of the dorsal horn [83]. Proprioceptive fibers terminate in lamina VI.

Motor nerves

Motor fibers leave the spinal cord as ventral spinal roots, where some fibers innervate skeletal muscles (extrafusal muscles) while other fibers innervate muscle spindles (intrafusal muscles). The motor nerve fibers are larger than sensory fibers belonging mostly to the Aα group of nerve fibers.

The cell bodies (α motoneurons) of axons that innervate skeletal muscles are located in lamina IX of the ventral horn of the spinal cord. The cell bodies of the nerve fibers that innervate the intrafusal muscle (γ fibers) are also located in lamina IX of the ventral horn of the spinal cord.

Autonomic nerves

Many nerve tracts include fibers that lead to and from the autonomic nervous system. Efferent preganglionic sympathetic innervation originates in neurons in the inter mediolateral column of the lower thoracic and upper lumbar segments of the spinal cord [83]. These preganglionic fibers leave the spinal cord as ventral roots and connect, through sympathetic cells in the sympathetic trunk, to effector organs.

The fibers of nerves of the autonomic nervous system are mostly unmyelinated (C fibers) or myelinated fibers of small diameter (Aδ fibers) and enter the spinal cord through dorsal roots. From the dorsal roots, they make contact with cells in the dorsal-most parts of the dorsal horn with their cell bodies being in the DRG. Dorsal roots that enter the spinal cord at T_{11} and L_4, therefore, contain sympathetic fibers from the body.

Parasympathetic innervation of organs in the body

Parasympathetic efferents and afferents that innervate organs in the abdomen, the lungs and the hear originate in the vagus nerve. Parasympathetic efferents that innervate the bladder and some genital organs originate in the dorsal roots of the S_3 and S_4 segments of the spinal cord. The afferent sympathetic innervation of viscera (visceral afferents) in the abdomen forms the greater and lesser splanchnic nerves.

Afferent sympathetic nerve fibers that innervate the lower body pass uninterrupted through the sympathetic trunk enter the spinal cord at T_{11}-L_4 levels through dorsal roots and terminate in the dorsal-most part of the spinal cord while the vagus nerve (CN X) provides most of the parasympathetic innervation of a visceral organ. Afferents from visceral nociceptors follow sympathetic nerves, while autonomic afferents from other receptors tend to follow parasympathetic nerves [83]. This, however, would indicate that the vagus nerve does not carry nociceptor afferents – an implication which is contradicted by the finding that vagal stimulation has been shown to affect nociception [56].

Sympathetic innervation of the head involves the superior cervical ganglion, the fibers of which follow the internal carotid artery to innervate the dura and some large intracranial arteries.

Pathology of nerves

Many studies have shown that nerve injury, neuroma formation, and nerve fiber degeneration can cause spontaneous discharges in nerve fibers proximal to the injury level [698]. Such pathologies may cause pain because the generated neural activity is interpreted in the same way as the activity that is caused by stimulation of nociceptors.

Viral infection (Herpes)

The herpes zoster virus can reside dormant in the ganglia of sensory nerves without producing any symptoms, but occasionally it may cause pain and eruption of vesicles on the skin over some part of one, or more than one, dermatome. The pain is severe and may persist for a long time after the vesicular rash fades. Immediate treatment with antiviral agents such as Acyclovir or Famvir helps reduce the duration of the rash and the incidence of subsequent chronic pain. Herpes zoster oticus involves the eighth cranial nerve and is known as the Ramsey-Hunt syndrome. Herpes simplex is the cause of blisters and sores most common to occur around the mouth, nose, and genitals.

Appendix B

General Organization and Function of Sensory Systems

Abstract

1. Sensory systems can be divided into four separate anatomical structures, namely those that conduct the stimulus to the receptors, the sensory receptors, the sensory nerves, and the central sensory nervous system.

2. Structures that conduct physical stimuli to the receptors can attenuate or amplify specific properties of the stimuli and modify the stimuli that reach the sensory organs. The most extensive modifications of sensory stimuli by the medium that conducts the stimulus to the receptors occur in the cochlea.

3. Sensory receptors can be subdivided into two groups. One consists of an extension of the afferent axon where the membrane is specialized to respond to a specific stimulus. The other type consists of separate receptor cells, the output of which is conducted through a synaptic contact with either the afferent sensory axon (cochlear hair cells and taste receptors) or a network of neurons (the retina and olfactory organ).

4. Functionally, sensory receptors can be divided into two main groups: one consists of receptors that respond to innocuous stimuli (such as mechanoreceptors in the skin, sensory cells in the ear, nose, and eye), and the other group consists of receptors that respond to noxious stimuli (nociceptors such as chemical and heat receptors).

5. Outer hair cells in the cochlea constitute the third group of sensory cells, which have an active micromechanical role in conducting the stimulus to the receptors (the inner hair cells) that convert the stimulus into a neural code. The outer hair cells do not participate in transducing the stimulus into a neural code and may be regarded as being a part of the conductive apparatus of the ear.

6. The output of sensory receptors in olfaction and vision is processed locally in the sense organs before being coded in the fibers of their respective nerves (cranial nerve I for olfaction and cranial nerve II for vision).

7. Pain is usually not regarded as a sense. Pain receptors (nociceptors) are similar to somatosensory receptors but mediate sensation of pain from the body and internal organs.

8. The sensory pathways for hearing, vision, taste, and somesthesia have many similarities in that they consist of an ascending and a descending path.

9. Sensory nerves of somesthesia, hearing, and taste consist of bipolar nerve fibers that enter the spinal cord as dorsal roots, as the root of the sensory part of cranial nerve V, and the roots of cranial nerves VIII and VII for hearing and taste respectively.

10. There are two parts of sensory pathways, the classical and the non-classical pathways (also known as the lemniscal and extra-lemniscal pathways).

11. The sensory nervous system for olfaction is different from that of hearing, vision, taste, and somesthesia. The nervous systems of these four senses have many similarities.

12. All fibers of the classical ascending pathways are interrupted by synaptic contacts with cells in the ventral portion of the thalamus, the cells of which project uninterrupted by cells in the primary sensory cortices.

13. The non-classical ascending pathways are interrupted by synaptic contact with cells in the dorsal and medical thalamus. The cells of this part of the thalamus bypass the primary cortices and project to cells in secondary sensory and association cortices, and to cells in several subcortical structures such as the lateral nucleus of the amygdala.

14. Cells in the nuclei of the classical pathways respond distinctly to specific sensory stimuli, while neurons in the nuclei of the non-classical pathways respond to a broad range of stimuli and integrate information on wider spatial scales than the classical pathways.

15. Parallel processing implies that the same information is processed in different structures. Stream segregation implies that different types of information, for example, spatial ("where") and object ("what") information are processed in anatomically different parts of the sensory nervous system.

16. Descending sensory pathways are abundant particular along the cortico-thalamic pathways. Some of these descending pathways typically extend caudally as far as the receptors themselves. It may be more appropriate to regard the descending pathways as being reciprocal to the ascending pathways than to regard these two systems as separate.

Introduction

The five sensory systems, hearing, vision, tactile (somatosensory), olfaction, and taste provide conscious perceptions of physical stimuli from the environment. In addition to these five senses, temperature receptors in the skin and the mouth mediate the sensations of warmth and cool and nociceptor pain. These senses, together with motor systems, serve the purpose of communications between an organism and the environment. In fact, all input that the central nervous system (CNS) receives from the environment comes through sensory systems.

Sensory systems consist of:
   a. the media that conduct the physical stimuli to the receptors
   b. sensory receptors
   c. sensory nerves
   d. structures of the central nervous system that respond to sensory stimuli

We will discuss three of the five principle sensory systems (somesthesia, hearing, and vision) first and then briefly cover some aspects of gustation and olfaction because few disorders are associated with these two senses, and little is known about the role of plasticity in these two sensory systems. The signals from the receptors are processed in the central nervous system, and this extensive processing is determined by genetics and by plastic changes of the function of the neural networks involved.

Neuroplasticity that is controlled by environmental and internal sensory signals interacting with innate programming is essential for normal sensory function. Neuroplasticity is most influential early in life, but plastic changes can occur at all ages [334].

The vestibular system, which monitors head movements, and the proprioceptive systems, which monitor motor activity, may be regarded as extensions of the sensory systems, but many authors consider them to belong to the motor system. The balance system and proprioception, together with vision and somesthesia, contribute to our perception of our body position.

Proprioceptive somatosensory systems, the receptors for which are found in muscles, tendons, and joints, monitor the motor systems and other bodily functions.

This Appendix also includes discussions of the afferent portion of the vagus nerve because of its important role of carrying sensory information from organs in the abdomen and the chest. The sensory information transmitted through the vagus nerve influences the cholinergic system of the brain and can modulate neuroplasticity and influence immune function. The vagus nerve has come into recent focus because electrical stimulation of the vagus nerve has been shown to be beneficial in the management of chronic neuropathic pain, depression, and severe tinnitus.

Sensory organs

Sensory organs consist of the receptors and the media that conduct sensory stimuli to the receptors. Auditory, visual, and olfactory receptor cells are located in special sensory organs that also contain a medium to conduct the physical stimulus to those receptors. Also, the eye contains some of the neural structures that process visual stimuli. The conductive structures in the auditory system are more complex than that of other sensory organs (for details see [460]).

Media that conduct the stimuli to the receptors

The media that conduct the physical stimulus to the receptors can modify the stimulus, attenuate it or enhancing it.

The ear

In hearing, the structures that conduct sound to the sensory receptors are complex, consisting of the middle ear that acts as an impedance matching device that improves sound transmission to the cochlea [460]. The media that conduct stimuli to the receptors in the ear are the sites of frequent causes of disorders.

The middle ear improves sound conduction to the fluid-filled cochlea by approximately 30 dB, and it provides a large difference between the forces that act on the two windows of the cochlea (round and oval windows). This difference causes the cochlear fluid to move and thus, provides the basis for activating the sensory cells of the cochlea. The acoustic middle ear reflex provides some amplitude compression [460].

Many of the disorders of the auditory system are related to the middle ear and the cochlea, with disorders of the middle ear being the only ones that can be successfully treated via surgical or pharmacological means. The cochlea separates sound according to their frequency (the cochlea performs spectral filtering), and it is regarded as a part of the conductive apparatus that leads the sound to the sensory cells (hair cells).

The eye

The structures that conduct light to the visual receptors provide the ability to focus an image on the retina (at least in young individuals) and some intensity compression through the action of the pupil. Tactile information is conducted through the skin that functions as a relatively simple mechanical system, but some receptors, i.e., the Pacinian corpuscles, have a more complex mechanical structure that filters the stimuli with regards to their frequency. (For more details, see [460]).

Receptors

Sensory receptors convert physical stimuli into a neural code. The receptors can be divided into two groups based on their morphology. One group consists of transformed axons, the membranes of which are specialized to sense specific mechanical stimuli. These transformed axons still function as regular axons and transmit their signals to the appropriate sensory nerves.

Mechanoreceptors in the skin belong to this type of receptor. The other type of sensory receptor cell is more complex and consists of a complete cell to which the afferent axon connects via synapses or synapse-like structures. Such receptor cells are found in the ear and the eye. (Taste and olfactory receptors also belong to this type of receptor). Protuberances on the receptor cell, such as the stereocilia of the hair cells in the cochlea or the outer segments of visual receptor cells, are sensitive to a specific physical stimulus. Visual receptors have an elaborate structure with discs that contain a light-sensitive substance. These receptor cells connect to a complex neural network in the retina, the last stage of which are ganglion cells that give rise to the axons of the optic nerve.

Auditory receptors are located along a structure in the cochlea known as the basilar membrane, which winnows sounds according to frequency. There are the two types of auditory receptor cells (inner and outer hair cells), which have completely different functions. Only the inner hair cells convert sound into a neural code, whereas the outer hair cells have a mechanical function that makes them work as "motors" that amplify the motion of the basilar membrane, increasing the sensitivity by approximately 50 dB. (This means that loss of function of outer hair cells causes hearing loss of approximately 50dB).

This action of outer hair cells may also be regarded as a part of the conductive apparatus. The action of the outer hair cells is non-linear, and their effect on the motion of the basilar membrane is greatest at low sound intensities. This process as well as the other compression process initiated by the stapedius reflex allows sounds within a large range of intensities to be coded in the discharge pattern of auditory nerve fibers that have a narrow dynamic range (For details, see [460]).

Both types of hair cells receive inhibitory input from the central nervous system but in different ways. The efferent fibers from the central nervous system terminate on the cell bodies of outer hair cells through a synapse, while most efferent fibers that target the inner hair cells terminate on the afferent dendrites that become the axons of the afferent nerve [646].

Since the outer hairs are an integral part of the mechanical system of the cochlea, the efferent innervation of outer hair cells makes it possible for signals from the central nervous system to affect the mechanical properties of the cochlea.

The outer hair cells are more vulnerable to insult than inner hair cells. Thus, noise exposure and ototoxic substances affect outer hair cells and often leave inner hair cells intact. This is the reason that hearing loss more than 50 dB is rare. A cochlear hearing loss is often accompanied by changes in the central nervous system, adding hearing loss and difficulties in the understanding of speech [721]. Exposure to sounds (augmented auditory environment) can also reduce age-related hearing loss [721].

Sensory nerves

Sensory nerve fibers travel in both cranial and peripheral nerves. The sensory nerves enter the central nervous system and make synaptic contact with target cells in the gray matter of the spinal cord for pain and the sensory nuclei of the brainstem and thalamus for vision. The axons that innervate receptors in the skin, muscles, joints, and tendons are bipolar cells that enter the spinal cord as dorsal roots, with their cell bodies located in the dorsal root ganglia. These axons travel in the dorsal column of the spinal cord to reach cells in the dorsal column nuclei in the medulla.

Before reaching this point, these axons give rise to collateral axons that terminate on cells in the dorsal horn of the segment where the axons enter, as well as in other segments of the spinal cord.

Sensory nerves of the face are also bipolar, and most belong to the sensory trigeminal nerve (portio major of CNV), the axons of which enter the pons and terminate on cells in the sensory part of the trigeminal nucleus. Some nerve fibers that innervate receptors of the face travel in the glossopharyngeal and vagus nerves but also terminate in the trigeminal nucleus.

CNII and CNVIII are purely sensory nerves, innervating visual and auditory-vestibular sensory organs, respectively. The axons of the optic nerve terminate in cells in the visual portion of the thalamus (the lateral geniculate nucleus, LGN). Auditory nerve fibers form collaterals that terminate in all three divisions of the cochlear nucleus. The cell bodies of the auditory nerve fibers are located in the spiral ganglion.

The axons that innervate the vestibular organ have their cell bodies in Scarpa's ganglion, and the axons terminate on cells in the vestibular nucleus.

All sensory nerves except the olfactory and the optic nerves terminate in nuclei that are ipsilateral to the sensory organs. The axons that innervate the sensory cells in the eye terminate in a network of neurons within the retina that gives rise to the optic nerve, the axons of which make synaptic contact with cells in the LGN.

In humans, approximately half of the axons terminate on cells in the ipsilateral LGN. The other half makes contact with cells in the LGN on the contralateral side. The nerve fibers of taste receptors travel in portions of cranial nerves VII, IX, and X, and terminate on cells in the nucleus of the solitary tract (NST). The nerve fibers of the olfactory nerve terminate in the olfactory bulb, the morphology of which is similar to that of the retina.

Neural pathways

Sensory neural pathways consist of ascending and descending pathways. Much more is known about the ascending pathways than the descending pathways. Ascending sensory pathways connect sensory organs with specific regions of the cerebral neocortex through a series of nuclei arranged hierarchically. The number of such nuclei is different for different sensory systems.

All sensory information, except olfaction, is relayed to the thalamus. Descending pathways connect cells of the cerebral cortex to various nuclei of the ascending pathways, and in some systems, even connect to the respective sensory receptors.

Some descending pathways originate from subcortical nuclei. Descending pathways are, for the most part, reciprocal to ascending pathways and may form loops in which information can circulate. That may be one of the bases for iterative interpretation of sensory information.

In general, the olfaction differs from the other sensory system, and the pathways of the somatosensory system differ from those of the auditory, gustatory, and visual pathways. As the somatosensory system also involves pain, we will discuss the somatosensory system separately (for more details about sensory pathways, see [460]).

Ascending sensory pathways

For hearing, gustation, and somesthesia, the first nucleus to receive input from the sensory organ, is located ipsilateral to the sensory organ but most of the axons of the cells of the nuclei cross the midline to make connections with other nuclei. In the auditory system, there are many connections between the ascending pathways of the two sides at most levels, including the cochlear nucleus but not the thalamus [460]. This cross communication allows input from one ear to reach thalamic nuclei on both sides in almost equal quantities, providing a bilateral representation of a sound that reaches one ear only.

Both the thalamus and the cerebral cortices are, thereby, always activated bilaterally. In the visual system, a neural network in the retina performs the first stage of information processing of visual inputs that is similar to that of the first nuclei of the auditory and somatosensory pathways.

The human optic nerve projects to the thalamic visual nuclei (lateral geniculate nucleus, LGN) bilaterally. Olfaction is different from all other sensory systems, and the olfactory bulb may be regarded as the first nucleus. Anatomically, the olfactory bulb has similarities with the neural network of the retina.

The axons of the cells in the dorsal column nuclei form the medial lemniscus, cross to the opposite side, and terminate on cells in the ventral thalamus (ventral posterior lateral nuclei, VPL).

The axons from the neurons of the trigeminal nucleus ascend in the medial lemniscus together with those from the dorsal column nuclei.

The fibers of the medial lemniscus enter the thalamic nuclei that are involved in somesthesia (the ventrobasal nuclei, VB); the ventral posterior medial (VPM) nucleus for the face region, and the VPL for the body. The fibers of the medial lemniscus have many types of collateral fibers that terminate on neurons of the brainstem reticular formation.

Two different ascending pathways

The fact that at least two parallel tracts of ascending sensory pathways project to the sensory cortices have been known for a long time [189, 199, 225]. These tracts have been variously named and defined by different investigators.

The two main sensory tracts that originate in the dorsal and the ventral portion of the thalamus respectively have been referred to as the lemniscal and the extralemniscal pathways [10], the specific and non-specific pathways [83] [460]}, and as the classical and non-classical pathways. This dichotomy is most relevant for the auditory, visual, and taste systems.

The auditory and visual systems have the most complex classical ascending sensory pathways. The fibers of the ascending sensory pathways have many types of collateral capable of making connections to and receiving input from many sensory nuclei cells at once, facts that usually are not apparent from the traditionally simplified drawings of ascending pathways. There are many connections between the two sides of the auditory pathways, but similar connections are absent in vision and the somatosensory systems.

The classical pathways are also known as the "slow and accurate" pathways, and the non-classical pathways are known as the "fast and dirty" pathways. The main distinction between the pathways occurs in the thalamus where the classical pathways use the ventral part of the thalamic sensory nuclei whereas the non-classical pathways use the dorsal-medial portions of these nuclei. The non-classical pathways bypass the primary sensory cortices.

Of the two different ascending pathways in the somatosensory system, one carries innocuous sensations, and one carries noxious (painful) information.

The one that carries innocuous information (touch, vibration, etc.), corresponds to the classical pathways, and the one that carries noxious information makes use of mainly the dorsal and medial thalamic nuclei and thus resembles the non-classical pathways. Noxious information can also reach the ventral thalamus and thereby, reach the primary cerebral sensory cortex.

Classical pathways

Most neurophysiologic studies of the sensory systems have concerned the classical sensory systems; only a few studies have concerned the functional involvement of the non-classical pathways [10], and only a small percentage of these have been performed in humans [446]. Incomplete knowledge of the anatomy of the non-classical pathways has hampered understanding of both their normal and pathological function.

Hearing

Auditory information enters the brainstem through the auditory nerve (part of CN VIII). Axons bifurcate twice, and each one of the axons of the resulting three branches makes synaptic contact with neurons in separate divisions of the cochlear nucleus (anterior ventral cochlear nucleus, AVCN, posterior ventral cochlear nuclei, PVCN, and dorsal cochlear nucleus, DCN) [460] (Figure B.1).

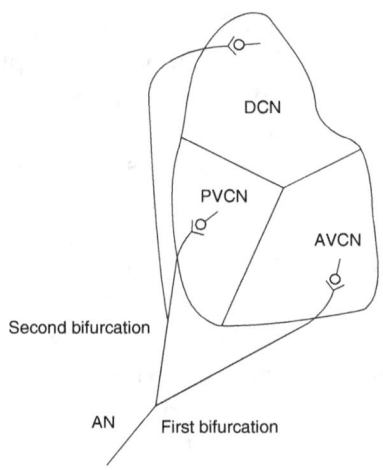

Figure B.1 Schematic of the cochlear nucleus showing the two bifurcations of an individual auditory nerve fiber that makes one nerve fiber innervate neurons in all three major divisions of the cochlear nucleus. (Artwork by Monica Javidnia).

Some of the axons of the cochlear nucleus cells are interrupted by synaptic connections in cells in the nuclei of the superior olivary complex (SOC), and some collateral fibers of these axons make synaptic contact with cells in the nuclei of the SOC. Some of the cells in the nuclei of the SOC receive input from both ears, and these cells are important for directional hearing. The axons of the neurons of the three divisions of the cochlear nucleus form the lateral lemniscus that crosses the midline to reach the midbrain relay of auditory information (the central nucleus of the inferior colliculus, ICC).

The axons of the cells in the SOC join the lateral lemniscus and terminate on cells in the ICC. The axons of the lateral lemniscus project to neurons in the central nucleus of the inferior colliculus (ICC), where almost all fibers are interrupted by synaptic contact. Some collateral fibers of the lateral lemniscus make synaptic contact with cells in the nuclei of the lateral lemniscus, the cells of which project to the ipsilateral and contralateral inferior colliculus (ICC) (Figure B.2).

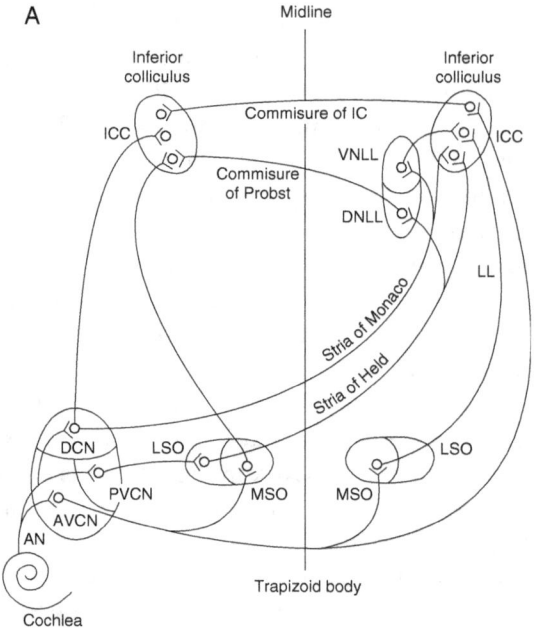

Figure B.2A Schematic of the ascending pathways from the left cochlea to the inferior colliculus. (Artwork by Monica Javidnia).

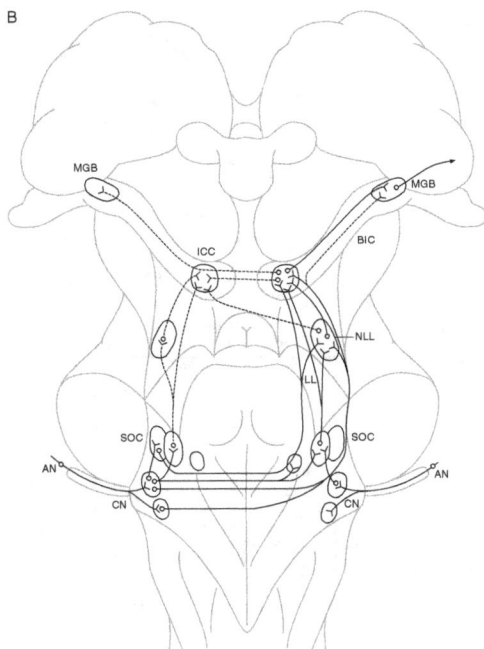

Figure B.2B Anatomical location of the major components of the ascending auditory pathways. Pathways from left auditory nerve to MGB are shown. (Artwork by Gailey).

The axons of the ICC form the brachium of the IC that ascend to the thalamus where all fibers make synaptic contact with the cells of the medial geniculate body, MGB, the thalamic relay of auditory information. The axons of the cells of the MGB project to the primary auditory cortex (A1) secondary auditory cortex (A2) and association cortices (for details see [460]).

Somatosensory system

The pathway of the somatosensory system that carries innocuous information is the dorsal column pathway. Nerve fibers that carry innocuous somatosensory information from the body are large myelinated fibers (mostly $A\beta$). These fibers travel as parts of mixed peripheral nerves to the spinal cord where they divide. A major branch of the somatosensory pathways travels on the dorsal surface of the spinal cord on the same side of the spinal cord as the dorsal column. The fibers terminate on cells in the gracilis and cuneatus nuclei in the dorsal column of the medulla oblongata [83, 476] (Figure B.3).

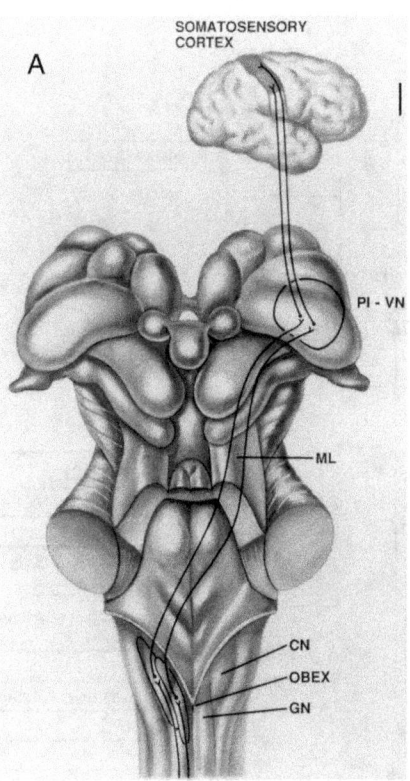

Figure B.3A Diagram of the somatosensory system. (Artwork by Coulter).

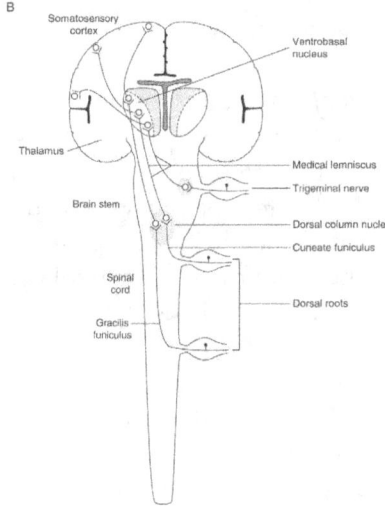

Figure B.3B Schematic of the somatosensory system. From: (Artwork by Monica Javidnia).

A more detailed diagram of the somatosensory system is shown in Figure B4.

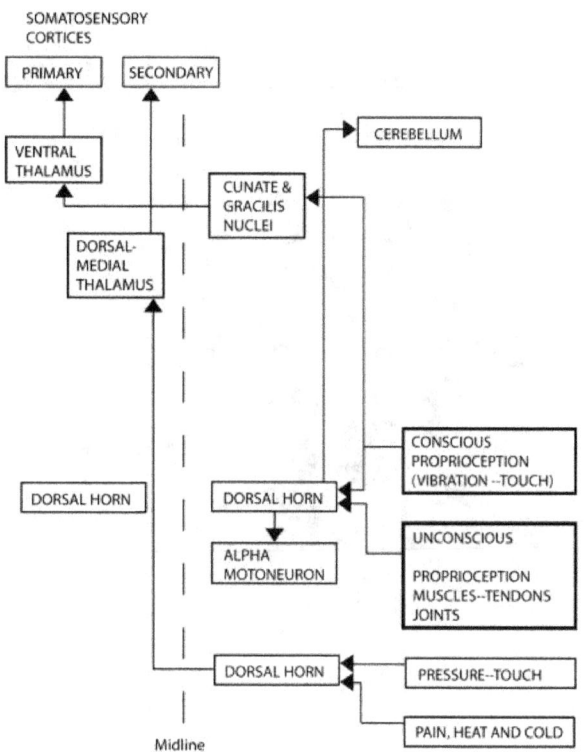

Figure B.4 Simplified diagram of the most important ascending pathways of the parts of the somatosensory system that mediate innocuous sensations and proprioception. (Modified from Møller: Intraoperative neurophysiological monitoring, 3rd edition).

Pathways of noxious information

The pathway that carries noxious information is known as the anterolateral system and consists of several separate pathways mediating pain, temperature, and some deep touch. We will describe the anatomy of the anterolateral system in detail later in Appendix C.

The trigeminal system

The nerve fibers that innervate pain receptors in the skin of the face and inside the mouth, including the teeth, travel mainly in the fifth, ninth, and tenth cranial nerves and make synaptic contact with cells in the trigeminal nucleus (Figure B.5). The sensory fibers of the trigeminal nerve that mediate innocuous stimulation enter the most rostral parts of the nucleus. Pain fibers enter the more caudal parts of the nucleus, which extend into the upper part of the spinal cord. From the trigeminal nucleus, axons cross the midline and ascend to the thalamus.

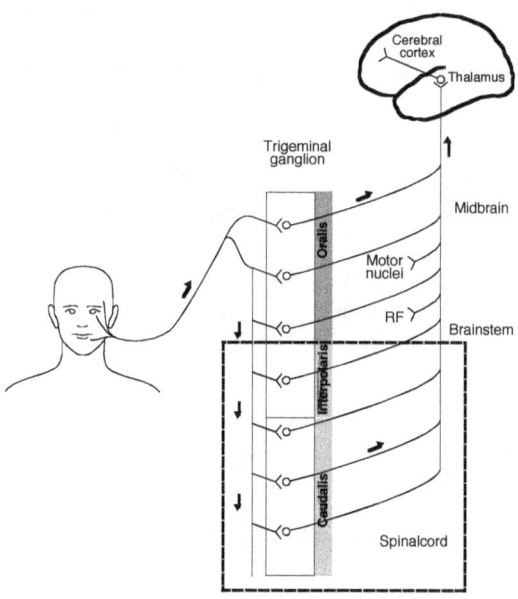

Figure B.5. The pathways of the trigeminal system. The upper part is the sensory part, and the lower (shaded) part is mainly involved in processing noxious stimuli. (From [460]) after Sessle, 1986 [610]).

Visual system

Information from visual receptors is transmitted synaptically to a neural network within the retina before entering in succession, the optic nerve, the optic chiasm, the optic tract, the visual thalamic nucleus (LGN), and the primary (striate) visual cortex (V1) [83] (Figure B.6). In humans and in animals with forward pointing eyes, the part of the optic nerve that carries information from the medial (nasal) part of the retina (the temporal visual field) crosses the midline at the optic chiasm and continues along the contralateral optic tract to the contralateral LGN as part of the optic tract (Figure B.6). The portion of the optic nerve that innervates the lateral retina continues uncrossed through the optic chiasm and travels as the ipsilateral optic tract.

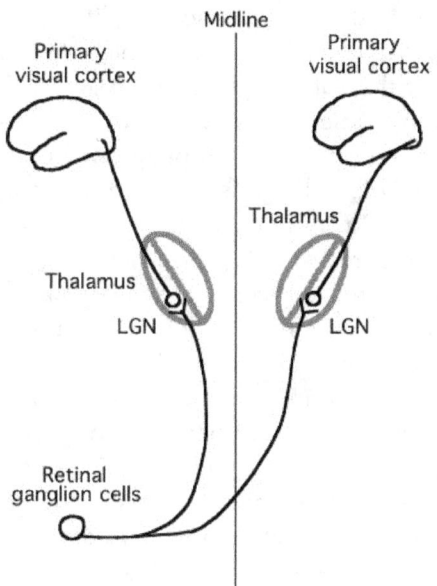

Figure B.6 Simplified schematic of the classical (reticulo-geniculo-cortical) visual pathways. (Artwork by Monica Javidnia).

Gustation

The classical pathways of gustation are similar to those of the hearing (Figure B.7), and somatosensory system. The main target of ascending taste fibers is the nucleus of the tractus solitarius (for details see [460]).

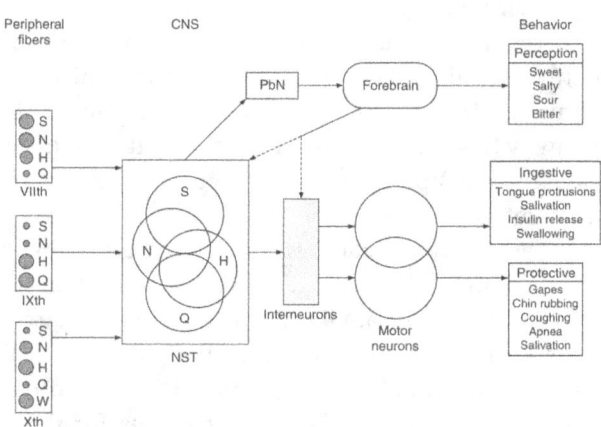

Figure B.7. Taste pathways.

Olfaction

Olfaction is different from the four other senses. Whether there are any sensory neo-cortical projections from olfaction is questionable as and few disorders are known to be related to olfaction. There are, however, connections to the entorhinal cortex. One aspect of olfaction, namely the heavy projection to the amygdala and other limbic structures, allows odors to invoke strong emotional reactions in addition to eliciting conscious perceptions.

The vomeronasal (pheromone) pathway may be of clinical interest [460] because of its direct connection to the nuclei of the amygdala through the olfactory bulb without any known projections to cortical sensory regions [234, 402] (Figure B.8). As no cortical structures are involved, a vomeronasal input will never produce a sensation of which a person is consciously aware. Pheromones can this influence vital functions such as sexual attraction and perhaps behavior unconsciously [460].

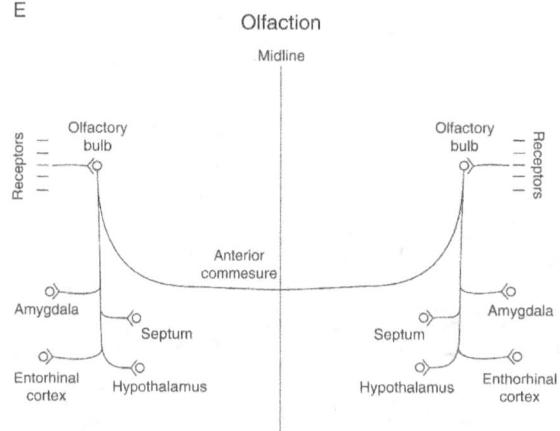

Figure B.8 Schematic diagram of olfactory pathways. (Artwork by Phillip Gilley).

Non-classical pathways

Each one of the three sensory systems, hearing, vision, and somesthesia, has distinct non-classical pathways. The axons of these non-classical pathways connect to the medial and dorsal divisions of the thalamus, as opposed to ventral, divisions of the thalamus that are used by the classical system.

From the thalamus, the axons project to many different subcortical structures such as the amygdala, anterior cingulate, hippocampus, and the hypothalamus. Projections are also made directly to the secondary and association cortices, bypassing the primary sensory cortices.

Auditory system

Some of the axons of cells in the ICC or their branches terminate on cells in two other divisions of the IC, the external nucleus (ICX) and the dorsal nucleus (DC). These nuclei belong to the non-classical pathways, and these cells send axons to cells in the dorsal and medial parts of the MGB [10, 460] (Figure B.9). Many of these neurons also receive input from somatosensory and visual systems, as indicated by the fact that they are also sensitive to those kinds of input.

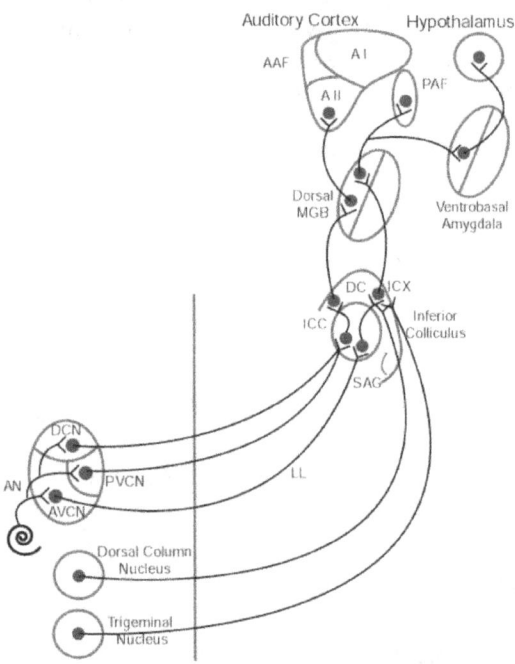

Figure B.9. Schematic drawing of the non-classical pathways for the auditory system. (Artwork by Monica Javidnia).

Unlike the cells in the classical pathway between the receptors and the primary cortices, many cells in the non-classical pathways respond to more than one sensory modality, and there is considerable interaction between non-classical auditory pathways and other sensory systems, mostly the somatosensory system [706]. There are also interactions between the visual and the auditory system in the thalamus [267].

The fact that the somatosensory system interacts with the non-classical auditory system makes it possible to determine if the non-classical pathways of the auditory system are active. It has been used in studies the activation of non-classical pathways in children [446] in people with tinnitus [438] and people with autism spectrum disorders. People who do not have tinnitus of autism spectrum disorders do not have signs of involvement of the non-classical sensory pathways. In these studies, a (nonsense) sound was presented to the ear, and the participants in the study were asked if the sound changed when electrical stimulation of the median nerve at the wrist was applied.

Using such tests have revealed that cross-modal interaction between the auditory and the somatosensory system occurs as a constant phenomenon in young children, indicating that the non-classical auditory pathways are active in children, but rarely in adults [438, 446]. This indicates that suppression of certain connections occurs during normal childhood development.

Other studies have shown evidence that these connections may have re-appeared in individuals with severe tinnitus [92, 438] and that is taken as a sign that re-routing of information has occurred. Involvement of the non-classical sensory systems may be an important part of the pathology of some disorders such as some forms of tinnitus and chronic neuropathic pain.

The visual system

In the visual system, the non-classical pathways also known as the non-geniculate pathways [83] (Figure B.10). The non-geniculate pathway has at least two parts, namely the superior colliculus (SC) pathway and the pulvinar thalamus pathway [83].

The parvicellular and the magnocellular channels are parts of the lemniscal system that are anatomically integrated with the pulvinar thalamic system. These are referred to as the paralemniscal pathways by some investigators [151] while other investigators have used different names for these two separate pathways, such as the classical and the non-classical systems.

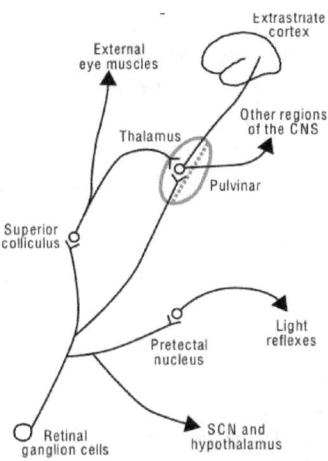

Figure B.10 Simplified schematic of the non-classical visual pathways. LGN: Lateral geniculate nucleus; SCN: Superchiastric nucleus. (Artwork by Monica Javidnia).

The pulvinar pathway involves the pulvinar and lateral posterior nucleus of the thalamus. Connections from the dorsal medial thalamic nuclei bypass the primary visual cortex, and their axons make synaptic contact with neurons in the MT/V5 association region of the visual cortex. This means that visual information that travels in the non-classical visual pathways arrives at the MT/V5 cortex earlier than information that travels in the classical pathways which must first pass through the V1 and secondary cortices (V2-V4).

Information that travels through the classical visual pathways may, therefore, interact in the MT/V5 cortex with an older version of the information that reached the area through the non-classical pathways.

The pulvinar thalamus is very large in humans, its volume is as much as 40% of the volume of the thalamus. The functions of the pulvinar thalamus is poorly known. Recent studies indicate that some cells in the pulvinar connect to cells in both hemispheres of the brain thus may have a role in connecting the two hemispheres, similar to that of the corpus callosum.

Processing in the two sensory pathways

Processing of sensory information that occurs in the classical and non-classical pathways is different. There is evidence that some symptoms and signs of disease, such as some forms of dyslexia, are related to an abnormal activation of non-classical ascending sensory pathways.

The paralemniscal branch of the pathway from the ventral thalamus also provides facilitatory input to the cortex. The two different pathways that constitute the ventral thalamic-cortical connections are separated anatomically in rodents but are integrated anatomically in other animals and appear as the thalamocortical pathway that originates in the VPL and VPM.

It is known that the non-classical pathways, at least those of the auditory system, provide subcortical connections to many structures in the brain that are otherwise only reached by sensory information through long cortical routes. The cells in the medial and dorsal thalamus project directly (subcortically) to limbic structures [352] such as the amygdala and other subcortical structures. The lateral nucleus of the amygdala can also be reached through the ventral thalamus, but only after passing through a long stream involving primary, secondary, and association cortices [353, 460].

The fact that the low route provides a subcortical connection to the amygdala [353] is important because this route may be re-activated in adults due to neuroplastic disorders such as some forms of tinnitus and central neuropathic pain. Limbic structures are normally only reached in adults through cortico-cortical connections (the "high route" [353]).

The subcortical connections mentioned above form the "low route" stream and project unprocessed and raw sensory information directly to the amygdala, bypassing the primary and secondary sensory cortices and association cortices.

These cortices comprise the "high route" that pass only highly processed information amygdala [353] whereas the low route passes more or less raw information to the amygdala and other subcortical structures.

In the auditory systems, these same regions of the association cortices also receive auditory information through the classical auditory pathways via the primary auditory cortex. That means that there exists an anatomical basis for an interaction between the auditory information that travels in the two ascending pathways.

Information that travels in the classical pathways may arrive earlier at the association cortices than the information that travels in the classical pathways, and that may cause unwanted effects.

Important differences between the two ascending routes

It is an important difference between the classical and non-classical pathways that the thalamic cells do not project to cells in the primary sensory cortices and that the subcortical parts of the non-classical pathways respond to more than one sensory modality while the classical pathways only respond to one modality of stimulation up to and including the cells in the primary cortices. In the classical pathways, the primary cerebral cortex is the last structure where cells only respond to one sensory modality, but in the non-classical pathways, even cells in subcortical nuclei respond to more than one sensory modality. Neurons in non-classical auditory systems and paralemniscal somatosensory systems have a poor spatial resolution [9] but can encode temporal patterns of stimulation into a rate code.

Both the classical and the non-classical pathways have collaterals that project to other systems. Of particular importance are the collaterals of the lemniscal tracts in the auditory and somatosensory systems that project to neurons in the reticular formation. The axons terminate in one segment of the spinal cord but and send collaterals to adjacent segments. Collateral connections play important roles in both the physiological and pathological aspects of the sensory systems, but these relatively minor extensions of major pathways are rarely documented sufficiently in neuroanatomical textbooks. The non-classical sensory pathways are phylogenetically older than the classical pathways.

Limbic system

Sensory systems have a plethora of anatomical connections to nuclei of the limbic system (Figure B.11). The lateral nucleus of the amygdala (AL) is the main limbic recipient of input from the auditory, somatosensory, and visual systems.

The lateral nucleus projects to the basolateral nucleus, which connects to the central nucleus of the amygdala. The central nucleus is the main output nucleus of the amygdala, and its neurons connect to endocrine, behavioral, and autonomic centers of the brain.

The central nucleus also projects to the nucleus basalis, which plays an important role in controlling arousal of the cerebral cortex.

The input to cortical cells from the nucleus basalis facilitates plastic changes in cerebral sensory cortices [36].

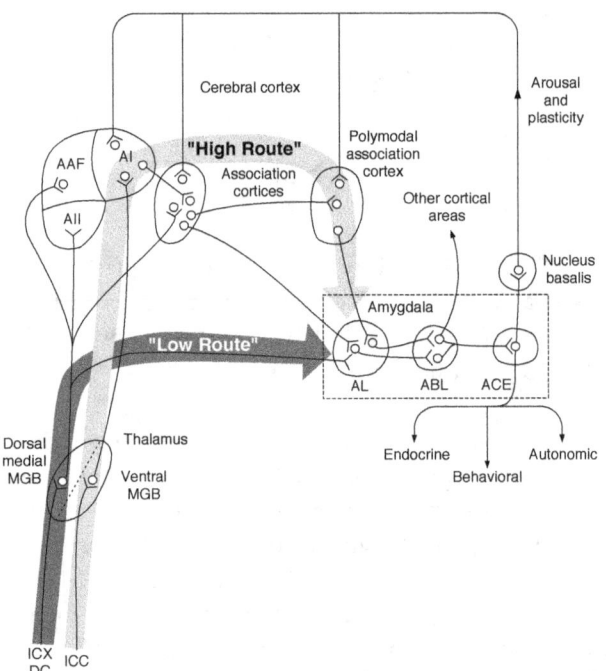

Figure B.11 Schematic illustrating the "high route" and the "low route" from the auditory system to the lateral nucleus of the amygdala. The drawing shows connections from the auditory system to the lateral nucleus of the amygdala. ABL: Basolateral nucleus of the amygdala; ACE: Central nucleus of the amygdala; AL: Lateral nucleus of the amygdala. Connections between the different nuclei of the amygdala and connections from these nuclei to different parts of the central nervous system are also shown. (Adapted from [460], based on [353]).

Sensory projections to limbic structures

The involvement of limbic structures in sensory functions including pain, especially the anterior cingulate gyrus, is supported by the beneficial effect of cingulotomy. The fact that recordings from subdural electrodes placed over the cingulate gyrus show responses to experimentally induced painful stimulation of the skin indicates that nociceptive input reaches the anterior cingulate gyrus (Brodmann's area 24).

The involvement of the cingulate cortex can explain some of the emotional components of pain, particularly central neuropathic pain.

Sensory routes to the amygdala

All sensory systems, except the olfactory nerve, project to the lateral nucleus of the amygdala. Olfaction has little cortical representation and the major target its pathway is the central nucleus of the amygdala.

This means that all sensory systems project to the amygdala and it would therefore be possible for the amygdala to serve the role to integrate information in all the different sensory systems. The amygdala may be important especially for the integration of taste and smell to create a holistic perception of the flavor of food.

While the anatomy of the connections from sensory systems to the amygdala is relatively well known, the functionality of these connections is much less well understood. Some studies have shown evidence that the non-classical auditory pathways may not be activated by sensory information in adult humans [438, 446] and consequently, the subcortical route to the amygdala may not be functional under normal conditions in adults. There is evidence that the non-classical auditory pathways are active in children [446].

The finding that some people with severe tinnitus have signs of activation of the non-classical auditory pathways [438] indicates that a subcortical route to the amygdala can become functional under pathological conditions, opening the possibility of subcortical sensory activation of the amygdala. Functional imaging studies have also provided evidence of increased activation of limbic structures in some individuals with tinnitus [368], which may occur through the "low route." (There is also evidence that the non-classical auditory system may be abnormally active in some developmental disorders such as autism [447]).

Certain sounds can cause affective reactions and that indicate involvement of the amygdala. Whether that occurs through the classical or non-classical pathways in unknown.

Proprioception

The somatosensory system is also responsible for proprioception a function essential for maintaining posture, performing fine motor tasks, and for accomplishing any motor task that requires bodily awareness.

Nerve fibers that carry proprioceptive input from the body also travel in mixed peripheral nerves and enter the spinal cord as dorsal roots.

Such fibers from the lower parts of the body together with fibers that carry some input from low threshold skin receptors are not interrupted in the dorsal column nuclei, but rather in the nucleus Z, which is located slightly more rostral and medial than the gracilis nucleus [346]. The axons of the cells of the nucleus Z cross to the opposite side and join the medial lemniscus [83].

Sensory input to spinal motor systems is mainly proprioceptive acting as feedback, but also visual and tactile input play important roles in motor control. Reaching for an object and knowing where one's hand is involved in motor control. Nociceptors also supply input to motor systems, as occurs in the withdrawal reflex.

The proprioceptive system's input to the motor system is especially important. Sensory stimulation can elicit general motor activity such as the startle reflex. Eye muscles are activated by sound as are neck muscles in righting reflexes. Loss of normal proprioception causes severe motor deficits.

Descending sensory pathways

Descending sensory pathways provide feedback to modulate information in the corresponding ascending pathways. In the sensory systems, the descending pathways are almost entirely reciprocal to the ascending pathways.

Both classical and non-classical ascending sensory pathways have reciprocal descending pathways. In that way, ascending and descending pathways build loops where information can circulate.

The best-known of such loops is the cortico-thalamic loop first described in detail by Per Andersen [27]. This study was followed by many studies that concerned this and other similar loops.

The descending pathways from the sensory cortices to the thalamic sensory nuclei are especially abundant, but many descending connections to more caudal sensory nuclei are also extensive [724]. Recently the cortico-thalamic connections have been implicated in the generation of the neural activity that is perceived as chronic neuropathic pain and tinnitus [367].

Some descending pathways reach as caudal as the first nucleus (spinal cord and cochlear nucleus [241]), and even the sensory cells in the cochlea have been shown to receive abundant efferent innervation [702] (for details, see [460]).

Little is known about the function of the descending sensory systems, and their role in pathologies remains uncertain. Recently, it was proposed that these pathways do more than providing central feedback to peripheral structures.

It has been suggested that the function of modulation of ascending activity, though important, could not justify the extensiveness of the descending pathways, which often have more fibers than the ascending pathways. It was recently proposed that the descending pathways send sensory information after being processed in central structures back to more peripheral structures where the awareness to a sensory stimulus is created [417].

Interaction: between the autonomic nervous system and sensory systems

The autonomic nervous system can be activated by sensory input in several ways. Autonomic activation of the autonomic system is most pronounced for the chemical senses, where taste can control secretion in the mouth and the digestive organs. Sensory systems connect to autonomic systems through the limbic system by which sensory input can change the function of the vascular system (blood pressure and heart rate) and cause sweating. In individuals with misophonia, trigger sounds can cause autonomic reactions such as salivation and contraction of muscles in the skin. Bright light can elicit sneezing in most people. Some of these reactions may occur without any conscious awareness, while others elicit distinct perceptions and can be aborted by conscious efforts.

Many of the connections from sensory systems to non-sensory systems are reciprocal. Just as the sensory systems influence the autonomic nervous system, the autonomic nervous system modulates sensory function. For example, sympathetic nerve fibers that terminate near mechanoreceptors in the skin can secrete norepinephrine, which increases the sensitivity of sensory receptors.

Sympathetic nerve fibers also terminate close to other receptor cells such as the hair cells in the ear [147] and the vestibular organs [175], but the function of these connections is unknown. The autonomic nervous system can also affect the function of sensory receptors by its effect on the blood flow to sensory organs.

Adrenergic nerve fibers terminate in sensory nuclei [341] where they can alter the processing of sensory information. Anatomically, these adrenergic fibers are different from those innervating blood vessels. The functional significance of the adrenergic innervation of the sensory ganglia is unknown, but it is reasonable to assume that this innervation plays a role in sensitizing sensory receptors during stress. There is also autonomic innervation of cells that process innocuous and noxious sensory information in the dorsal horn of the spinal cord, which is known to influence the neural processing of pain signals.

While bifurcation of nerve fibers is the anatomical basis for parallel processing, not all fibers that bifurcate form functional connections because some connections terminate in dormant synapses [697]. When dormant synapses become unmasked, processing may be altered, or new routes for information may be opened neuroplasticity. This means that not all routes that can be verified anatomically are functional. Dormant routes may, therefore, offer redundancy that can be activated after injury, or because of a change in demand by expression of neuroplasticity.

The term "dormant synapses" was coined by Patrick Wall in 1977 [697] to describe synapses that were anatomically present, but which could not activate the neurons on which they terminate. Such "dormant" synapses can be "unmasked" through the expression of neuroplasticity or a change of the input from, for example, low rate to high rate or from continuous firing to burst to fire.

Changes in the neural representation that occur in response to changes in demand often include an increase in the response area. Extension of response areas has been demonstrated in the somatosensory cortex in humans in studies by Edward Taub and his colleagues [670]. The cortical representation of the body to which pain is referred also increases as a result of expression of neuroplasticity [115, 158, 731]. Activation of such dormant connections may also cause symptoms of diseases. (For details see [460]).

Organization of cerebral sensory cortices

Sensory cortices consist of primary, secondary, and higher-order cortices that connect to association cortices and other parts of the central nervous system. The sensory cortices receive input from the ascending sensory pathways, process this information, and then send it to other regions of the cerebral cortex and other parts of the brain.

The cells in the primary cerebral cortices are the last cells in the ascending classical sensory pathways where cells respond only to on sensory modality. From there, information is distributed to higher cortical regions and to other parts of the brain where it is processed with information from other sensory pathways. Cells in primary cortices respond to only one modality of sensory stimuli, while cells in higher order cortices (including secondary (auditory) cortices [197]) may respond to more than one modality. The dorsal and medial thalamic nuclei are the final common relays for the non-classical sensory pathways. From this point, the information branches out to higher cortical regions, such as the secondary and association cortices, bypassing the primary sensory cortices. Axons of the thalamic non-classical nuclei target many subcortical structures in different parts of the brain.

Extensive processing occurs within cerebral sensory cortices (primary and secondary sensory cortices and association cortices). For example, the majority of the synapses on cells in cerebral cortices are connections from other cells in the same or different regions of the cerebral cortex. Association cortices coordinate input from different sensory systems and mediate sensory information to motor centers and other parts of the central nervous system.

The primary sensory cortices also send information to more peripheral parts of the sensory nervous system through extensive descending pathways that are parallel to the ascending sensory pathways.

Cells in primary cortices respond to only one modality of sensory stimuli, while cells in higher order cortices (including secondary (auditory) cortices [197]) may respond to more than one modality.

Cells in the sensory cortices are organized according to the spatial organization of sensory receptor surfaces. If one were to project the basilar membrane of the cochlea onto the surface of the auditory cortex and observe both as stimuli were presented, he would find that the hair cells that respond best to a frequency are overlaid on top of the most responsive neurons for that frequency. The auditory cortex is anatomically organized according to the frequency of sounds to which the neurons respond best; it is organized tonotopically.

Similarly, a representation of the body (homunculus) can be laid out over the surface of the somatosensory cortex, and the receptor surface of the retina can be projected onto the visual cortex. The primary visual cortex (V1) is also organized according to the visual field (for details, see [460]).

The earliest quantitative information about the somatotopic organization of the somatosensory system was published by Penfield [513]. Penfield was a neurosurgeon who became interested in neurophysiology while training in Oxford under Sherrington, an eminent physiologist. Penfield became the first to make extensive use of the opportunities that are available in the neurosurgical operating room for studies of the functioning nervous system in humans.

Specifically, he used the knowledge and understanding of nervous system function he had acquired under Sherrington to study the somatosensory cortex in patients on whom he operated. Penfield's functional mapping of the somatosensory cortex has not been significantly improved upon, or repeated to the extent that has replaced the maps he published in the 1930s. Penfield's maps still currently appear in modern textbooks. Additions have been made subsequently, and it is now recognized that there are many subdivisions of the somatosensory cortex that have separate maps, see [460]).

The extent of the correlation between spatial mapping of the cortices and nuclei and the anatomical configuration of the receptor surfaces as well as the extent that these representations are influenced by the stimulation intended to objectively elicit them are interesting questions.

It has been known for a long time that the mapping of the auditory cortex based on response to frequencies can be molded by sound stimulation [168, 316] and it has been difficult to study to what extent such mapping exists in the absence of stimulation [243].

Published studies, however, show that deaf animals deprived of stimulation of the auditory nerve have a rudimentary cochleotopic organization in brainstem nuclei [251] and the auditory cortex [243, 617]. Thus, there is no question that sensory stimulation is important for the organization of the nervous system [334]. How fast such organization occurs after sound exposure is not known, but experience from individuals who have received cochlear implants seems to show that it occurs rapidly. A similar question can be applied to the mapping of the somatosensory system and the retina onto their respective cortical areas.

The advent of cochlear implants has not only elevated the question to the level of practical importance with regards to the auditory system, but it has also made possible the study of the origin of tonotopic organization of the auditory cortex [154]. Thus, sound input is necessary for proper development of the auditory nervous system [334]. Cortical maps in the adult organisms are not static either, and they can be modified by various means such as through the expression of neuroplasticity. The response of individual cells depends on the convergence of input and the balance between inhibitory and excitatory input. Increased convergence widens a cell's response area; lateral inhibition makes cells' response areas narrower. Furthermore, other complex interactions between the inputs to different cortical cells affect their response to sensory stimuli and the appearance of cortical maps.

In the auditory system, sound stimuli, or their absence, may activate expression of harmful neuroplasticity, causing tinnitus and hyperacusis [454]. Cortical maps of other sensory systems can also be altered through the expression of neuroplasticity as shown in animal research [316, 559].

In addition to spatial organization, cells of sensory cortices are organized anatomically according to the properties of sensory stimuli. Cortical maps that reflect functional properties of stimuli are known as functional maps, or computational maps. An example of computational maps is the mapping of auditory space [460] [599]. Computational maps are equally dynamic and modifiable by expression of neuroplasticity as well.

Subcortical interactions between different sensory systems

It is well known that interactions between different sensory inputs occur in the secondary sensory cortices and in association cortices where cells respond to more than one sensory modality, especially in the polymodal cortices. There are also similar connections between different sensory systems that can provide similar integrations subcortically. Anatomical studies have shown that neurons in the cochlear nucleus connect to the somatosensory system through the trigeminal nucleus [619, 749] and dorsal column nuclei [282]), thus providing the basis for some integration of and interaction between somatosensory activation from the skin around the ear and the auditory system [457].

There are also other anatomical locations where similar interactions may occur. One place is the midbrain [143] where information from the caudal trigeminal nucleus and auditory information in the inferior colliculus can interact [750]. Another is between cells in the inferior colliculus and cells in the deep layers of the superior colliculus [725]. There are also other, more centrally located, sites for interaction and integrations of activity in different modalities.

Organization of neural processing

Neural processing of the same information occurs in anatomically different parts of the brain, referred to as parallel processing. Different kinds of sensory information are processed in different parts of the brain, referred to as stream segregation.

Parallel processing

In parallel processing, the same sensory information is processed in different populations of neurons in sensory systems, or that information can follow several routes as it travels in ascending sensory pathways. The anatomical basis for parallel processing in the auditory system is repeated bifurcation of fibers in the ascending sensory pathways. For example, each auditory nerve fiber innervates neurons in three different parts of the cochlear nucleus, which is the first relay nucleus for auditory information.

A similar anatomical basis for parallel processing occurs at more central locations of ascending sensory pathways. Examples are the lateral lemniscus and the medial lemniscus that send collaterals to several structures of the brainstem, such as the reticular formation, before reaching the thalamus [460]. Axons that carry somatosensory input to the spinal cord and the trigeminal nucleus give off many collateral axons that make synaptic contact with cells in many different locations in the spinal cord and brainstem.

The separation of pathways in classical and non-classical pathways is also an example of parallel processing, where the same information is processed in different populations of nerve cells.

Stream segregation

Stream segregation is distinct from parallel processing in that different kinds of information are processed in different populations of neurons. While parallel processing is evident at peripheral levels of the ascending sensory pathways, stream segregation has been associated with only the higher levels of the nervous system. For example, the processing of information that occurs in association cortices is divided into streams, where different kinds of information are processed in different parts of the association cortices.

This separation based on modality was first described in the visual system [421, 683] where it was observed that spatial information was processed in a dorsal stream but object information was processed in a ventral (or temporal) stream, (Figure B.12). These two categories have become known as the "where" and "what" types of information.

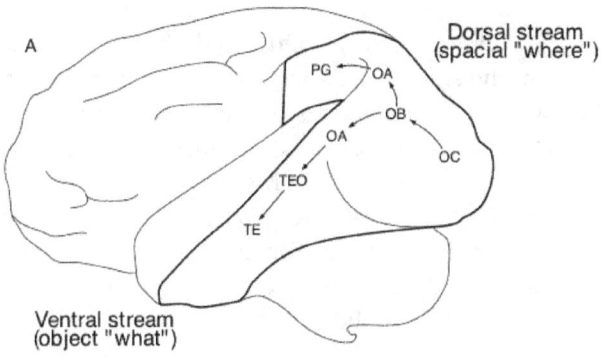

Figure B.12. Illustration of stream segregation in the visual system in the monkey brain. OC, OB, OA, TEO, TE, and PG: different areas of the visual cortex [69]. (Artwork by Monica Javindia).

Similar forms of stream segregation have been found to occur in the auditory system [549] where it was found that object ("what") matters are processed in an anterior-ventral region of the cerebral cortex in humans, and non-human primates and place ("where") information is processed in a posterior dorsal stream [549]. As studies of stream segregation have progressed, it has been clear that segregation of several different qualities of sensory stimuli occurs, and that stream segregation is not simply limited to separation of spatial and object information [460].

The streams of visual information in the association cortices that are involved in the feedback of hand movement (reaching) are different from those streams that concern visual perception [219]. Injury to even one of the two streams of visual information, causes deficits either of visual feedback (when the dorsal stream is injured) with intact perception of visual images, or deficits in visual perception, leaving visual feedback for hand movements intact (when the ventral stream is injured).

These studies [219] were done in persons with strokes limited to the anatomical regions that processed one of the two main visual streams.

Connections to non-sensory parts of the central nervous system

Sensory systems connect to many different parts of the central nervous system that are not anatomically regarded as sensory regions: autonomic centers of the brain and motor system.

We have already mentioned that the limbic system (the emotional brain) receives sensory input. Likewise, the reticular system of the brainstem receives sensory input that is important for the control of wakefulness. More recently, it has become evident that the insular lobe plays an important role in sensory functions, especially those associated with internal organs and relates to the perception of the "self."

The vagus nerve

The anatomy of the vagus nerve is complex, and it has both descending and ascending sensory fibers and pain fibers, in addition to its major content of parasympathetic fibers that innervate the lower body. Parts of the vagus nerve have been shown to be involved in pain and pain control. There is evidence that the vagus nerve carries information from pain receptors in various parts of the body and connects to afferents in the cervical spinal cord [56]. Vagal afferents project to neurons that can exert both inhibitory and excitatory influence on nociceptive processing in the spinal cord via bulbospinal pathways [56].

The main function of the vagus nerve was formerly regarded to be supplying parasympathetic influence to internal organs. Its descending fibers, however, comprised only 20% of the total fibers of the vagus nerve. Only recently has the research focus shifted to the previously understudied 80% afferent, and mostly sensory, fibers.

These afferent fibers mediate sensory information from many internal organs. Some of these pathways may mediate the suppression of pain that can occur from electrical stimulation of the vagus nerve that has been observed [270]. Electrical stimulation of the vagus nerve suppresses experimental pain.

It is important to note that the target of these afferent fibers is the nucleus tractus solitarii (NTS) that connects to many different brain structures including many brainstem nuclei important for peripheral control of pain through the locus coeruleus-nucleus raphe magnus system (NA-serotonin system [56, 404].

Many investigators now agree that the vagus nerve is very important in many normal functions and many diseases. For example, it is important in signaling disorders in the body.

It is believed that activation of vagus afferents produces unspecific sensations such as feeling ill in response to signals from the abdomen rather than distinct pain sensations. It has been estimated that about half of common myocardial infarctions do not have pain as a symptom, but instead cause a feeling of illness similar to the influence. These feelings are probably mediated by the vagus nerve. The vagus nerve can substitute for the spinal cord in mediating sensory input from the lower body, including sensations from genitalia [636].

Other investigators emphasized the importance of the connections between the NST and the locus coeruleus, either directly or via the paragigantic (PGi) nucleus [404]. Facilitatory influence on spinal cord pain neurons is probably mediated through a longer and more complex route from the NST through the forebrain to the dorsal horn neurons, probably involving the RVM system of ON and OFF cells (Figure B.13) [56].

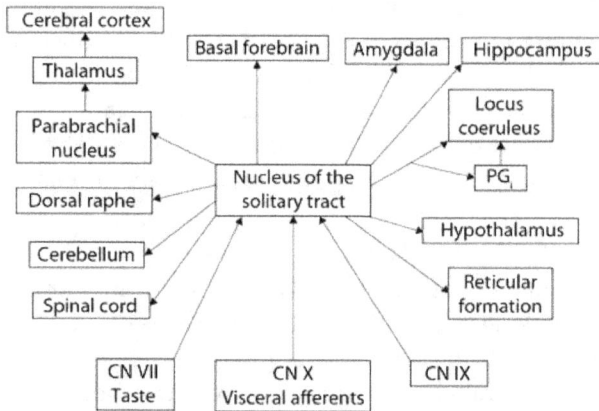

Figure B.13 Composite drawing of the pathways from and to the NTS.

PGi: Paragigantic nucleus. The connection between the NST and the locus solitarius is unclear; it may consist of a direct connection, or it may go through the paragigantic nucleus (PGi). The lateral PGi has many functions related to the brainstem cholinergic system [618] and parasympathetic system such as related to the heart and REM sleep [148]. (Artwork by Monica Javidnia).

The wideness of the range of functions performed by the regions that receive input from the vagus nerve implies that the modulation of the vagus nerve can produce an equally extensive range of effects.

Electrical stimulation of the vagus nerve has been used for many years to control epileptic seizures [170] and is now being investigated for the use in the treatment of pain and severe tinnitus [168] [169], pain [320], and depression [489]. Indeed, vagus nerve stimulation has been in clinical use for many years, and the FDA approved it 1997.

As the NTS neurons convey information to structures that process memory, such as the amygdala, hippocampus, and frontal cortex, (via a polysynaptic pathway to the locus coeruleus, the primary CNS source for norepinephrine), the vagus nerve can participate in memory and neuromodulation. Vagus nerve stimulation could thus offer a potential treatment for disorders such as Alzheimer's disease, other forms of dementia, and also post-traumatic stress disorders (PTSD) for which one of the treatment goals is the extinction of memory [404].

It was mentioned above that the vagus nerve receives input from organs of the reproductive system. For example, stimulation of the vagina can modulate activity in the vagus nerve and reduce the perception of pain from other sources in both animals [126] and in humans [709]. The vagus nerve can be stimulated by implanted electrodes in the portion of the vagus nerve that travels in the neck close to the surface.

This means that electrical stimulation of the vagus nerve can be performed without major invasive surgical procedures [460].

It has been shown earlier that stimulation of the nucleus basalis promotes activation of neuroplasticity [36, 316] and promotes cortical arousal. There is recent evidence that stimulation of the vagus nerve may have similar effects [168, 492].

Neural control of the immune system

There are two main divisions of the immune system, the innate and the adaptive. The innate system is the first responder to intruders such as viruses and bacteria. It always responds in the same way. The adaptive immune system takes over after the innate system and can learn. It will respond stronger to the same pathogen when repeated. The adaptive immune system has similarities with neuroplasticity. We have both immune systems and both afferent and efferent parasympathetic activity is thought to play a role in immunomodulation [672].

The innate system is the oldest phylogenetically. Studies of the innate immune system in a one-millimeter long nematode have shown evidence of neural control of the immune system in this phylogenetic very early version of the innate immune system (Figure B.

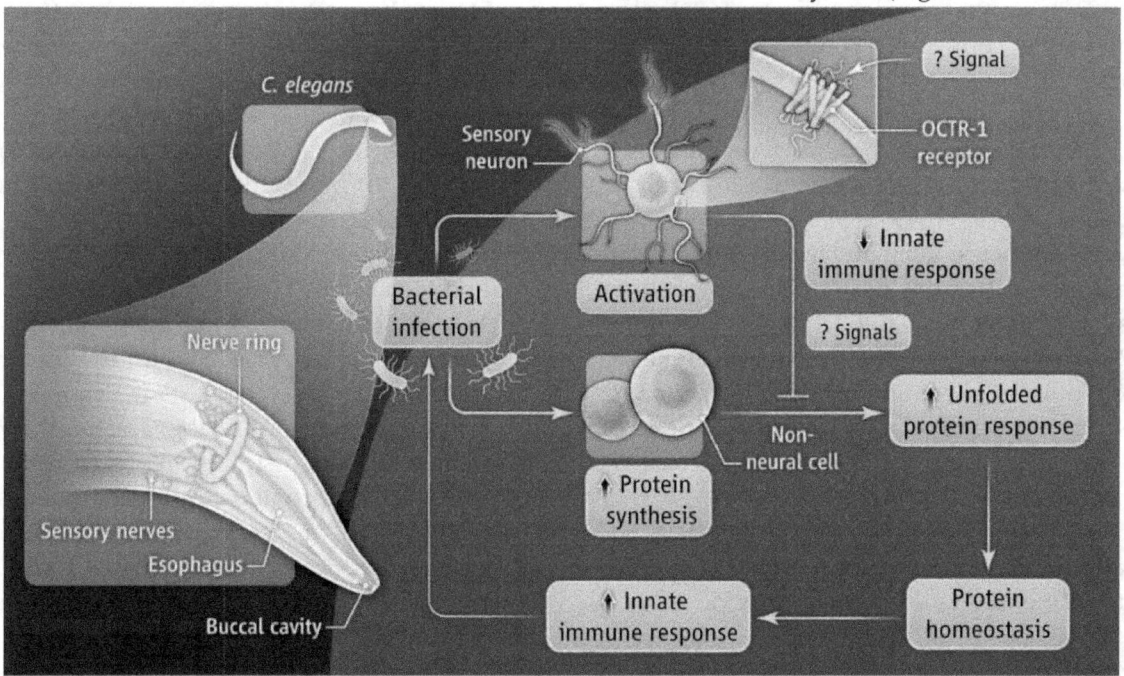

Figure B.14 Illustration of how an infection of a nematode, *C. elegans,* is fended off by the innate immune system. (From Tracey, K. J. (2011). "Ancient Neurons Regulate Immunity." Science 332: 673-674).

The immune system plays fundamental roles in many mental illnesses such as depression, chronic fatigue and Alzheimer's disease [242]. Microglia is the brain's equivalent to macrophages and serves important immune roles within the central nervous system such as in dendritic pruning, and it is involved in neuroplasticity. There is evidence that cytokines, which are the innate immune system's proteins, are responsible for coordinating the bodily response to infections also play an important role in learning processes such as long-term potentiation (LTP) in the brain. Some hypotheses state that some of the signs of Alzheimer's disease are manifestations of immune reactions. Some studies have indicated that depression is an inflammatory condition [246].

There is also evidence that the immune system and thus, the vagus nerve and the cholinergic system of the brain are involved in a wide range of diseases, such as Alzheimer's disease, neurodegenerative disorders, and such seemingly different diseases as chronic pain [384] and disorders of the cardiovascular system [672].

This makes the vagus nerve an attractive avenue for possible therapeutic interventions to a wide range of disorders. Through the NTS the vagus nerve can activate the brain's cholinergic system [477, 678], which is anti-inflammatory [565] and has effects on the immune response [672]. The vagus nerve has control of cholinergic activity in many parts of the central nervous system, and it thereby affects the immune system, mostly enhancing it, but increased vagal tone can also suppress the immune systems such as can occur in individuals with brain injuries [672].

The vagus nerve activates the nicotinic anti-inflammatory pathway [682]. This signaling requires α7 nicotinic acetylcholine receptors (nAChR) expressed on non-neuronal cytokine-producing cells. A7 nicotinic acetylcholine receptor agonists inhibit cytokine release and protect animals in a variety of experimental lethal inflammatory models [200].

It has been shown in animal models of intestinal inflammation that vagus nerve stimulation ameliorates such inflammation.

This was ascribed to the effect of the vagus nerve activity on the cholinergic nervous system, which attenuates the production of pro-inflammatory cytokines and inhibits inflammatory processes [565].

Some studies suggest shown evidence that the vagus nerve may be an indirect modulator of innate inflammatory processes, exerting its anti-inflammatory effects via postganglionic modulation of immune cells in primary immune organs. Gallowitsch-Puerta and colleagues have discussed advances in the possible mechanisms by which the vagus nerve can mediate the immune response, and the role of nAChR activation and signaling on macrophages and other immune cells [200].

The natural (physiological) anti-inflammatory mechanisms that control the immune system these have caught recent interest because they may induce pharmacologically to treat diseases of an overreacting immune system. The α7-nicotinic acetylcholine receptor (α7nAChR) pathway is one such possibility, and there is evidence that nicotine has beneficial effects, though its toxicity is an obstacle. Receptor agonists for the α7nAChR would be another possibility [682]. This system is activated through the vagus nerve by events in the viscera.

Overactive central nervous system immune systems also cause damage such as after ischemic strokes where much of the second phase damage is due to the effect of the immune reaction to debris from the initial cell death. Overproduction of tumor necrosis factor (TNF α) and other cytokines are involved in many disease processes including inflammation.

Medications such as minocycline have been found beneficial in reducing post-stroke deficits [345, 746]. However, so far, this treatment has not found general clinical use in the treatment of strokes. Clot-dissolving medications (tissue plasminogen activators, TPA) are still the standard treatment although studies in stroke patients have found that it provides little advantages, while administration of minocycline has been found to effectively reduce post-stroke neurological deficits [345]. Other immunosuppressive agents seem to have similar beneficial effects [231].

Reticular formation

The axons of the ascending sensory tracts that pass through the brainstem send collaterals to the reticular formation. The reticular formation controls wakefulness and excitability of cortical neurons, and sensory activation of the reticular formation is necessary to elicit from cortical cells responses to sensory stimulation.

This means that perception of sensory stimuli requires activation of sensory receptors *and* activation of the sensory cortices from the reticular formation. Non-classical pathways provide more extensive input to the reticular formation than do the classical pathways. Arousal of the cerebral cortex can also occur through the amygdala via the nucleus basalis, which means that emotional activation and attention can also increase the excitability of sensory cortices. The vagus nerve, through its target nucleus, the nucleus tractus solitarius (NTS), has a similar capability.

Dynamic organization of sensory systems

Textbook descriptions of the structure of the sensory pathways such as also in this book are based mostly on anatomical studies. Anatomically verified connections may not be functional, however, under normal conditions because they terminate in synapses that are ineffective at a given time. The efficacy of synapses can increase or decrease because of the expression of neuroplasticity.

Unmasking of normally dormant synapses can alter the processing of sensory information and can open connections within sensory systems; thereby, re-routing information to neurons that normally do not receive such information.

Similarly, masking of functional synapses can interrupt connections that are normally functional and eliminate processing of sensory information in neurons that normally perform such processing. Connections from sensory systems to other systems in the central nervous system are also subjected to changes in the expression of neuroplasticity.

Neuroplasticity can be initiated by changing demands of sensory systems, or as compensatory measures after injuries.

The information that flows in some parts of sensory pathways can be consciously modulated; whereas other ascending information is subject to unconscious control. We have already mentioned that there are connections to the limbic system from different nuclei of sensory pathways ("low route") and the cerebral cortex (association cortices, the "high route") [353].

The classical pathways provide the most central connections, and the non-classical pathways provide subcortical connections to the amygdala and other subcortical structures, but these (anatomically verified) connections may not always be functional. There are indications that the "low route" of auditory information is active in children up to about the age of 15 [446] and that it can be active in adults in connection with diseases such as tinnitus or autism [438, 447].

The flow of information in the "high route" to the amygdala can be modulated consciously, whereas information that reaches the amygdala through subcortical connections is probably not subjected to similar conscious modulation. Activation of the amygdala through the "high route" that may mediate fear can be controlled consciously while the flow of information in the "low route" is largely beyond such conscious control.

Many studies have been based on what is known as functional imaging (fMRI, PET scan). More recently, other methods that aim at more direct measures of neural activity, such as MEG [597, 642, 708] and recordings of various forms of electrical activity from the brain (EEG), have been used in studies of the pathology of non-nociceptor pain and tinnitus [597, 642].

Descriptions of the structure of the sensory pathways are based on anatomical studies. Anatomically verified connections may not be functional, however, under normal conditions because they terminate in synapses that are ineffective at a given time. The efficacy of synapses can increase or decrease because of the expression of neuroplasticity. Unmasking of normally dormant synapses can alter the processing of sensory information and open connections within sensory systems and thereby re-route information to neurons that normally do not receive such information.

Similarly, masking of functional synapses can interrupt connections that are normally functional and eliminate processing of sensory information in neurons that normally perform such processing. Connections from sensory systems to other systems in the central nervous system are also subjected to changes in the expression of neuroplasticity. Neuroplasticity can be initiated by changing demands of sensory systems, or as compensatory measures after injuries.

The information that flows in some parts of sensory pathways can be consciously modulated; whereas other ascending information is subject to unconscious control. We have already mentioned that there are connections to the limbic system from different nuclei of sensory pathways ("low route") and the cerebral cortex (association cortices, the "high route").

The classical pathways provide the most central connections, and the non-classical pathways provide subcortical connections to the amygdala, but these (anatomically verified) connections may not always be functional. The flow of information in the "high route" to the amygdala can be modulated consciously, whereas information that reaches the amygdala through subcortical connections is probably not subjected to similar conscious modulation.

Activation of the amygdala through the "high route" that may mediate fear can thereby be controlled consciously while the flow of information in the "low route" is largely beyond such conscious control. Expression of neuroplasticity may cause reorganization of the nervous system that can change neural processing of sensory stimuli, or re-routing of information and cause symptoms of disease ("Plasticity diseases"). Such functional changes may cause the generation of sensations without any physical stimuli reaching sensory receptors.

The phantom limb sensations are examples of sensations that are generated in the central nervous system but referred to a peripheral anatomical location (that no longer exists) [475]. Another example is tinnitus in individuals with a severed auditory nerve, where the sensation of sound is referred to the ear but obviously not generated in the ear.

Interpretation of sensory information

Little is known about the interpretation of sensory information. It has been hypothesized that some sensory stimuli may be interpreted according to the principles of analysis by synthesis. Morris Halle at MIT (1965) suggested that spoken words were interpreted by mentally mimicking words and then comparing the mimicked words with the words that were heard.

It was assumed that the process of interpreting words was localized to Wernicke's area of the association cortex. However, recent studies have shown evidence that much larger areas of the cerebral cortex are involved in interpreting spoken words [677]. Comparison of freshly acquired sensory information against stored information seems to be important for interpreting sensory information.

Much sensory information is heavily distorted. The retina, for example, has a blind spot, where the optic nerve exits, devoid of the visual receptors. The portions of the image that is projected onto that spot will be absent in the neuronal message that the eye provides to the brain.

The density of the sensory cells in the retina varies over the surface being less dense (fewer cells per square millimeter) in the periphery compared with the center of the retina where images are projected. This would cause the image sent to the brain to be distorted. It is not known how that is corrected to obtain an undistorted picture. It has been hypothesized that we do not perceive the picture that is sent to the brain by the eye directly but instead a stored picture that matches the one that is sent by the eye. That does not seem to solve the problem because the stored pictures would have similar distortion because it must have been created from images that are sent to the brain from the eye. These are some of the interesting challengers for the neuroscientists of the future.

Where in the brain is awareness of a sensory stimulus generated? Most descriptions of the central nervous representation of sensory stimuli are limited to the cerebral cortices, often in fact only to the primary and secondary sensory cortices. One might suggest the most centrally located structure as being a candidate for where the conscious awareness is generated.

Recently, however, it has been suggested that it might be a much more peripheral location [417]. The reason for that hypothesis is related to the abundant descending pathways that accompany all ascending sensor pathways.

It has been claimed that although it is assumed that the descending pathways have modulatory effects on the ascending activity, they are just too abundant to explain that function.

It has been suggested that the descending pathways may transport processed information about sensory stimuli to an anatomically more peripheral level of sensory nervous system and that it is at these peripheral levels that the conscious awareness of a sensory stimulus is achieved. Awareness of sensory stimulation is important and can be beneficial in many ways, but some forms of awareness are not beneficial. (For details see [460]).

Appendix C

Neuroscience of Pain

Abstract

1. Pain may be classified into two categories: Pain that is evoked through direct stimulation (physical or chemical) of specific receptors (nociceptors), and pain that is not caused by stimulation of nociceptors.

2. Nociceptors are located to the skin, the cornea, tooth pulp, muscles, joints, peripheral nerves, the respiratory system, and viscera.

3. Stimulation of nociceptors causes acute pain that has a fast and a slow component.

4. Perception of acute and chronic pain is affected by many circumstantial factors such as expectation, stress, and emotional state.

5. (Transmission of pain in the dorsal horn of the spinal cord (or trigeminal nucleus) can be modulated by input from skin receptors (Aβ fibers), and by descending activity from supraspinal sources such as the periaqueductal gray.

6. Pain can be modulated through endorphins and medications such as NSAID and opioids.

7. The sympathetic nervous system can modulate the sensitivity of nociceptors and the transmission of pain signals in the spinal cord and the trigeminal nucleus.

8. Itch is caused by stimulation of receptors similar to those that evoke acute pain.

Introduction

Many forms of pain are both purposeful and beneficial to a person, such as pain that warns not to move an injured limb. Some warnings may be purposeful, but not beneficial because there is no remedy to avoid the danger that the pain correctly has signaled. Pain is an important diagnostic sign of many disorders. Pain receptors (nociceptors) detect many of the events that pose a danger to the organism in various ways. Non-nociceptive pain does not seem to be beneficial to an individual, nor does it seem to be purposeful.

Chronic neuropathic pain, is an example non-nociceptive pain (covered in Chapter 6).

Pain is an important indicator of diseases or trauma. Pain should only be treated if it can be excluded that the pain is caused by a treatable condition or if the underlying cause is not treatable. The high prevalence pain and its enormous toll on the quality of life heighten the importance of understanding the function of the pain systems for all who are active in the field of healthcare. The International Association for the Study of Pain (IASP) defines pain as "an unpleasant sensory and emotional experience associated with tissue damage or potential damage or described in such terms."

The emotional component of pain can be highly subjective, and there are great individual differences in the way pain is perceived. The reaction to pain often varies from time to time within the same person. Pain that persists for a long time reduces the quality of life, a factor that unfortunately has not attracted the attention of the medical community that it deserves. The quality of life considerations is important in medical treatment (or lack of treatment), and likewise, play an important role in pain management. Pain can be the cause of suicide, an indication of the enormity of its effect on quality of life.

Pain has two main components: One is the sensation ("it hurts"), and the other is an expression that can best be described as suffering (or distress). This is the component that reduces the quality of life most.

The intensity of pain and a person's perception of it are difficult to measure objectively. A person's perception depends on a combination of factors such as emotional state, the circumstances under which the pain was acquired, and whether it is perceived as a threatening signal. The perception of pain is also affected by factors such as arousal, attention, distraction, and expectation. The amount of control a person believes he or she has over a situation of pain is a very powerful factor affecting the emotional component of pain.

Visceral pain, originating from inside the body is perceived as being more inescapable than pain referred to the surface body and, as such, is often perceived to be more severe than the pain that originates from the surface of the body.

Pain is a more complex sensation than other somatosensory sensations, and the sensation and perception of pain are much more variable than that of ordinary sensory stimuli. Pain is not commonly regarded as a sense and textbooks often cover it in sections separate from those that deal with the more traditional senses. The sensation of pain can be modulated by drugs such as the common kinds of painkillers including opioids. This the main difference between pain and somatosensation.

The diversity of the expression of pain and its cause is a severe obstacle for effective diagnosis and treatment of pain. Current physician training is often insufficient to fulfill the goal of effective treatment and care for patients with severe pain.

Pain plays an important role in medicine and is the most common reason for visits to the emergency room. Paradoxically, the efforts to treat patients experiencing pain, and the basic research that is devoted to its study, is much less than what could be justified by the degree of suffering and the number of people who are affected by pain. Pain is in many ways an enigma, available treatments are often ineffective, and some treatments cause severe side effects.

Pain seldom exhibits any detectable morphological or chemical abnormalities. That means that the physician is often left to treat pain disorders based on the patient's description alone. Compounding this difficulty is the fact that the anatomical location to which pain is referred may be different from the actual anatomical location of the malady that caused the pain.

The sole mechanism through which pain is experienced has historically been regarded to be neural activity in the central nervous system (CNS) elicited by stimulation of pain receptors and transmitted in distinct pathways through the central nervous system. We now know that pain signals undergo far more complex processing in ascending and descending pathways. It is now established knowledge that expression of neuroplasticity plays an important role in many forms of pain.

Pain that is caused by activation of nociceptors is subjected to change through the expression of neuroplasticity in the neural circuits that transmit and process pain signals and pain can be caused by neural activity that is generated in the central nervous system without any peripheral input.

Pain that is caused by activation of neuroplasticity is discussed in Section 3, Chapter 6. This Appendix describes the basic anatomy and physiology of pain. A more detailed description of pain is provided in a separate book (Møller, A.R., *Pain: Its Anatomy, Physiology, and Treatment.* 2014, Dallas: Aage R. Møller Publishing [461]).

Classification of pain

Pain can be divided into two main groups, nociceptor pain, also known as physiological pain, and non-nociceptor pain, which approximates the term "pathological pain." The International Association for the Study of Pain (IASP) has defined different forms of pain. The term "physiological pain" is used to describe pain caused by stimulation of pain receptors (nociceptors) in normal tissue whereas the term "pathological pain" is used to describe the pain that occurs in association with pathologies with or without stimulation of pain receptors. Pain has been divided, into two large groups that are sometimes considered a hybrid of the others [150]. Nociceptive, or physiological, pain is caused by stimulation of nociceptors that respond only to stimuli of a certain modality that reach an intensity that is typically unsafe for an organism. Peripheral nerve fibers pass these signals to the central nervous system and the limbic system, producing emotional effects. Physiological pain is sometimes referred to as acute pain, and although it is not in the category of pathological pain, if it is allowed to persist, it may transition into a chronic and pathological pain. Acute pain can thus be a precursor to more serious conditions.

Inflammatory pain is associated with peripheral sensitization imitated by tissue damage and the infiltration of immune cells. It does involve stimulation of nociceptors and can be described as a subset of nociceptive pain, but as the sensitivity of the nociceptors is caused by a disease state, inflammatory pain can also be categorized as pathological.

For this reason, inflammatory pain is sometimes classified as a hybrid of physiological and pathological pain and sometimes as its category. Each of these two groups of pain has several subcategories [731] (Figure C.1).

Acute pain is elicited by activation of pain receptors in normal tissue, and that is known as physiological pain [121].

Pathophysiological pain, or clinical pain, is pain elicited by inflammatory processes and which is associated with peripheral and central sensitization. Central (neuropathic) pain includes pain caused by lesions or dysfunction in the central nervous system [413].

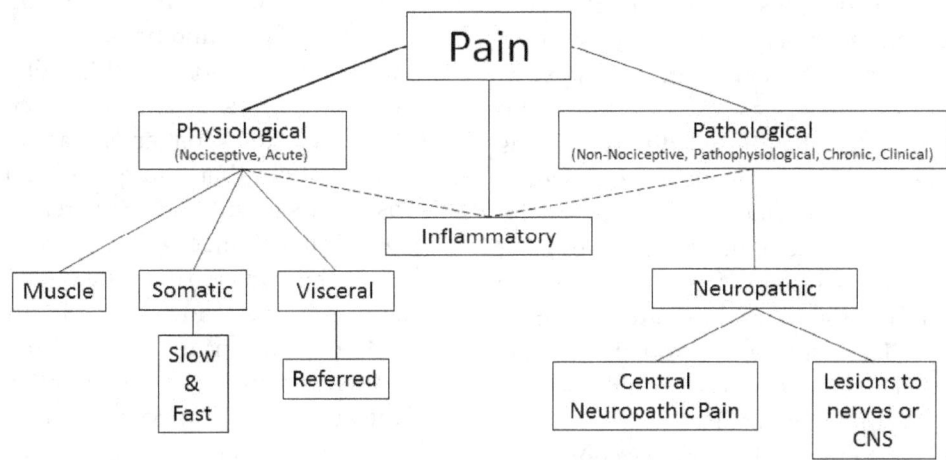

Figure C.1. The dotted lines to inflammatory pain now indicate that inflammatory pain is sometimes considered a hybrid and sometimes considered a regular subdivision. (Artwork by Michael Wiseman).

Other investigators [150] have defined three main types of pain namely:

1. Physiologic
2. Inflammatory and
3. Neuropathic pain.

Physiologic pain is the result of normal stimulation of nociceptors; inflammatory pain is caused by varying kinds of inflammation, of different kinds and by tissue damage (Figure C.2). Nociceptive pain and pathophysiological pain overlap, in that nociceptive pain, includes both the normal condition of stimulation of nociceptors and inflammatory pain. Inflammatory pain may be classified as a type of pathophysiologic pain together with neuropathic pain [150].

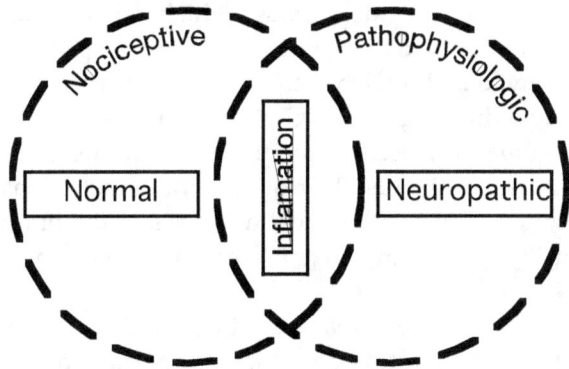

Figure C.2 A classification of pain that defines two main overlapping groups of pain, namely:

1. Nociceptive pain that can occur as a normal condition and as a result of inflammatory processes;

2. Pathophysiological pain that includes neuropathic pain and pain caused by inflammatory processes [150].

Neuropathic pain is not caused by activation of specific pain receptors but instead, is caused by abnormal neural activity.

(The term neuropathic pain theoretically relates to pain from the nervous system in general. However, people in different professions use the term differently. Neurologists, for example, seem to restrict the use of the term to describe different forms of pain from peripheral and cranial nerves and use modifiers such as central or chronic to describe other forms of pain from the nervous system).

Also, investigators have used different terms to describe pain from the nervous system. Devor has defined neuropathic pain as pain caused by lesions to the nervous system such as to nerves [150] or the central nervous system (central neuropathic pain or chronic neuropathic pain). According to Merskey and the IASP chronic neuropathic pain is pain caused by a lesion or dysfunction in the central nervous system [413] by the IASP.

Pain may cause many different reactions and activate other parts of the nervous system such as the autonomic nervous system. Pain can often cause emotional (affective) reactions such as anger and fear, anxiety and depression, which relate to an abnormal activation of limbic structures, especially the amygdala but also the cingulate gyrus and the periaqueductal gray (PAG). This activation of the amygdala may occur through cortical routes from the dorsal thalamus [353], see [460]). Evidence has mounted that dysfunctional networks in the brain contribute to many of such complex symptoms [354].

In this Appendix, we will first discuss the anatomy and physiology of the systems that process acute pain. We will discuss some treatments for pain and their mechanisms of action, as well as their side effects. Pain in which activation of neuroplasticity plays an important role is covered in Chapter 6 in this book. A more detailed description of the biology of pain can be found in the book: [461]. (See also [460]).

Clinical assessment of pain intensity

In the office setting, it is common for physicians to ask patients to grade their current pain level on a 0-10 scale with 0 representing no pain and ten the worst pain they have ever experienced, to provide a rough index of the severity of pain and track relative levels of pain over time. In addition to this subjective rating, the examiner assesses the effect that the pain has had on limiting the patient's activities under the assumption that more severe pain tends to be associated with greater relative reductions in physical activities.

The clinician may evaluate the psychological effects of pain including depression to obtain a better picture of the severity and the effects of the patient's pain. However, quantitative evaluations of the suffering from pain are not common. The fact that pain can be regarded as having two components, one being the sensation of pain "hurt" and the other being the degree of suffering is not recognized and a person's evaluation of pain may not represent the suffering component.

The fact that pain sensation is regulated through cortical and limbic structures may explain how psychological factors can modulate the sensation of pain.

For people who have difficulty communicating, other measurements such as of autonomic functions such as heart rate, blood pressure, sweating and, restlessness, and agitation, etc. are also been used as indices of pain. For instance, it is common for anesthesiologists to use acute elevations in the patient's blood pressure as an indicator that the patient may be experiencing pain and hence require deeper anesthesia.

Somatic pain

Tissue damage, such as that caused by injuries due to accidents, is a common cause of acute pain. Most forms of postoperative pain are due to tissue damage produced by the surgical procedure. Ischemia can cause pain through stimulation of specific pain receptors and is probably the cause of an aspect of muscle pain that occurs after strenuous exercise.

Inflammation of the peripheral nerves, nerve roots, joints, tendons, and muscles are also common causes of pain. Muscle and joint pain such as in rheumatoid arthritis, are common causes of chronic pain. Tooth pulp contains C-fibers but not A fibers, so dental pain lacks the "fast phase" and is often poorly defined and is this perceived as a broad ache.

Nerve compression and entrapment

Mechanical irritation and compression of peripheral and cranial nerves can cause pain either through stimulation the mechanoreceptive nociceptors in the *nervi nervorum* or through generating impulses in the nerve proper, where unmyelinated fibers (C-fibers) and small myelinated fibers (Aδ fibers) become mechanosensitive through an inflammatory process or other pathology that changes the membrane properties. Without the presence of one of these latter processes, only large myelinated fibers (Aα and Aβ fibers), are sensitive to mechanical compression. This means that compression of peripheral nerves or their roots does not normally cause pain and if it does, the nerve is usually inflamed. The common back pain can therefore often be treated successfully by administration of an anti-inflammatory agent such as ibuprofen.

Compression of sensory fibers typically causes paresthesia, described as tingling, or "pins and needles" sensations. Compression of the smaller C or Aδ fibers due to spinal stenosis will only produce pain if the nerve root is inflamed or otherwise injured. Compression of motor nerves usually causes muscle weakness.

Acute or chronic back pain is a typical example of a pain condition with complex causes [369]. Acute back pain is known as sciatica because it often involves the sciatic nerve. Symptoms typically consist of bursts of shooting or stabbing pain that limits motion and often interferes with posture. The pain may "radiate" down a leg. It is caused by acute damage to spinal nerve roots and lasts from a few days to a few weeks. It is mechanical in nature often caused by trauma endured during work or sports.

Chronic, often diffuse, low back pain is the most common medical complaint in industrial countries. Back or leg pain is often associated with structural spine abnormalities such as compression of spinal roots, and bulging or herniated vertebral disks.

This association, however, is loose; there have many different forms and actual the cause often is unknown. While compression of spinal nerve roots can cause back pain, not all back pain is caused by compression of spinal nerve roots [369, 705] and much is musculoskeletal in origin. In fact, similar abnormalities often occur in asymptomatic persons [260]. In fact, only inflamed nerve roots cause pain when compressed.

Various kinds of spondylotic diseases can cause back pain [705]. Spinal stenosis is a frequent cause of back pain, but the stenotic abnormalities that are revealed from MRI or CT scans are poorly correlated with the pain that a person experience [369] as many people with spinal stenosis do not have pain. (Spinal stenosis: Decrease in size of spinal foramina with subsequent compression of spinal nerves). A similar paradox occurs in other situations, such as in connection with vascular contact (compression) of cranial nerves [439].

Back pain and traumatic nerve injuries are frequent causes of disability and early retirement and, as such, have enormous economic implications. Due to the difficulty in establishing a causal relationship pain and morphological abnormalities, insurance companies have room to question the credibility of the patients in question and refuse them adequate treatment.

It is believed that the pain in the carpal tunnel syndrome is caused by pressure on or entrapment of the median nerve [394, 639]. Carpal tunnel syndrome is the second most common industrial injury in the U.S.A. [639]. The pain and tingling can often be relieved by surgically decompressing the nerve, but the symptoms can also be relieved by splinting, cortisone injections, massage, and immersion of the hand in water. Resting the limb or change of activities can also relieve the symptoms.

Like many other pain conditions, the pain from carpal tunnel syndrome is worsened by psychosocial factors such as boredom, stress, job dissatisfaction, monotonous routines, and insecurity.

Ulnar nerve entrapment is the second most common entrapment neuropathy [394, 639], carpal tunnel syndrome being the first with symptoms of numbness and tingling in the distribution on the hand of the ulnar nerve (the fifth digit and the lateral aspect of the fourth). Other peripheral nerves such as the sciatic and common peroneal nerves are subject for similar entrapment (for an overview of mononeuropathies, see [394]).

Again, if entrapment of a mixed nerve causes pain, the nerve is often inflamed. Compression of healthy nerves does not produce pain, but instead, it may cause other sensations such as tingling.

The fact that treatments that do not relieve the presumed entrapment are effective in disorders such as many forms of low back pain and the carpal tunnel syndrome support the hypothesis that inflammatory processes are a prerequisite for nerve compression causing pain. These forms of pain, particularly when lasting a long time may also have a central component.

A more benign form of compression of peripheral nerves occurs when the sciatic nerve is compressed while sitting with crossed legs or while resting the upper parts of the legs on a hard surface. Symptoms include tingling in the leg and foot, but not pain, supporting the hypothesis that mechanical compression of a peripheral nerve mainly affects large diameter myelinated fibers leaving smaller (pain) fibers unaffected.

Such compression interferes with the axoplasmatic flow in the axons, and cause ischemia which may be the cause of the specific sensations that are associated with acute compression of large peripheral nerves [339].

Muscle pain manifests in two main forms: Pain that is associated with muscle contractions and pain that occurs independently of muscle contractions. Naturally, muscle spasm and excessive exercise may cause pain in muscles from exhaustion, but many forms of muscle pain are not related to muscle contractions. Several disorders involving muscle referred pain are not even accompanied by any detectable muscle pathologies. To complicate this issue, the descriptions that patients provide of such pain vary greatly [490].

The term myalgia is used to describe muscle pain of many etiologies, including some that have cerebral involvement such as encephalomyelitis and chronic fatigue syndrome (fibromyalgia). Chronic fatigue syndrome is an ill-defined disorder that is more likely a group of disorders that involve many unknown factors together with stress, boredom, unsatisfying work or troublesome home conditions, etc.

Myalgia (pain from muscles) can have many causes, and it may be difficult to differentiate it from a pain that originates from other tissues such as joints, tendons, ligaments, and bones.

For example, headaches that are caused by contraction of neck muscles may not be easily distinguished from pain due to other causes. The muscle contractions that cause or contribute to severe pain are often tonic and therefore not as easy to detect as tremor or spasm.

Painful muscle contractions may be associated with EMG activity, which is a sign that the contractions are caused by α motoneuron activity, but muscle contractions may also have chemical causes such as electrolytic imbalance or changes in the extra cellular fluid [351].

There are three different forms of contractile activation of muscles: (1) electrogenic stiffness caused by activation of motoneurons and neuromuscular endplates (have observable EMG activity); (2) electrogenic spasm (pathological and involuntary electrogenic contraction), and (3) contracture (occurring within the muscle fibers independent of EMG activity) [629].

The tension or the tonus of a muscle depends both on the activation of the contractile apparatus and on the basic viscoelastic properties of the muscle tissue. Only the first mentioned form of activation is associated with EMG activity; the other form of contraction causes an increased mechanical stiffness of the muscles that is not induced by activity in the motor nerve that innervates the muscle in question. Muscle contraction can, therefore, occur without any measurable electrophysiological signs, a factor that has clinical diagnostic importance. Such increased mechanical stiffness can be determined through physical examination and can be measured quantitatively as resistance against a slowly applied force.

Words like, muscle tone and muscle tension, are sometimes used synonymously, but some authors [629] define muscle tone to mean only viscoelastic changes in a muscle that occurs in the absence of contractile neural activity.

The resting muscle tone has been assumed to be caused by a low rate of firing of motor nerves thus caused by the activity of α motoneurons. However, this assumption seems to rest on a misconception according to Simons and Mense [629] who described methods to measure muscle tone mechanically and credited Walsh 1992 [699] for clarifying the misconception that muscle tone was normally caused by electrical activation of the contractile apparatus of muscles.

Increased muscle activity (spasm) contributes to such forms of pain as back pain and tension headache. The form of spasm of muscles that causes pain is usually tonic contractions.

Hyperactivity of α motoneurons from increased excitatory input or decreased inhibitory input of segmental or supraspinal origin may cause spasm.

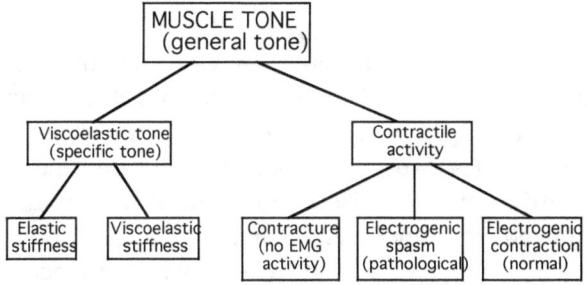

Figure C.4. The relationship between terms commonly used to characterize muscle tension: tone, stiffness, contracture, and spasm. Based on [629].

Muscle Pain

Pain from muscles may be caused by stimulation of nociceptors, but many forms of muscle pain such as myofascial pain and fibromyalgia have a complex pathophysiology, most of which is unknown.

There is considerable evidence that altered function of central nervous system structures is involved in producing muscle pain. Proprioceptors, such as tendon organs and receptors in joint and ligaments and muscle spindles, may be involved in signaling pain due to excessive muscle contractions.

The output of proprioceptors may cause pain Often initiate from trigger zones in the temporalis muscle, in suboccipital, sternocleidomastoid, and upper trapezius muscles from where pain attacks can be elicited. Based on Simons and Mense1998 [629]).by activating neural circuits that are normally not activated by proprioceptors, thus similar to the cross-modal interaction that occurs in neuropathic pain causing allodynia. Local processes in the spinal cord that affect muscle tone can also affect the sensation of muscle pain.

Studies have shown that there are specific nociceptors throughout muscles that may mediate pain [490]. These nociceptors are free nerve endings that are mostly located near muscle endplates. They are innervated by Aδ fibers like the nociceptors found in the skin, and they may play a role in causing pain from excessive muscle contractions [224]. Several kinds of noxious stimuli such as chemicals and mechanical stimulation can activate the same nociceptors [224], which are also sensitive to endogenous substances, such as those released during inflammatory processes and injury. Exposure to chemical and mechanical stimuli can sensitize these receptors.

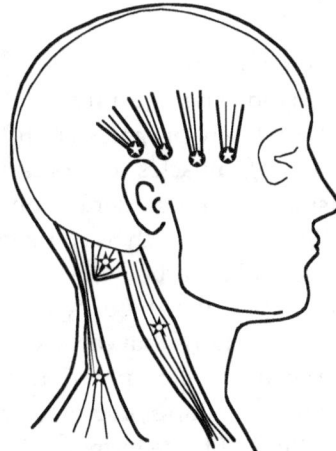

Figure C.3 Tension-type headaches are often initiated from trigger zones in the temporal muscle, in suboccipital, sternocleidomastoid, and upper trapezoid muscle from where pain attacks can be elicited. Based on Simon and Mense 1998 [629].

It has been debated whether tension headaches are forms of myofascial spasm [684]. The involvement of temporomandibular joint disorders, or a combination of that and some other factors have been suspected to a contributing factor in what is often called tension headaches. Anyhow, despite the frequency and the socioeconomic consequences of tension headaches [296], little is known about the pathophysiology of the disorder, and consequently, the search of treatments have been mostly of empirical nature [129].

Muscle tension as a cause of pain

Muscle tension plays an important role as a cause of pain. Abnormally increased muscle tone can be caused either by changes in the viscoelastic properties of muscles or by contractile activity mediated by the motor nerve and the motoneurons (Figure C.4)

Animal experiments have shown that serotonin combined with bradykinin [412] can produce muscle hyperalgesia from mechanical stimuli (pressure) [224]. The peripheral sensitization of muscle nociceptors is rapidly followed by functional changes in dorsal horn neurons, similar to that which occurs in acute myositis. (Myositis: Inflammation of muscles).

Input from the sympathetic nervous system increases α motoneuron excitability. Since pain increases sympathetic activity, a vicious cycle may be initiated.

This cycle may increase or maintain pain after the original cause of the pain dissipated. For example, if we assume that back pain is initiated by a transient compression or injury to a dorsal root, and then the initial pain may cause increased sympathetic activity that further increases the activity of α motoneurons causing pain.

That pain may become self-sustaining and persist after the injury to the dorsal root has healed. This process can only be interrupted if the pain is eliminated totally for some time. Incomplete relief of acute pain may facilitate pain by further activating the sympathetic nervous system.

The term muscle spasm is usually used to describe involuntary muscle contractions that are accompanied by EMG activity. Examples of pain from involuntary muscle contractions are spasmodic torticollis, trismus, stiff-man syndrome and nocturnal leg cramps, but even tension headaches belong to this group of disorders. Trismus is an involuntary closing of the jaw due to tonic spasm of muscles of mastication. Spasmodic torticollis [524] was discussed in the chapter on motor disorders. It is a source of pain because of the persistent muscle contractions. Nocturnal leg cramps that involve mainly contraction of the gastrocnemius muscle are painful.

One likely pathway for maintaining pain from muscle contractions consists of neurons in the dorsal horn (or trigeminal nucleus) that receive input from nociceptors in muscles and which activate neurons in the sensory regions of the cerebral cortex through a thalamic pathway. These neurons in the sensory cortex then activate neurons in several regions of the brain such as limbic structures and SMA the neurons of which can activate neurons in the motor cortex, and subsequently α-motoneurons, completing a circle that can maintain muscle contractions.

Interrupting that vicious circle at any point can relieve the pain. Inducing paresis of the afflicted muscle for instance by Botulinum toxin is one way of doing that.

The finding that the effect of Botulinum treatment increased gradually over a 60-day observation period supports the hypothesis that neuroplasticity of proprioception is involved.

The "stiff man" syndrome

The "stiff-man" syndrome is a rare condition that is characterized by slowly progressive stiffness of axial and proximal leg muscles and occasional painful muscle spasms. It is a disorder of spinal or brainstem origin [351] and is characterized by antibodies to glutamic acid decarboxylase (GAD) in a majority of people with these symptoms. Involuntary muscle contractions that cause pain are often loosely described as cramp, contracture, spasm, or tetanus without making precise reference to the accurate definitions of these terms [264, 490].

Myofascial pain

Myofascial pain is closely related to painful muscle contractions (muscle spasm). Myofascial pain is a complex disorder, the pathophysiology of which is poorly understood. The presence of trigger points is typical for the disease, and much research has been devoted to studies of the basis for such trigger points.

We mentioned trigger zones in connection with trigeminal neuralgia. Myofascial pain syndrome often has trigger points from which pain attacks can be elicited [73, 264].

Myofascial trigger points are described as being sensitive spots on a muscle where a palpable "taut" band of muscle fibers can be identified [264]. These trigger points can be identified by finger palpation. Trigger points can be located not only at the place to which the pain is referred but also to locations that are distant to that of the perceived pain.

Studies have shown that various kinds of treatment directed to such trigger points can alleviate the pain. Other studies have indicated that the trigger points represent a spinal reflex [238, 264] (Figure C.5). Reduced range of motion, local pain, and muscle tenderness are common symptoms that occur together with pain in the myofascial pain syndrome.

The cause is not known but may be inflammatory, though some investigators believe it is psychosomatic. The myofascial pain syndrome is often associated with trigger points from where pain attacks can be elicited. Referred pain is common in disorders of myofascial pain [264].

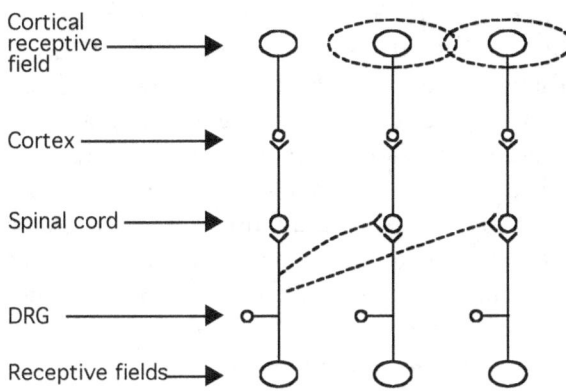

Figure C.5. Hypothesis about the expansion of a receptive field and creation of trigger points by the unmasking of dormant synapses. (Adapted from Hong and Simons (1998)[264]).

Other investigators have hypothesized that the trigger points are regions of a muscle with a "local twitch response" (LTR) associated with loci of high sensitivity that have developed as a result of minor injuries. It has been shown that such "latent trigger points" [679] occur in 50 % of asymptomatic individuals [271]. These loci can be converted into active trigger points by some external event which causes them to sensitize their nociceptors. Leakage of calcium and other substances may activate nearby muscle fibers resulting in the formation of a taut band. The EMG activity that can be recorded from these "taut bands" is very localized and is not caused by endplate potentials [271]. It has therefore been hypothesized that the EMG activity at the trigger points is caused by contractions of intrafusal muscles caused by sympathetic activity [271] (Figure C.6). That means that the LTR may be a polysynaptic reflex.

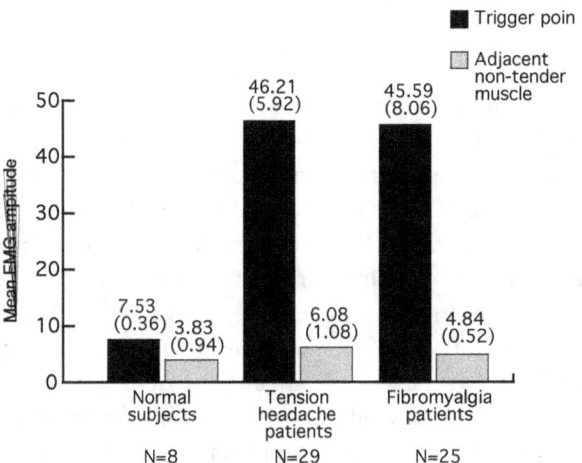

Figure C.6 Mean EMG amplitudes (and standards errors) recorded from a muscle at a trigger point and an adjacent non-tender muscle. (Data from [271]).

Fibromyalgia

Fibromyalgia [51] presents with a wealth of more or less diffuse symptoms, one being chronic and widespread muscle pain (see chapter 5). Fibromyalgia has therefore been regarded as a muscle disorder (hence the name), but little evidence of abnormalities (pathologies) of muscles has been found despite great efforts. Criteria for a definition of fibromyalgia have been proposed, but it seems clear that the disorder called fibromyalgia is not a single entity but rather a complex basket of pathologies. The symptoms may differ from person to person and from time to time. While the main symptoms of fibromyalgia are muscle pain, depression is an important component as is fatigue.

Fibromyalgia and myofascial spasm are no longer regarded as disorders of the muscles. It has recently been suggested that maladaptive neuroplasticity together with activation of the immune system are involved in fibromyalgia [487] [246] and likewise in the chronic fatigue syndrome [113, 469].

These hypotheses are also supported by the fact that pain management aiming at chronic neuropathic pain using psychotherapy, exercise, and psychoactive drugs are effective means of treatment for this disorder.

Headaches

Headaches are forms of pain that affect many people. The category includes migraines, cluster headaches, and tension headaches. The term primary headaches refer to headaches that have no clear cause [52]. Migraines are forms of primary headaches. Migraines are of two kinds; one form presents with an aura (classic migraine) and one does not have an aura (common migraines) [58]. While headaches occur in approximately 91% of men and 96% of women, migraines are about three times as frequent in in women as in men (about 6% of men and 18% of women). Migraines are most common in the third decade of life and in lower socioeconomic groups. Migraines are associated with an increased prevalence of depression and panic attacks [582, 624].

Migraines involves the trigemino-vascular system and sensitization of the trigeminal nucleus and nociceptors in the meninges [738] as well [68]. Migraines are often accompanied by allodynia, indicating the involvement of expression of neuroplasticity [88].

There is also evidence that migraines are neurogenic disorders [76, 582] and that the insula lobe may be involved in creating the symptoms of migraines [76]. There are indications that female reproductive hormones are involved in creation of the symptoms of migraines. Migraines are frequent in women during fertile age but decreases after menopause. The "footprints" of migraines in the brain persist and after menopause common headaches are common on the side where the migraines were.

Mild increase in blood pressure can aggravate the pain in migraines because of sensitization of peripheral nociceptors that innervate intracranial blood vessels.

Sensitization of second-order neurons in the spinal cord on which input from intracranial structures and skin in the ophthalmic skin converge may explain the allodynia that often accompanies migraine attacks and the referred pain in the periorbital region [88]. Allodynia outside the area of referred pain may be explained by sensitization of third order trigemino-vascular neurons that receive input from the head and the upper limb in addition to input from intracranial structures.

The developments of drugs in the triptan family (e.g. Sumatriptan), which are selective 5-HT1B/1D receptor agonists, were a considerable the improvement in treatment of migraine and cluster headache. Non-specific pain-relieving drugs [129] and some unconventional treatments, such as application of capsaicin in the nose, have been shown to have beneficial effects in relieving these symptoms.

Cluster headaches and migraines are complex disorders with other symptoms than pain such as tearing and stuffy nose on one side. Cluster headaches are caused by pathologies of the brain [129]. Recent studies seem to support the hypothesis that vascular pathologies are involved in causing the symptoms of migraine, in that it has been shown that the individuals with migraine have a higher incidence of strokes than individuals who do not have migraine headaches [337]. Cluster headaches are cousins to migraines that often respond to the same treatments.

Symptoms of myocardial infarction

It has been shown that specific cells in the thalamus are dedicated to pain from ischemia of the heart [503]. Ischemia of the heart often occurs without specific pain sensations and presents as a general feeling of being unwell, and it may be associated with other diffuse symptoms such as nausea [488]. These expressions of cardiac ischemia may be communicated by the vagus nerve.

In many cases, myocardial infarction does not present with any pain symptoms, but rather gives diffuse symptoms such as a feeling of illness, nausea, etc. In a large population study (Framingham study) it was found that as much as 25% of the incidences of myocardial infarction was unrecognized by the individuals, and in one-half of these, the episodes were truly silent [531].

Visceral pain

Visceral pain is not perceived in the same way as somatic pain, and the location of the pain is less specific than somatic pain, and it often has an emotional component being inescapable [60]. Pain that originates in the viscera and the heart is often referred to locations on the surface of the body [531], and such pain is known as referred pain.

Most visceral nociceptors are free nerve endings that are chemoreceptors or stretch receptors [105]. The chemoreceptors are sensitive to substances secreted from an inflamed or ischemic tissue.

Stretching of smooth muscles and ischemia are common causes of visceral pain from the gut. Cutting, crushing, or burning of the bowel does not evoke pain but distension of muscles and hollow organs, stretching of organs, ischemia, and necrosis generates pain. Chemical irritation of the gut can result in pain as can inflammation. It is debated whether visceral pain is caused by activation of non-specific wide dynamic range receptors rather than specific nociceptors [105, 546].

Referred pain

Referred pain is an example of redirected (misdirected) spatial pain information. Pain that which may occur during myocardial infarction is not always localized to the heart but instead, referred to a different location on the body, usually on the surface [531]. The locations to which the pain is referred varies among individuals. Pain from the heart is referred to the left arm, jaw, and epigastrium; whereas pain from the gallbladder is often referred to right shoulder, hip and knee. Pain from organs in the pelvis is referred to dermatomes of T_{12}-L_1 (and perhaps L_2 and L_3), often bilaterally.

No secondary neuron in the spinal cord receives only visceral input, and there are much fewer visceral than somatic afferents [105]. The visceral pain system thus has a little-dedicated infrastructure, which may be why pain from viscera is so poorly localized.

Pain from the nervous system

Neuropathic pain theoretically includes all forms of the pain originating in the nervous system caused by morphological changes in the nervous system, or by functional changes such as those that result from expression of neuroplasticity. Neurologists, however, usually only use the term neuropathic pain to describe pain that is associated with nerves.

In this book, we will use the term central neuropathic pain to describe the pain that is generated by abnormal activity in the central nervous system without input from nociceptors (see Chapter 6).

Pain associated with peripheral nerves is common, and its causes can be compression, trauma, or inflammation. Compression and trauma (including surgically induced trauma) usually affect a single nerve, as do some forms of viral-induced inflammation.

Many peripheral and cranial nerves may be affected in diabetes and alcohol-related neuropathies. Age-related changes may also cause pain that is related to nerves. Pain from the central nervous system may be caused by trauma or ischemia such as from strokes (infarcts or bleeding). Since subdural bleedings do not usually produce pain, pains that occur together with intracranial bleeding (approximately 15% of all strokes are hemorrhagic) may be caused by the accompanying vasospasm. (For details see [460]).

Central nervous system pain

There are two main categories of CNS pain. One is related to morphological changes such as trauma and strokes, and the other is related to functional changes such as those induced by expression of neuroplasticity.

Injuries to the central nervous system such as those arising from trauma (traumatic brain injuries, TBI) or ischemia can produce pain, but little is known about how such pain is related to the insult in question. Strokes may cause pain depending on which regions of the brain are affected. Tissue damage and ischemia are assumed to cause the pain.

A specific kind of pain is related to injuries of the thalamus (thalamic pain) (Dejerine-Roussy syndrome) [259]. It is noteworthy that lesions to specific structures of the thalamus can cause relief of pain.

Nerve injuries may be associated with transsynaptic degeneration of cell bodies in the dorsal horn [652], and sprouting of Aδ fibers to the superficial lamina of the dorsal horn [730], which may cause pain sensations and pain from innocuous stimulation ("allodynia").

The pathophysiology of pain that is related to insult to the central nervous system such as strokes, other forms of ischemia, or iatrogenic lesions is poorly understood. It is interesting that lesions to the thalamus can give specific pain syndromes (thalamic pain), while lesions in other parts of the thalamus are effective in treating pain [744]. Paradoxically, strokes that affect specific parts of the thalamus produce pain and analgesia and loss of temperature sensation at the same time.

Pain pathways

Pain pathways are usually regarded as belonging to the somatosensory system [460], but the central nervous system pathways of pain (the anterolateral system) have both similarities and differences with the part of the somatosensory system that mediates innocuous sensations. In this book, we regard the pain pathways to be the non-classical somatosensory pathways. Like sensory systems, chronic neuropathic pain pathways consist of ascending and descending pathways.

The ascending pathways communicate information from the periphery to central structures that provide the conscious reactions to pain stimuli, as well as unconscious reactions.

The pathways for nociceptor pain are known as the anterolateral system and consist of the anterior and the lateral tracts of the spinothalamic tract (STT), the spinomesencephalic tracts, and the spinoreticular tract. The STT is regarded as the most important one. The STT and the spinomesencephalic tracts are mainly crossed pathways while the spinoreticular tract is bilateral. Pain information from the face and the inside of the mouth [299] enters the brainstem through the trigeminal nerve. These fibers make synaptic contact with cells in the caudal division of the trigeminal nucleus [299].

The spinothalamic tract (STT) has two parts, the ventral and the lateral STT. The lateral tract originates in cells in lamina I (substantia gelantinosa) and the anterior tract originates in cells in lamina IV and V of the spinal (dorsal) horn.

The descending pathways communicate information from central structures to neurons along the ascending pathways, including the dorsal horn of the spinal cord and sensory nuclei of the brainstem (mainly the trigeminal nucleus). The descending pathways can modulate the neural traffic in these ascending pathways.

In addition to these ascending and descending pathways, the autonomic nervous system plays a role in the processing of pain information in the spinal cord. The sympathetic nervous system can modulate the sensitivity of nociceptors (mainly sensitize), and it can affect the synaptic threshold and synaptic efficacy of neurons in the spinal cord.

Diffusion of neuroactive substances in the gray matter of the spinal cord can affect spinal cord synaptic transmission of pain. (For information about the pharmacology of the dorsal horn, see [736, 737]).

Neural circuitry in the spinal cord

Pain fibers that enter the spinal cord in dorsal roots make synaptic contact with cells in the dorsal horn (Figure C.7), and most of the axons of these cells cross the midline at the segmental level and ascend in the anterolateral tracts [83]. Most C-fibers terminate on cells in lamina II of the dorsal horn.

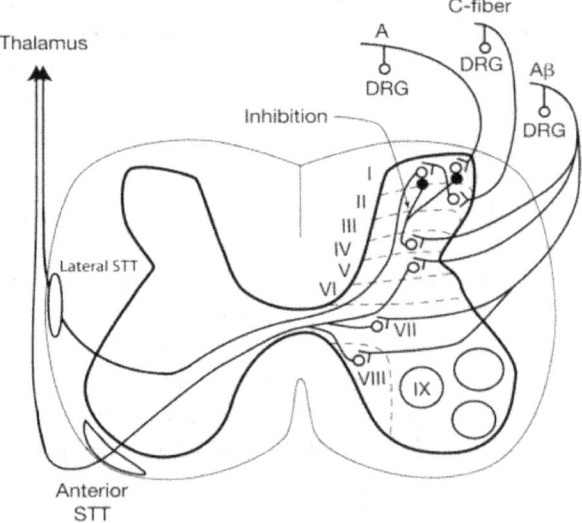

Figure C.7. The termination of the Aβ, Aδ, and C fibers in the dorsal horn of the spinal cord and their ascending connections that carry innocuous information to the dorsal column nuclei and the two tracts (lateral and anterior) of the pain pathways (spinothalamic tract, STT). DRG: Dorsal root ganglion. (Artwork by Monica Javidnia).

Aδ fibers terminate on cells in layer I but have collaterals that terminate in laminae IV and V [83]. The short axons of the cell in lamina II make synaptic contact with cells in lamina I. (Lamina I is also known as the substantia gelatinosa). Some of the interneurons in lamina I send collaterals (secondary branches) to more rostral or more caudal segments traveling in the tract of Lissauer (dorsolateral fasciculus).

Some cells are modality specific, and others are polymodal, (Figure C.8) meaning that they receive input from nociceptors that respond to different modalities of noxious stimuli.

The simultaneous connection of incoming pain fibers to cells in multiple segments is important for understanding some of the pathologies of the spinal cord and peripheral nerves.

Studies of how plastic changes can affect the way these collaterals can activate cells in other segments was one of the first solid proofs of the importance of activation of neuroplasticity. Normally, axons that enter a certain segment can only activate cells in that segment and a few neighboring segments (Figure C.8). Patrick Wolf showed ([697]) that when the dorsal root to a segment of the spinal cord was severed, the input to that segment from a distant segment could activate cells that such input was unable to activate before the root was severed.

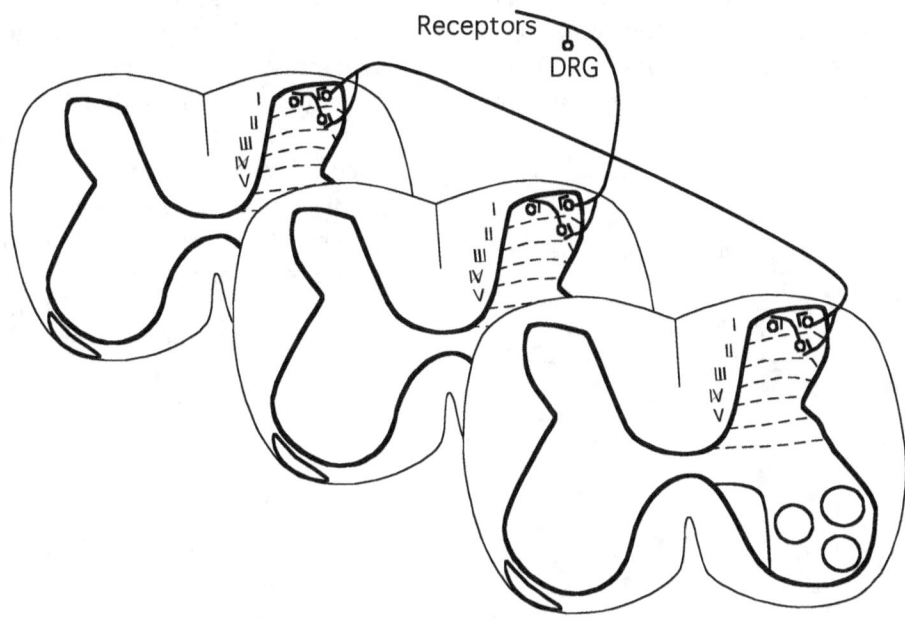

Figure C.8. Collateral interneurons in lamina I terminate in spinal segments above and below the segment where their innervation enters (the tract of Lissauer). (Artwork by Monica Javidnia).

One branch of the large diameter (Aβ) fibers that innervates innocuous sensory receptors ascends to dorsal column nuclei. Another branch of these fibers terminates on cells in laminae III, IV, and V of the dorsal horn of the spinal cord (Figure C.7). Some of these cells send axons that terminate in inhibitory synapses on cells in lamina I of the spinal cord horns. Innocuous sensory information can thus have an inhibitory effect on the transmission of nociceptive information in the dorsal horn.

The spinal cord circuitry illustrated in Figures C.7 and C.8 has been highly simplified. It shows mainly connections from receptors to the spinal cord and from the spinal cord to supraspinal structures and omits most of the internal connections in the spinal cord.

Each cell has many inputs, both inhibitory and excitatory, and in fact, most of the synaptic connections to cells in the spinal horns originate in other cells in the spinal horn of the same or other segments of the spinal cord. This internal circuitry is very important for processing of pain information.

The spinothalamic tract

The pathways for nociceptor pain are known as the anterolateral system consisting of the anterior and the lateral tracts of the spinothalamic tract (STT), the spinomesencephalic tract, and the spinoreticular tract.

The STT and the spinomesencephalic tract are mainly crossed pathways while the spinoreticular tract is bilateral. Pain information from the face and the inside of the mouth [299] enters the brainstem through the trigeminal nerve.

These fibers make synaptic contact with cells in the caudal division of the trigeminal nucleus [299].

The spinothalamic tract (STT) has two parts, the ventral and the lateral STT. The lateral tract originates in cells in lamina I (substantia gelatinosa) (Figure C.9) and the anterior tract originates in cells in lamina IV and V (Figure C.10. The fibers of the STT in humans, originate mostly in interneurons in lamina I and V ([83] but additionally the axons of WDR neurons in deeper layers of the spinal horn contribute. These axons cross the midline at the segmental level and ascend as the STT towards the thalamus.

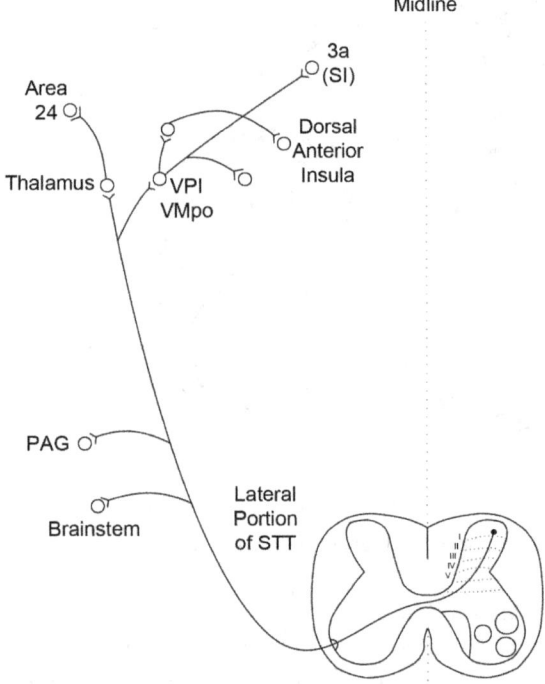

Figure C.9 Connections from the lateral portion of the STT from cells in lamina I of the dorsal horn. VPI: Ventral posterior inferior (nuclei of the thalamus); VMpo: Ventromedial posterior oralis (nuclei of the thalamus); SI: Primary somatosensory cortex. (Modified from Møller, A. R. (2006) Neuroplasticity and disorders of the nervous system. Cambridge University Press Cambridge. Reprinted with permission from Cambridge University Press [448][288].) Artwork by Monica Javidnia.

The fibers of the lateral part of the STT mainly originate in cells in lamina I of the dorsal horn and project to the medial and posterior thalamus. The axons of these cells project to the insula and some extent to area 3a of the SI.

The dorsomedial thalamic neurons also connect to neurons in the reticular formation and the periaqueductal gray (PAG).

The PAG (also known as the central gray) surrounds the aqueduct interconnecting the third and fourth ventricle. It is involved in (suppression of) pain, and it has many other functions. The PAG connects to the amygdala, hypothalamus, thalamus, locus coeruleus, and other structures [461].

The targets of the anterior STT are cells in the lateral, medial and intermediate parts of the ventral thalamus (ventral posterior lateral (VPL), the ventral posterior medial (VPM), ventral posterior inferior (VPI) nuclei and several nuclei in the mediodorsal thalamus (Figure C.10). The anterior portion of the STT gives off collateral fibers to several structures in the brainstem such as to cells in the reticular formation.

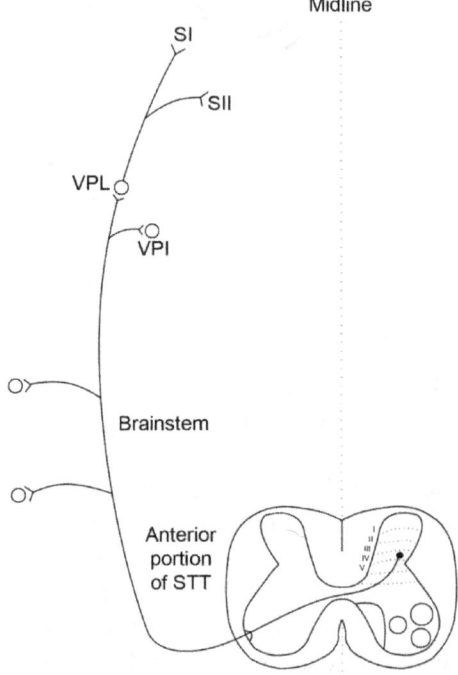

Figure C.10 Connections from the anterior STT from neurons in lamina IV-V. VPI: Ventral posterior inferior (nuclei of the thalamus); VPL: Ventral posterior lateral (nuclei of the thalamus). (Modified from Møller, A. R. (2006) Neuroplasticity and disorders of the nervous system. Cambridge University Press Cambridge [448][288]). (Artwork by Monica Javidnia).

Before reaching the thalamus, STT gives off collateral fibers to several structures in the brainstem, such as to cells in the reticular formation.

The cells of the VPL and VPI project to the primary somatosensory cortex (SI) and this pathway is likely responsible for the fast phase of pain that is localized.

The dorsomedial thalamic neurons connect to neurons in the reticular formation and the PAG also known as the central gray. The PAG is a small group of cells that surrounds the aqueduct interconnecting the third and fourth ventricle. It is involved in suppression of pain, and it has many other functions. The PAG connects to the amygdala, hypothalamus, thalamus, locus coeruleus and other structures (Figure C. 11).

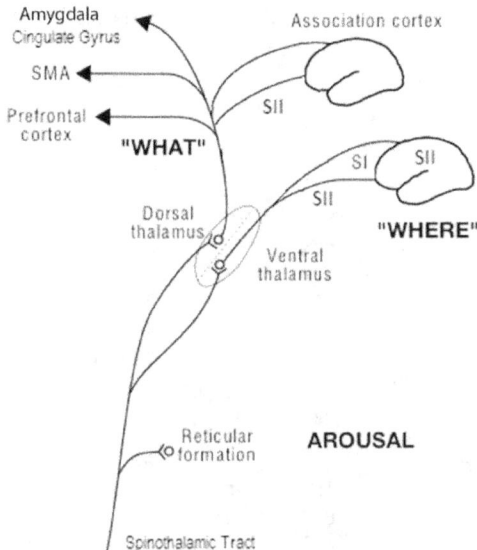

Figure C.11 A simplified summary of the ascending central portions of pain pathways, emphasizing that stimulation of nociceptors produces two kinds of information, namely objective ("what") and spatial ("where") information. The figure also shows some of the regions of the brain that can be reached by neural activity that is elicited by painful stimuli. The nuclei of the ventral thalamus also receive input from the somatosensory system via the medial lemniscus, providing spatial information regarding skin stimulation. (Artwork by Monica Javidnia).

Some fibers of the anterior STT originate in cells in lamina IV of the spinal cord. The cells of laminae VII and VIII that send fibers in the anterior STT are polysensory and, therefore, more complex than cells in another lamina of the spinal cord.

These cells have polysynaptic innervation by converging sensory fibers that respond to both innocuous and noxious stimuli. Some of these cells probably also integrate motor and sensory information.

The cells of the VPL and VPI project to the primary and secondary somatosensory cortex (SI and SII) and this pathway is likely responsible for the fast phase of pain that is localized. This means that only the anterior STT (Figure C.10) has connections to the ventral thalamus and from there, fibers connect to the SI. The ventral thalamus provides spatial information ("where"), while the part that uses the dorsal-medial thalamus mainly provides information about the character of the pain ("what").

Targets of unmyelinated fibers

In humans, the activity in unmyelinated (C-fibers) has been shown to reach both SI and SII cortical areas on the contralateral side, and SII on the ipsilateral side [306]. The fact that pure C-fiber activation reaches the SI cortex may imply that activation of C-fibers may produce a sensation of pressure or touch in addition to a sensation of pain (Figure C. 12).

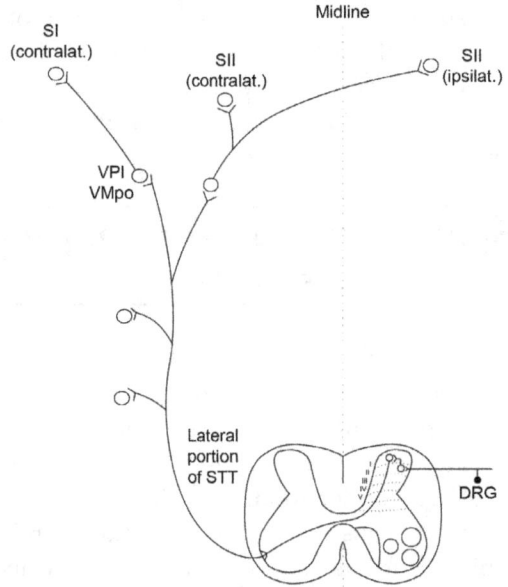

Figure C.12 Schematic illustration of the projection of unmyelinated C-fibers through the lateral portion of the spinothalamic tract (STT). Notice that the projections to SII are bilateral, but SI only receives input from contralateral receptors. (Artwork by Monica Javidnia.

Other ascending pain tracts

Of the other ascending tracts of the anterior lateral system, the spinoreticular tract (Figure C.13) is largely bilateral, and its main target is the reticular formation of the brainstem.

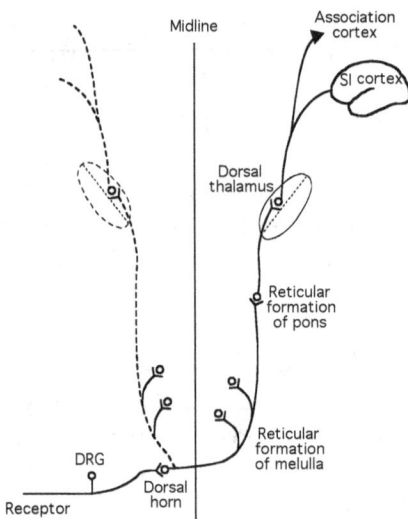

Figure C.13. The spinoreticular tract [461]. (Artwork by Monica Javidnia).

It should be remembered that each of the anterior lateral tracts gives off collateral fibers at many levels, many of which terminate in the reticular formation of the brainstem, affecting wakefulness.

Spinal cord processing of pain signals

The network of neurons in the dorsal horn that is involved in the transmission of pain signals to supraspinal structures is complex, and the processing that occurs in these neurons is incompletely understood. It is known, however, that interneurons in the dorsal horn and the trigeminal nucleus play an important role in the modulation of transmission of pain impulses because they receive inhibitory as well as excitatory input from supraspinal sources (for details see [460]).

Input from sensory receptors in the skin can modulate the transmission of pain signals in the dorsal horn of the spinal cord and the trigeminal nucleus.

The function of these interneurons is affected by chemicals such as SP and other potent neuroactive substances (such as norepinephrine and serotonin) that reach these interneurons through diffusion in the gray matter of the spinal cord or the trigeminal nucleus.

Wide dynamic range neurons

Some of the cells in laminae IV and V are known as the wide dynamic range (WDR) neurons [83] because the outputs from these cells reflect a large range of intensities of their inputs. Some fibers of the anterior STT originate in the WDR neurons in lamina IV and V of the spinal cord. These WDR cells (Figure C.14) receive input from both mechanoreceptors and nociceptors in the skin. The cells of laminae VII and VIII that send fibers to the anterior STT are polysensory and are therefore more complex than cells in other laminae of the spinal cord.

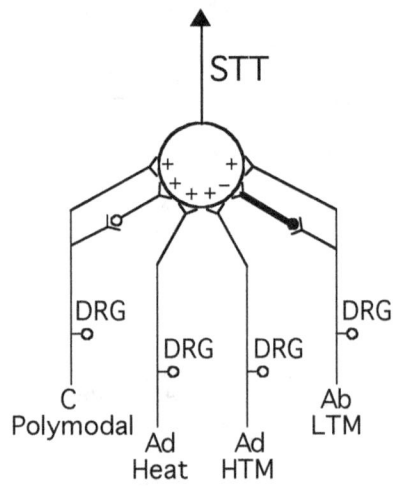

Figure C.14. A WDR and its multimodal inputs. LTM: Low threshold mechanoreceptors; HTM: High threshold mechanoreceptors. (Artwork by Monica Javidnia. Adapted from Price [528])

WDR neurons receive input from several types of receptors including high and low threshold mechanoreceptors through Aδ and Aβ fibers, heat receptors (Aδ fibers) and polymodal receptors that are innervated by C fibers and responding to different kinds of noxious stimulation (Figure C.14) [628]. The axons of the WDR neurons cross the midline and ascend in the anterior STT. The WDR neurons are important for mediating pain signals.

Due to their involvement in the generation of chronic neuropathic pain, and their ability to change neuroplastically the way they respond, WDR neurons have received significant attention.

Sensory fibers for both innocuous and noxious stimuli converge on to these cells. Some of these cells probably also integrate motor and sensory information.

Ascending visceral pain pathways

The visceral afferents that enter the spinal cord through dorsal roots ascend in the spinothalamic and the spinoreticular tracts [83]. Many afferents travel in the vagus nerve (CNX), the fibers of which terminate in the nucleus tractus solitarii (NST). Visceral afferents participate in autonomic reflexes such as the vomiting reflex generated from irritation of the gastric mucosa (or the vestibular system). Similarly, the emptying reflexes of the bladder and the rectum are controlled by stretch receptors, the afferents of which enter the spinal cord at S_2-S_4 [83]. Since these reflexes can be suppressed voluntarily, their pathways must receive input from high central nervous system centers. This is contrary to many other autonomic reflexes that cannot be modulated voluntarily.

Some of the mechanoreceptors in visceral organs are Pacinian corpuscles, but their exact anatomical role and functions are not yet fully known [83]. Activation of these receptors is perceived as deep touch. Some of the axons from these receptors terminate on cells in the dorsal horn; others travel in the vagus nerve and terminate on cells in the NST.

No secondary neurons in the spinal cord receive only visceral input, and there are much fewer visceral afferents than somatic afferents [105]. These facts are most likely the reason why pain from viscera is poorly localized. Some activation of visceral receptors does not produce pain, but a sensation of general illness. This is most likely mediated by the vagus nerve.

The nerve fibers that innervate nociceptors in visceral organs in the lower abdomen, including the reproductive organs, follow sympathetic nerves and enter the spinal cord as dorsal root fibers in the T_{12}-L_4 dorsal roots (Figure C.15). Pain fibers from visceral organs send collaterals to several segments of the spinal cord, therefore, complicating a determination of exactly where the pain originates.

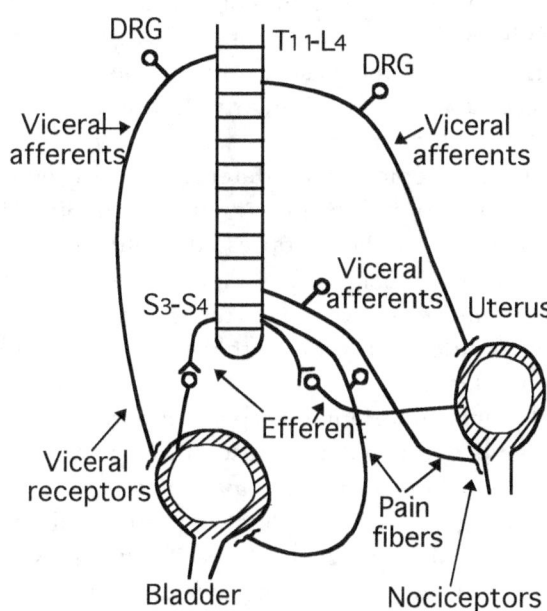

Figure C.15. Visceral afferent innervations in the lower body and motor (efferent) innervations. The afferent pathways of visceral nociceptors in the bladder and those of the neck of the bladder (including the prostate gland and the uterus) are shown together with motor innervations of the bladder and the uterus. (Artwork by Monica Javidnia).

At each segment of the spinal cord, visceral pain fibers make collaterals that terminate on the same cells in lamina I of the dorsal horn that receive input from pain receptors in the skin (through $A\delta$ fibers). Other collaterals of the visceral pain fibers terminate on cells in the intermediolateral column of the spinal horn [83]. These cells connect to sympathetic efferents and to motoneurons that innervate skeletal muscles. The intermediolateral column is only present from T_{12} to L_2 [83].

There is one exception to this pattern of innervation of visceral nociceptors, namely the nociceptive innervation of the neck of the bladder, the prostate, the cervix of the uterus, and the distal rectum. The fibers of these nociceptors travel together with parasympathetic pelvic nerves and enter the spinal cord as sacral spinal dorsal nerves (S_2-S_4) [83] (Figure C.15).

The visceral afferents of the cranial nerves terminate in the solitary nucleus, and those entering the spinal cord through dorsal roots ascend in the spinothalamic and the spinoreticular tracts [83].

Visceral afferents participate in autonomic reflexes such as the vomiting reflex generated from irritation of the gastric mucosa (as well as the vestibular system). Similarly, the emptying reflexes of the bladder and the rectum are mediated by stretch receptors, the afferents of which enter the spinal cord at S_2-S_4 [83] (Figure C.15). Since these reflexes can be suppressed voluntarily, their pathways must receive input from high central nervous system centers. This is contrary to many other autonomic reflexes that cannot be modulated voluntarily.

It is important to keep in mind that most of the knowledge about these ascending pain pathways was obtained using anatomical methods of investigation. Much less is known about the functional importance of specific tracts, which is partially dependent on synaptic efficacy. The synaptic efficacy is subjected to changes through the expression of neuroplasticity that can be initiated in many different ways. Neural connections (sprouting and elimination of axons and synapses) may also occur because of expression of neuroplasticity.

Differences between visceral and somatic pain circuits

Visceral pain and other forms of pain that are not under the control of the person who has the pain seems to mostly project to of the ventrolateral parts of the PAG whereas brief pain that is caused by stimulation of superficially located pain receptors mostly project to the dorsolateral and lateral parts of the PAG.

While the dorsolateral and lateral parts of the PAG mediate reduced responsiveness to noxious signals, excitation of the sympathetic nervous system and increased motor activity (Fight-or-flight response) the neurons in the ventrolateral column of the PAG coordinate instead inhibit sympathetic activity and decrease motor activity [474].

The reaction to pain stimuli that activate the ventrolateral parts of the PAG is associated with recuperation such as after intense exercise or in connection with chronic pain that is perceived to be an inescapable stressor [312]. Inescapable pain is also related to depression or depression-like symptoms, and it activates the hypothalamo-pituitary-adrenal axis [60]. Dysfunctional networks in the brain may also be involved in causing some of these symptoms [354].

Peripheral control of pain

It was mentioned above that activity in large fibers (Aβ) that innervate low threshold sensory receptors in the skin exert an inhibitory influence (through an inhibitory interneuron) on the cells in lamina I and II of the dorsal horn of the spinal cord that processes pain information.

Activity in collaterals of large diameter (Aβ) sensory fibers also provides inhibitory influence on WDR neurons in the dorsal horn, likely via an inhibitory interneuron.

Loss of input from Aβ fibers can occur, for example, in connection with skin lesions from trauma or from surgical treatment, where the outer layers of the skin are removed, (e.g. in tattoo removal).

Decreasing or elimination of the normal spontaneous input from large (Aβ) fibers may, therefore, increase the pain from stimulation of pain receptors, and in some situations, it can even cause the sensation of pain without stimulation of the specific pain receptors in the skin.

Blowing air on a spot that has been hurt by heat is a natural way of accomplishing inhibition of pain pathways from stimulation of sensory receptors in the skin and activating Aβ fiber.

Transdermal electric nerve stimulation (TENS) [718], using electrical impulses of a low intensity but high frequency, likely alleviates acute pain in a similar way. Electrical stimulation (TENS) can provide inhibitory input from Aβ fibers to pain circuits in the dorsal horn, and thereby alleviate such pain. TENS is also beneficial in the long-term treatment of pain through the expression of neuroplasticity.

Central control of pain

The processing of pain signals in the spinal cord is under considerable influence from supraspinal structures. This function is important as it offers a way to reduce nociceptor pain. The central influence on the transmission and processing of pain signals in the spinal cord is much more extensive than the processing of innocuous sensory information. Several different supraspinal structures exert strong control of pain transmission at the segmental level of the spinal cord. Similar control of pain transmission occurs in the trigeminal nucleus.

There are at least three separate descending systems that can modulate the transmission of pain signals, and which originate in supraspinal structures. Primarily this modulation occurs by influencing neurons in laminae I and II of the dorsal horn. Two of these pathways involve the PAG and connect to dorsal horn neurons through at least one interneuron in the rostral ventromedial medulla (RVM), and in the dorsolateral pontomesencephalic tegmentum (DLTP) [182]. The vagus nerve may also be regarded as a descending pathway that can modulate pain [206, 320]. (For details see [460]).

The PAG is an important source of descending activity that can modulate transmission of pain signals elicited by nociceptors. Descending activity from the PAG can modulate transmission of pain impulses at spinal segmental level (or brainstem level) [182]. Descending monoaminergic (serotonin and norepinephrine) connections from the reticular formation to the dorsal horn may suppress pain impulses in the dorsal horn, and thus prevent pain impulses from reaching higher central nervous system structures [121].

Some investigators perceive this complex descending system that controls transmission of nociceptive information in the spinal cord as a part of a negative feed-back system that may be activated by noxious stimulation and exert an inhibitory effect on some forms of nociceptive input [47]. This mechanism is thus similar to lateral inhibition that increases contrast in sensory systems [460], and it may explain how pain can inhibit pain.

It is well known that pain in one part of the body can suppress pain in another part of the body [209] and the saying that one can only have pain in one place at a time is generally true, although it may mean that the central nervous system focuses on the worst pain. If that pain is gone, the next worst pain becomes "the worst pain." This is another way that pain is different from the perception of innocuous sensory stimulation.

Periaqueductal gray pathway

The PAG, in addition to receiving ascending input from pain receptors through the mesencephalic system, also receives input from the amygdala and the frontal lobe via the hypothalamus (Figure C.16 and C.17).

Brainstem structures, such as the nucleus cuneiforms, pontomedullary reticular formation, locus coeruleus, and other catecholaminergic nuclei, also provide input to the PAG [254].

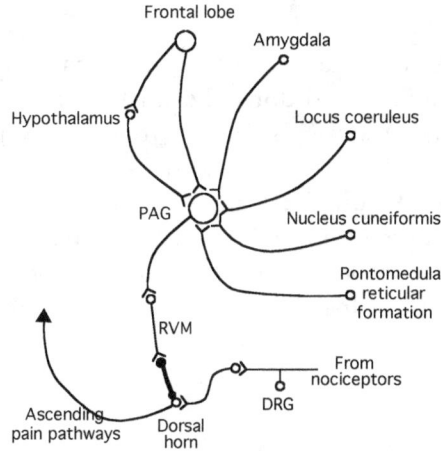

Figure C.16. Input to the PAG and pathways through which modulation of transmission of pain signals by the PAG can occur through the RVM pathway. (Artwork by Monica Javidnia).

The PAG plays an important role in modulation of pain. The cells in the PAG receives its input from the frontal lobe, the limbic system, and the forebrain, and there is a direct connection from the medial prefrontal and insular cortex to the PAG [41]. The amygdala provides input to the PAG [22] as well as the hypothalamus [182] (Figure C.17). The hypothalamus is important in connection with pain, and it has been shown that electrical stimulation or infusion of opioids (natural morphine or synthetic morphine-like substances) in specific parts of the hypothalamus can produce analgesia. Electrical stimulation of prefrontal cortex can also alleviate pain.

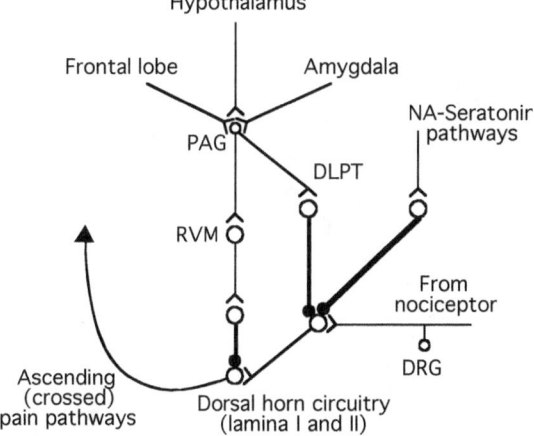

Figure C.17. Summary of the three different descending spinal tracts to cells in lamina I and II of the dorsal horn (RVM, DLPT, and NA-Serotonin pathways), showing the sources of input to the PAG. (Artwork by Monica Javidnia).

There are a few direct connections between cells of the PAG and dorsal horn neurons, but the cells of the RVM act as interneurons between the PAG and the neurons in the dorsal horn of the spinal cord (Figures C.16 and C.17). PAG cells that activate interneurons in the RVM can influence interneurons in lamina II of the dorsal horn, and thereby control the flow of neural activity that is elicited by noxious stimulation. Endogenous opioids (endorphins and enkephalins) act on local circuits in the RVM, and electrical stimulation of the RVM nuclei or injection of opioids in these structures produces analgesia and inhibits the response of dorsal horn neurons from stimulation of nociceptors [182].

Appendix D

Anatomy and Physiology of Motor Systems

Abstract

1. The motor cortices, basal ganglia, thalamus, cerebellum, and spinal cord are the main anatomical components of the motor system within the CNS.

2. The descending motor pathways of mammals are organized in two systems, known as the lateral system and the medial system.

3. The lateral system consists of the corticospinal and rubrospinal tracts. Its axons originate in cells in the primary motor cortices, premotor, and supplementary motor areas. Some fibers originate in somatosensory cortices.

4. The axons of the lateral system terminate on interneurons in the spinal cord that send axons to α motoneurons (lower motoneurons), and some (few) axons terminate without interruption on α motoneurons.

5. The medial system consists of the vestibulospinal, the reticulospinal, and tectospinal systems. It originates in cells in the vestibular nucleus and the superior colliculus of the brainstem and cells in the brainstem reticular formation.

6. The lateral system innervates distal limbs and provides fine movement.

7. The medial system innervates proximal limbs and torso muscles and provides gross movements and is the basis for posture. These tracts also provide facilitation for α motoneurons.

8. The basal ganglia modulate motor commands from the cerebral cortex and return the information back to the cerebral cortices via thalamic nuclei.

9. The neural circuits in the spinal cord and the trigeminal motonucleus perform considerable processing of motor commands that arrive from the brain.

10. The axons of the descending motor tracts give off many types of collaterals within a specific spinal segment, and they reach several spinal segments.

11. The spinal cord can generate commands for movements such as standing, scratching, swimming, and walking without supraspinal input.

12. Normal conscious activation of α motoneurons requires simultaneous excitatory input from many sources.

13. Several supraspinal structures influence the excitability of α motoneurons. The inhibitory and excitatory input to α motoneurons and other spinal motoneurons comes from higher brain centers and other segments of the spinal cord.

14. Spinal reflexes such as the stretch reflex, the tendon reflex, the reciprocal (inhibition) reflex are important for normal motor control. Renshaw cells and segmental circuitry provide negative feedback to α motoneurons.

15. The organization of the motor system differs vastly between animal species, and that can render invalid the transfer of findings drawn from studies in subprimates. This is especially the case for the corticospinal system minimally developed in non-primates.

Introduction

The somatic motor system controls voluntary movement and posture; it is the output organ for all conscious communications. The somatic motor system is complex and features sophisticated control systems involving loops, most of which are integrated with one another. There is also a large degree of redundancy and plasticity. Motor systems can, therefore, undergo reorganizing easily in response to changing demands or injury.

Expression of neuroplasticity, however, can also cause symptoms and signs of disease.

Many of the basic principles of the motor systems were discovered by Eccles & Lundberg in the 1970s using cats, but not all of these findings are transferable to the human systems. The corticospinal system is the best example of a highly important human pathway that is poorly developed in subprimates. When extending published animal results to human physiology, it is important to know from which animals the results were obtained.

Disorders of the motor system may cause loss of voluntary movement, fine motor weakness, muscle spasm, tremor, twitches, synkinesis, involuntary movements (chorea, athetosis), and deficits in coordination (ataxia). Disorders may also cause symptoms such as increased reflexes and abnormal activity such as spasm and spasticity.

The motor systems interact with sensory systems at several levels. One is in the cerebellum, and one is the cerebral cortex where there is considerable interaction between the somatosensory cortex and the premotor cortices. Motor systems are dependent on the feedback they receive from the proprioceptive parts of the somatosensory system. The spinal reflexes are examples of such interactions.

There are several fundamental differences between the motor systems in primates and subprimates. Since much research on the function of the motor system originates from studies in subprimates, it is important to make a distinction between findings that can and cannot be applied to human neurophysiology.

Other marked differences between subprimates and humans concern the thalamus where the human pulvinar thalamus occupies 40% of the volume of the thalamus, greater proportion than in subprimates. Little is known about the function of the pulvinar thalamus; it seems to be involved in attention tasks [342]. It has recently been shown to provide connections between different parts of the cerebral cortices.

In this appendix, we will discuss the general organization and basic functions of the motor system. After that, we will discuss the causes and the pathophysiology of some common disorders of the motor system. Lastly, we will discuss movement disorders in which the expression of neuroplasticity plays an important role.

Anatomy of the primate motor system

Kuypers (1981)[340] distinguished between two different groups of descending pathways: the medial system and the lateral system. The (dorso) lateral pathways (Figure D.1) comprise the corticospinal and rubrospinal tracts, and the (ventro) medial system (Figure D.2) consists of the vestibulospinal, reticulospinal and tectospinal tracts.

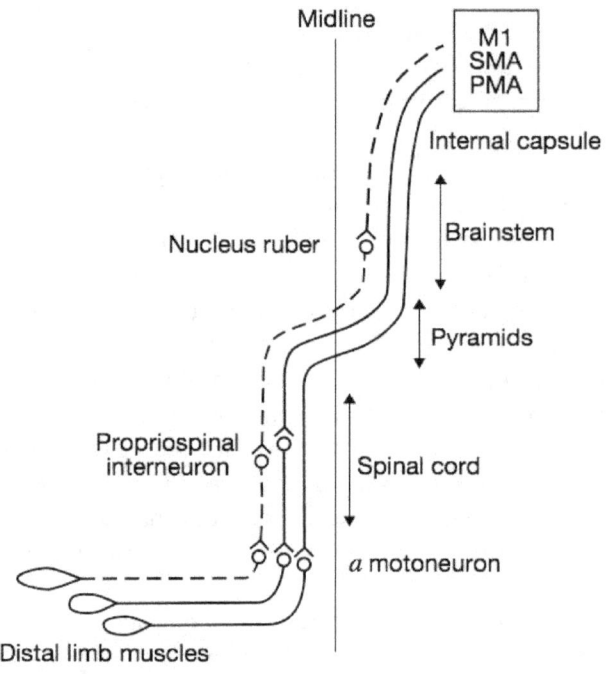

Figure D.1 Schematic drawing of the lateral motor system showing axons of the corticospinal tract that target α motoneurons directly and axons that reach the α motoneurons through and interneuron. The dashed line shows the connections of the rubrospinal tract (Based on [461]).

The lateral system provides sophisticated voluntary motor control for fine movements, mainly of distal muscles of the upper limbs. Flexors are activated more than extensors by the lateral system. The lateral system superimposes on the medial system, which mainly provides control of posture, breathing, ambulation, and orientation of the head (Figure D.2).

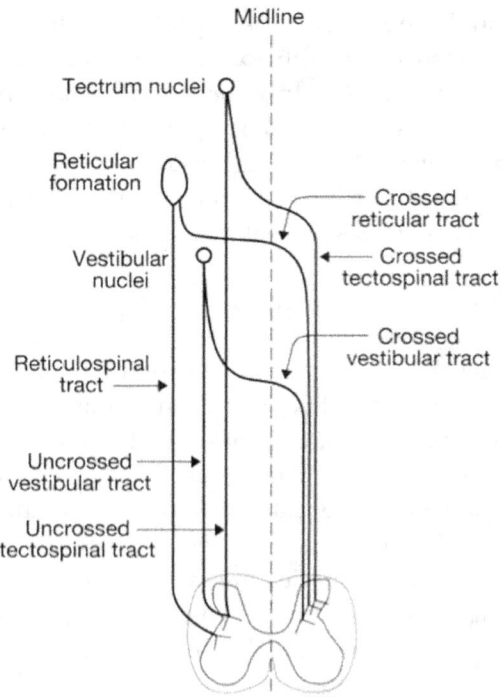

Midline

Tectrum nuclei

Reticular formation

Vestibular nuclei

Crossed reticular tract

Crossed tectospinal tract

Crossed vestibular tract

Reticulospinal tract

Uncrossed vestibular tract

Uncrossed tectospinal tract

Figure D.2. Simplified schematic diagram of medial descending motor pathways of the medial system showing the vestibular, tectospinal, and reticulospinal tracts (Based on [461]).

While the lateral pathways (corticospinal and rubrospinal tracts) control finer movements of extremities, the medial group of descending tracts controls locomotion, posture, and reaching. The medial tracts supply both voluntary and involuntary control of muscle activity. Since the activity in these tracts can modulate spinal reflexes, they are important for automatic functions such as posture, and many other functions that do not require conscious attention.

The two most direct pathways from the MI, PMA, SMA and somatosensory cortex to the α motoneurons are the corticospinal (also known as the pyramidal) and the rubrospinal tracts (Figure D.1). The rubrospinal tract originates in the red nucleus (nucleus ruber), which receives input from the MI. The tracts of the medial system are less direct (Figure D.2).

The tectospinal tract originates in the tectum (mainly the superior colliculus, SC) and the reticulospinal tract originates in the pontine and medullary reticular formation; the vestibulospinal tract originates in the vestibular nuclei (Figure D.2).

The eponymous nuclei from which these tracts originate all receive input from the MI through more or less direct pathways.

It is important to point out that the fibers of all descending pathways have many collateral fibers. These collateral fibers not only connect to neurons in the parts of the spinal cord that are directly related to motor control, but they also supply input to neurons that control spinal reflexes. In fact, much control of movement is mediated by supraspinal control of spinal reflexes.

Some types of stereotyped movements such as walking and breathing can be performed without supraspinal input and can thus be controlled by neural circuits in the spinal cord.

Some collaterals of descending motor fibers (possibly corticospinal tract fibers that originate from the sensory cortex) can control sensory functions, particularly the sensitivity of neurons in the dorsal horn of the spinal cord that is involved in the transmission of pain signals to the central nervous system.

Collaterals also terminate on neurons in the different parts of the basal ganglia and cerebellum. The involvement of the basal ganglia and the cerebellum in motor control is complicated and shall be discussed last in this section.

Lower α and γ motoneurons

The α and γ motoneurons are the targets of the descending motor tracts. These motoneurons are located together in the different parts of layer IX of the ventral horn of the spinal cord. Their axons form the ventral spinal roots that innervate skeletal (extrafusal) muscles and the (intrafusal) muscles of muscle spindles.

The α motoneurons are also found in the motonuclei of cranial nerve motonuclei. α motoneurons are among the largest nerve cells in the body, and each cell has many synapses that connect input from different sources (estimated to be approximately 10,000-50,000). The α motoneurons are known as the "final common pathway" (Sherrington) of the motor system.

The α motoneurons receive convergent input from propriospinal neurons and other local segmental interneurons (excitatory and inhibitory). These interneurons receive their input from supraspinal sources through long descending pathways (corticospinal, rubrospinal, vestibulospinal, and reticulospinal tracts), and from local spinal sources.

As mentioned above, some of the fibers of the corticospinal tracts (pyramidal tracts) provide monosynaptic input to α motoneurons directly from cells in the M1, PMA, SMA and the somatosensory cortex [26, 525] (Figure D.1), but most corticospinal fibers activate α motoneurons through propriospinal interneurons.

These interneurons provide a means of modifying input from supraspinal sources and cells in other spinal segments before it reaches the α motoneurons. The lateral system of descending pathways provides disynaptic and polysynaptic input from different parts of the cerebral motor areas and other supraspinal sources.

Brainstem motonuclei

The motor fibers of cranial nerves have cell bodies in the motonuclei of the respective cranial nerves. Although less is known about them, the organization of cranial nerve motonuclei is similar to the organization of the motonuclei of the ventral horns of the spinal cord.

Sensory and motor nerves connected ipsilaterally to nuclei and motonuclei respectively except the facial motoneurons. Muscles of the upper part of the face (forehead) receive bilateral innervation from the facial motor cortex and the motoneurons innervating muscles of the lower part of the face receive only unilateral contralateral innervation. The facial motonucleus receives separate input from limbic structures and the motor cortex. Often, emotional smiling can be evoked either voluntarily from the motor cortex or involuntarily through input from limbic structures [132]. The smile evoked by a command from limbic structures is distinctly different from those coming from the primary motor cortex (MI). A genuine smile cannot be produced on command. Lesions of the tract between the MI and the facial motonucleus do not prevent spontaneous facial expressions, and people with such lesions can smile in response to a good joke but cannot produce a polite social smile.

Central pareses such as capsular hemiplegia are often associated with exaggerated emotional facial expressions (smiling or crying) that the individual cannot suppress. People with disorders of the basal ganglia such as Parkinson's disease (PD) lack the capacity for spontaneous emotional facial expressions, whereas voluntary, social smiling is possible.

Signs of the complexity of cranial nerve motonuclei comes from animal studies of the facial motonucleus, which have shown the existence of dormant synapses that make interconnections between facial motoneurons that innervate different groups of facial muscles[575]. These studies showed that repeated electrical stimulation of the facial nerve caused the development of synkinesis of facial muscles similar to the abnormal muscle response that can be observed in persons with HFS. It was concluded that these changes were caused by expression of neuroplasticity that unmasked dormant synapses that connected different motoneurons in the facial motonucleus [575].

Lateral spinal pathways

The dorsolateral pathways are mostly crossed tracts that terminate mainly on propriospinal interneurons that are located anatomically in the intermediate zone of the spinal horn. These propriospinal interneurons connect by short axons to α motoneurons that supply muscle on distal extremities. Some (few) fibers connect uninterrupted to α motoneurons.

The rubrospinal tract is also usually included in the lateral motor system. It is small and less influential in humans compared to what it is in subprimates.

Evolution seems to have shifted from a focus on the red nucleus, and rubrospinal system to the cortex and corticospinal system subprimates have extensive rubrospinal tracts. The development of the lateral system increased through the evolution of primates; it is big and dominating in humans, but very small in subprimates. This is the main difference between the motor systems in primates and subprimates. In humans, the corticospinal system is large while the rubrospinal system is very small.

Corticospinal tract

The corticospinal system innervates muscles in the distal limbs in humans, it controls fine movements, especially of the fingers. The cortical representation of the hands, fingers and feet and toes is extensive, allowing fine movements. The cortical representation increases through the extensive use of specific movements.

The corticospinal tract originates not only in cells of the MI (Brodmann's area 4) as was believed earlier but also cells in PMA, SMA (Brodmann's area 6), and the somatosensory cortices (SI) also contribute (Figure D.1).

The fibers of this tract descend through the internal capsule and cross to the opposite side at the pyramids in the lower medulla. From there, most fibers travel in the lateral part of the spinal cord. Most of the fibers of the corticospinal tract cross the midline at the lower medulla (medullary pyramid), but some fibers travel to targets in the ipsilateral spinal cord. Some, mostly uncrossed fibers, travel ventrolaterally near the midline as the ventral corticospinal tract. Some fibers of cells in the MI innervate cranial motor nerve nuclei and other brainstem cell groups, the so-called corticobulbar pathways.

The descending spinal fibers terminate in the ventral horns of the segments of the spinal cord. Approximately 15 % of the fibers remain ipsilateral, not crossing the midline, but this proportion may vary wildly within the population [83]. For example, the fraction of crossed to uncrossed corticospinal fibers in humans varies from one individual to another.

The corticospinal tract is asymmetric in about 75% of the population [83]. Both the lateral and the ventral portions are typically larger on one side (most often on the right side) [83]. This is of importance for assessing the effect of spinal cord injuries (SCI), and individual variation may be responsible for some variety in symptomology.

A few of the fibers of the corticospinal tract terminate directly (monosynaptically) on α motoneurons (Figure D.1). This is particularly the case for motoneurons that control the small muscles in the hand.

Some authors claim that only 10 % of corticospinal fibers terminate directly on α motoneurons [602] in humans. In primates, the number of fibers that connect monosynaptic to α motoneurons has increased and includes motoneurons that innervate lower extremities. In the monkey, severance of the corticospinal tract mainly influences the ability to use hands for precision grips. However, the effect of lesions to the corticospinal tract in humans is wider and includes an effect on spinal reflexes. It is likely that there are more monosynaptic connections in humans than even in the chimpanzee. The monosynaptic innervation mostly regards motoneurons that innervate muscles in the distant limbs (hands, fingers).

Most corticospinal fibers, however, terminate on interneurons (propriospinal neurons), which in turn connect to α motoneurons through short axons [83, 541] (Figure D.1). The axons of these propriospinal interneurons terminate on α motoneurons, which are located in the different parts of layer IX of the ventral horn of the spinal cord. Input from motor cortices can be modulated by these propriospinal interneurons that receive input from many different sources in the spinal cord and the brain.

The corticospinal tract is more developed in primates than in non-primates and humans probably have the most developed tracts. In the monkey, the corticospinal fibers terminate on interneurons located in several layers of the ventral horn (especially layers VII-VIII) [83, 541].

In the great apes and humans, the corticospinal tract extends throughout the spinal cord and terminates in large parts of the spinal gray including the dorsal horn, but the projections are mostly segregated in the ventral horn area. The ventral shift of the projections of corticospinal tracts has occurred in higher animals, and these fibers connect either directly to α motoneurons or via propriospinal neurons with short axons (see Figure D.1 [525]).

The corticospinal tract is small and only slightly developed in subprimates such as the rat. In the cat, only a few corticospinal fibers in the neck terminate monosynaptic on α motoneurons (lamina IX of the ventral spinal horn) [525].

Although other pathways send information through the pyramids, the corticospinal tract does so most prominently, while the other descending motor tracts appear to pass primarily through other parts of the medulla. This broad distinction was the reason for classifying motor tracts as belonging to either the pyramidal or the extra pyramidal systems.

This division of the motor systems was regarded to reflect phylogenetic development, with the pyramidal system being the newer of the two systems. This distinction was commonly used in conjunction with movement disorders, where disorders related to the basal ganglia were known as "extra pyramidal" disorders.

The division into pyramidal and extrapyramidal motor systems were abandoned when it was found that the basal ganglia connect backward to the cerebral motor cortices, enabling the basal ganglia to provide input to what was earlier known as the pyramidal system. This division is therefore misleading because the basal ganglia provide input to the MI via the thalamus, and input from the basal ganglia can reach the spinal cord not only through pathways that do not pass through the pyramids but also through the corticospinal tract. The fact that the MI receives input from the basal ganglia means that disorders of the basal ganglia may affect the transmission of information in the corticospinal tract.

Corticospinal fibers make collateral connections with neurons in subcortical centers [340]. The collateralization of the fibers of the corticospinal tract is extensive and very complex [525]; some of these corticospinal fibers have collaterals that innervate neurons in different areas of the spinal cord.

Perhaps the most surprising findings are that micro-stimulation of a specific site on the cortex can evoke contraction of many different muscles, and it can cause descending activity in many different tracts due to connections from the MI to the basal ganglia and the red nucleus [525]. Morphological studies show connections to the striatum, specific and non-specific thalamic nuclei, the red nucleus, pontine nuclei, the mesencephalic, pontine and medullary parts of the reticular formation, dorsal column and trigeminal sensory nuclei, and the lateral reticular nucleus [717].

Again, it must be pointed out that the connections commonly shown in diagrams are based on morphological studies, and it is not known how many of these connections are active at any given time. The pool of non-conducting synapses represents the redundancy that may be activated through the expression of neuroplasticity that can be initiated by injuries of changes in demand.

Section of the pyramids fails to give spasticity, just weakness and lost fine motor skills. This is evidence that the pyramidal system also functions through the extrapyramidal system. (Pyramids: an anatomically distinct structure of the lower medulla). (The two-motor system hypothesis regards the extrapyramidal system to be a system that includes the basal ganglia, while the pyramidal system was the corticospinal system).

This means that a stroke in the motor cortex will cause spasticity due to its influence on both pyramidal and extrapyramidal systems.

It has been estimated that a motonucleus that consists of 300 motoneurons receives inputs from 4,500-6,000 last-order interneurons, some being excitatory and some inhibitory [525]. Again, as discussed earlier, these data are based on histological studies, and as Jankowska and her co-workers have pointed out, we know little about the synaptic efficacy in these pathways. There may be great differences in these different pathways.

Rubrospinal tract

The rubrospinal tract (Figure D.1) is a major projection pathway from the red nucleus, which is located in the midbrain and receives input from the MI [83] as well as other motor centers like the cerebellum. The rubrospinal tract terminates in the same parts of the spinal gray matter as the corticospinal tract, and it supplements the cerebrospinal tract in mediating voluntary movements. The rubrospinal fibers are few, estimated to be only 1 % of the number of the corticospinal tract in monkey and man, and its importance in humans has been questioned [83]. However, the red nucleus has a strong influence on the spinal cord via the cerebellum [83].

Medial spinal descending pathways

The medial descending pathways consist of the medial and lateral vestibulospinal pathways, the medial and lateral reticulospinal and the tectospinal pathways, which are phylogenetically the oldest motor pathways Figure D.2. These tracts all have their nuclei in the brainstem, while some, but not all of these nuclei, have input from the motor cortices.

The anatomy of the motor tracts that belongs to the medial system is poorly understood. Some investigators have found that normally these pathways have both crossed and uncrossed tracts (some sources state that only the tectospinal tract is bilateral, and this tract only extends to the cervical part of the spinal cord).

The medial system is important for control of posture, and it provides the facilitation of α motoneurons that allows the normal use of muscles.

The axons of the tectospinal tract mostly originate in cells of the superior colliculus, which receive input from the visual, and the auditory system, the somatosensory system, and from motor cortices. The axons of the vestibulospinal pathway originate in cells of the vestibular nuclei, thus receiving signals from the balance organs in the inner ears.

The vestibulospinal tracts have two parts, the lateral vestibulospinal tract, which reaches all parts of the spinal cord, and the much smaller medial vestibulospinal tract, which reaches only the cervical and upper thoracic parts of the spinal cord.

The fibers of the vestibulospinal tracts terminate on neurons in the medial part of the spinal horn and provide excitatory influence on both α and γ neurons. The reticulospinal pathway originates in cells in the reticular formation of the brainstem, mainly the pons and the medulla, which receive connections from many other structures such as the cerebral cortex.

The excitability of the motor system can be modulated by several systems. One system is the (noradrenalin) NA-serotonin system. The axons of the NA-serotonin pathways project to the spinal cord, modulating neural activity in the motor system including α motoneurons. The NA-serotonin system increases the excitability of α motoneurons [712] (for an overview, see [132]).

The tracts of the medial system (Figure D.2) terminate on cells in the ventromedial zone of the spinal gray, where they control propriospinal interneurons and the motoneurons that control muscle on the trunk and girdle, mostly extensor postural or "anti-gravity" muscles. The tectospinal and vestibulospinal fibers are crossed pathways [525] (Figure D.2) that terminate predominantly on propriospinal neurons and other interneurons.

Tectospinal pathways

Many of the fibers of the tectospinal tract originate in cells in the superior colliculus (SC), which receives input from the visual system and the auditory system, as well as the SI and MI cortices. The SC also receives abundant input from the vestibular system. This tract is especially involved in and coordinates movements of the head and eyes. The fibers from the SC also innervate neurons of the motor nuclei of the cranial nerves (CN) III, IV, and VI that control the external eye muscles.

The fibers of the tectospinal tract terminate mainly in the rostral spinal cord innervating muscles of the neck and upper body.

Vestibular spinal pathways

The vestibulospinal tract consists of the lateral vestibulospinal and medial vestibulospinal tracts. The lateral vestibulospinal tract originates in the lateral vestibular nucleus and reaches all parts of the spinal cord, where the fibers provide excitatory input to both α and γ motoneurons [83]. Its main influence, like the reticulospinal fibers, is on the motoneurons in the medial part of the ventral horn that control muscles on the trunk and the proximal muscles of the extremities.

These muscles are important for antigravity control of posture, so the main function of this tract is to control antigravity muscles (muscles that oppose the force of gravity). The medial vestibulospinal tract reaches only the cervical spinal cord, and it is therefore mostly involved in head movements in response to the vestibular input. Since the vestibular nuclei have few, if any, input from the cerebral cortex, the vestibulospinal tract mediates mostly automatic reflex movements that have to do with adjustment of muscle tone.

The vestibular nuclei have input from the reticular formation, which forms an indirect route to the vestibular nuclei from the cerebral cortex. A major input to the vestibular nuclei is the midline cerebellum.

While the vestibular system is important for posture, it is possible to maintain normal posture and locomotion without any input from the vestibular system. People without a functioning vestibular organ can have a normal life with little noticeable signs or symptoms, provided that the loss of vestibular function occurs early in life.

Since a loss of input to the vestibular system has little noticeable symptoms and signs, the function of the vestibulospinal tract may be regarded as redundant - at least partly - and its function can be replaced by that of other systems.

However, the vestibular pathways may also receive input from other systems than the inner ear balance organs, and it may, therefore, be active even where when there is no input from the inner ear.

Other descending pathways

In addition to these specific motor tracts described above, there are descending connections that have neuromodulatory functions on the motor system. The raphe nuclei [83] are the source of serotonin, and projects to the spinal cord through noradrenalin (NA)-serotonin pathways. The locus coeruleus is the source of norepinephrine, also projects to the spinal cord (both the raphe nuclei and the locus coeruleus also send connections to many regions of the brain) [83].

The cells in the raphe nuclei receive their input from many sources, including the cerebral cortex and the hypothalamus. The cells in the locus coeruleus receive most of their input from two groups of cells in the reticular formation. One such group of cells is located in the ventrolateral part of the reticular formation, and these cells provide excitatory input to the locus coeruleus cells. The input from the other group located in the dorsomedial part of the reticular formation is inhibitory [83]).

The fibers of the NA-serotonin pathways are slow conducting and terminate throughout the grey matter in the spinal cord, where they modulate segmental neural activity including the excitability of α motoneurons. Both serotonin and norepinephrine increase the excitability of α motoneurons [712] (for an overview see [132]).

These descending pathways are involved in adjusting muscle tone. Both of these tracts excite the interneurons of the locomotor central pattern generator (CPG). During REM sleep, these descending monoaminergic neurons have their lowest activity, which may explain the suppression of movements of muscles that are controlled by the spinal cord [83]. (These descending tracts have been included in the reticulospinal tract).

The fibers of the descending monoaminergic tracts have many collaterals, some of which reach the dorsal horn, where they can suppress pain impulses from reaching higher central nervous system structures by reducing the excitability of dorsal horn cells that respond to noxious stimulation [83]. These descending systems are activated during stressful situations when muscle tone is increased, and pain sensitivity is reduced.

Motor Cortices

Motor commands are mainly generated by the primary motor area (M1) (Brodmann area 4), supplementary, and premotor areas (SMA and PMA) (area 6). The SMA is also known as M2, and the PMA is known as M3. These premotor cortical areas are extensive and occupy more than 60% of the cortical area in the frontal lobe that projects to the spinal cord [159] and they have many other functions. Parts of the cingulate cortex (Brodmann's area 23 and 24) also contribute to motor control, as do parts of the somatosensory cortex.

Anatomically, the main motor cortical areas are different from sensory cortices in that they lack layer 4, the main input layer of sensory cortices. The fibers of the lateral spinal system [340] (corticospinal and rubrospinal tracts) originate not only in the primary (M1) cells, but cells in the premotor (PMA) and supplemental motor areas (SMA) also contribute to the descending corticospinal tracts and thereby, provide input to neurons in the ventral spinal cord that can control reflexes and activate α motoneurons. Input from the somatosensory system (S1) can also reach neurons in the ventral spinal cord (including the α motoneurons) through the lateral system.

Axons from the premotor areas terminate mainly in cells in the intermediate zone of the spinal cord, and some of these terminate in the ventral horn around motoneurons. Otherwise, the projection to the spinal cord of neurons in the premotor and supplemental cortical areas is similar to those from M1. The output of cortical neurons is the result of considerable intracortical processing [181].

The connections from to the cortex to others structures such as the basal ganglia, the thalamus, and the cerebellum build feed-back and feed-forward loops that provide considerable processing of motor commands that descend to the spinal cord and the nuclei of cranial motor nerves.

The internal organization of motor cortices is dynamic [525]. Many studies have demonstrated that connections in the motor cortex are not "hard-wired." Rather, its organization and function are subjected to changes by the expression of neuroplasticity in response to changing demands or from injuries to central nervous system structures such as may result from strokes or trauma [297].

(Early mention of neuroplasticity in the motor system by Eccles [161] seems to have been directed to ontogenetic development rather than to what we now understand to be neuroplasticity).

There is considerable evidence that ineffective synapses can be unmasked through the expression of neuroplasticity. Ineffective synapses that have become effective (unmasked) can establish new functional connections between adjacent cortical areas [525] and between neurons in MI and other regions of the central nervous system. Re-organization of the MI may occur in response to an extensive use of certain muscles such as certain fingers of string players [165], or as a result of amputations [233, 525]. The changes in the organization of the MI that occur after amputations seem to occur in response to altered sensory and proprioceptive input to the motor cortex (via SI).

In this connection, it is interesting to note that the transection of the facial nerve causes the cortical area of the forelimb to expand [157, 525, 580]. Donoghue et al. 1990 [157] showed that within 1-4 hours after facial nerve transection, electrical stimulation of the vibrissae area of the motor cortex elicited contractions of the biceps and wrist extensor muscles.

It is also interesting to note that this reorganization occurs with a short delay, which means that it cannot be due to new morphological changes. That expansion of the cortical territory of the forelimb muscles is more likely the result of changes in synaptic efficacy (unmasking of dormant synapses), or changes in protein synthesis in the cells [623].

The information about the severance of the motor nerve may reach the motor cortex through the sensory nervous system. The facial nerve, however, does not carry somatosensory or proprioceptive fibers (but taste fibers [460]), and the trigeminal nerve is regarded to provide proprioceptive feedback for face movements.

Jacobs and Donoghue [157, 283] showed that changes in the cortical representation occurring after sectioning of the facial motor nerve could be mimicked by injection of Bicuculline (a GABA$_A$ antagonist) in the cortex, which indicates that changes in GABAergic inhibition are involved in the creation of the observed cortical re-organization.

Animal experiments have shown evidence that changes in the function of neurons in the dorsal horn of the spinal cord occur after interruption of motor nerves [262].

The severing of the motor nerve fibers caused a decrease in response to stimulation of large myelinated fibers (A-fibers) from the cut nerve 2-5 hours after axotomy. The efficacy of C-fiber input to the lateral dorsal horn increased after axotomy, thus, a similar reaction as occurs in acute myositis [262]. This indicates that neuroplasticity can be an important factor in establishing muscle tone.

Cortical motor maps can also reorganize after SCI. It has been shown that the motoneuron pool recruited by magnetic stimulation of a particular location within the cerebral cortex, which activates muscles that are innervated by spinal segments immediately rostral to the injury, is larger in individuals after SCI than it is in control subjects [676]. This was taken to indicate that a (limited) flexible relationship exists between parts of the motor cortex and the muscles they innervate. Motor-evoked potentials were also different in persons with SCI than in normal individuals.

The motor evoked potentials recorded from people with SCI had a shorter latency than those recorded from normal individuals, indicating enhanced excitability and a reorganization of the motor pathways after SCI, with a possible expansion of the cortical territory occupied by muscles that are innervated from spinal segments immediately rostral to the injury. These results are convincing evidence in the role of neuroplasticity in generating some of the symptoms and signs that are present in people with SCI).

Activation of the primary motor cortex

Descending pathways can be activated by electrical stimulation of the MI, and motor activity can be initiated in muscles in different parts of the body.

Stimulation of the motor cortex in humans can be done by electrical stimulation from electrodes placed on the scalp [414] (transcranial electrical stimulation).

Recordings from the exposed spinal cord in animals have confirmed that such stimulation activates cortical neurons because of its ability to activate the corticospinal tract [321]. Stimulation of the somatosensory cortex (SI) can also elicit muscle contractions, but it requires a higher intensity than stimulation of the MI.

Transcranial electrical stimulation is associated with considerable pain and therefore cannot be used in awake individuals. Impulses of a strong magnetic field can induce an electrical current in intracranial tissue and thereby activate cells in the motor cortex in humans [23, 43, 569]. The magnetic impulses are generated by passing an impulse of electrical current through the coil [23].

The magnetic field is not attenuated by the skull bone (only by the distance), and this is why such stimulation can be applied non-invasively and without eliciting pain). Such stimulation is painless and can be applied to an awake person without any noticeable discomfort.

Transcranial electrical stimulation is often used in anesthetized humans for intraoperative neurophysiologic monitoring [144, 637] of motor systems when the spinal cord is at risk of injury in surgical operations. Transcranial magnetic or electrical stimulation of the motor cortex elicit responses in descending motor tracts that can be recorded from the exposed spinal cord. Recordings of such responses from the exposed spinal cord in cats, monkeys, and humans to electrical stimulation of the MI have contributed to our knowledge about the function of the corticospinal tract [144].

When recorded from the surface of the exposed spinal cord, at least six such waves can be identified in response to electrical or magnetic stimulation of the motor cortices (M1, PMA, SMA and the somatosensory cortex). The earliest wave occurs with a latency of approximately 5 msec [321].

This wave (the D-wave) represents the direct response from the corticospinal tract caused by direct activation of pyramidal cells in MI that sends their axons descending in the corticospinal tract, The D waves that are elicited by stimulation of axons of pyramidal cells of the motor cortex seems to be generated by descending volleys in the corticospinal tract. The D-wave is followed by a series of 5-6 negative waves, (I waves or indirect waves).

The I waves are generated by activity in the same tracts that are elicited by stimulation of other cells in the motor cortex. The direction (and thus the position of the stimulating coil) affects the waveform of the recorded potentials.

The I-waves occur with an interval of 1.5-2 msec in animals [321] and approximately the same in humans (Figure D.3) [144]. These I-waves are assumed to be caused by subsequent activation of interneurons within the different layers of MI.

The later (longer latency) I waves are probably generated in cells that are located closer to the surface of the cortex [321].

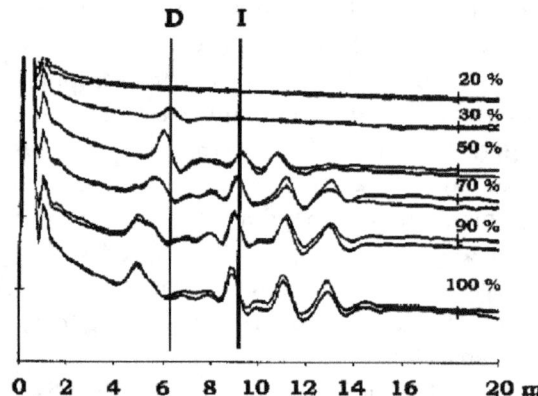

Figure D.3. Similar recordings as in Fig D.4, done in a person undergoing a scoliosis operation. D and I waves are shown from a 14-year-old child with idiopathic scoliosis. The stimuli were applied through electrodes placed at Cz and 6 cm anterior. 100%=750 volts (From Deletis, 2002).

The direction of the applied electrical current is important for the generation of the D and I waves, and if the electrode placement on the scalp is altered, the recorded wave pattern changes [144].

It appears that both the activity that is represented by the D wave and the I waves are necessary for activating α motoneurons.

Transcranial electrical stimulation acts slightly different on the motor cortex from electrical stimulation [321], and elicits I waves to a greater extent than magnetic stimulation [321]. The ventral corticospinal tract may contribute to the I waves, but the I waves are most likely a result of intracortical processing.

Brainstem control of motor activity

The brainstem, together with the basal ganglia, cerebellum and the spinal cord, coordinates basic voluntary motor programs that are issued by the motor cortex. The brainstem also generates commands for basic motor functions such as swallowing, chewing and breathing without input from the cerebral cortex. Some of the control circuitry for eye movements are also located in the brainstem.

The medial system together with the NA-serotonin systems adjusts muscle tone in awake persons by adjusting the amount of facilitatory that are applied to the α motoneuron. Relaxation of muscles is done by reducing the facilitatory input to α motoneurons. Skeleton muscles are paralyzed during sleep by not applying sufficient facilitatory input to α motoneurons in the spinal cord to allow input from motor cortices to activate the α motoneurons.

The brainstem reticular formation, through the reticulospinal tract, plays a central role in controlling muscle tone and in the ability to elicit spinal motor activity. It is known that activity of skeletal muscles of the body and head (except the eye muscles and those involved in respiration) are blocked during rapid eye movement (REM) sleep (also known as paradoxical sleep).

Blockage of skeletal muscle movement is apparent during REM stage of sleep while the eye muscles are active during that sleep stage, but other relaxed during other kinds of sleep. This means that the excitability of α motoneurons is controlled by varying the facilitatory input to α motoneurons. This "paralysis" of skeleton muscles occurs because of lack of facilitatory input from the reticular spinal tract and other parts of the medial system. Anesthetic agents, contributing to the muscle relaxation that is often induced during surgical operations, suppress the facilitatory systems.

If the facilitatory input to the somatic motor system is not interrupted during REM sleep as it is normally [82], the person may sleepwalk and become violent and attack his or her sleep companion. This is a specific disorder known as rapid eye movement behavior disorder (RBD).

The ability to activate skeletal muscles through transcranial magnetic stimulation of the motor cortex area is reduced during normal surgical anaesthesia because of reduced facilitatory input to α motoneurons. This thus another sign that the degree of wakefulness affects the ability to activate skeletal muscles.

Surgical anaesthesia may affect the excitability of cortical neurons in the motor cortices, but most of the depressive effect is likely to be caused by the reduction of descending facilitatory input to spinal motoneurons. In general, "blocking" of motor activity from the brainstem is mainly done by reducing the facilitating input to α motoneurons that are necessary for descending cortical signals to be able to activate the α neurons.

Central control of motor activity

That changing the attention can change the muscle response elicited by cortical stimulation (Figure D.4) demonstrates how activity from the central nervous system can modulate the excitability of motor systems. The effect of supraspinal activity on the excitability of muscles in the hand of an awake person is illustrated by the response to transcranial magnetic stimulation of the motor cortex (Figure D.4).

That activation of skeletal muscles through (magnetic) stimulation of the motor cortex is affected by attention (Figure D.4) mean that high brain structures can alter the excitability of motoneurons in awake persons as illustrated in Figure D.4.

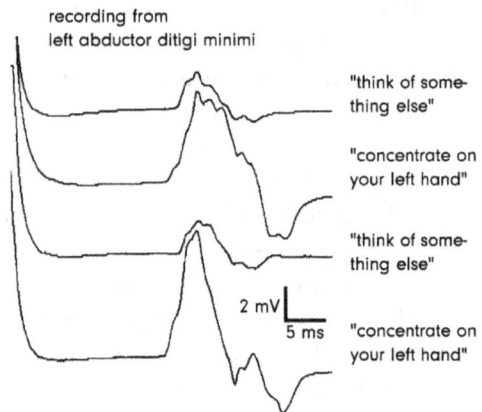

recording from
left abductor ditigi minimi

"think of some-
thing else"

"concentrate on
your left hand"

"think of some-
thing else"

2 mV

5 ms "concentrate on
your left hand"

Figure D.4. Illustration of facilitatory and inhibitory influence from the conscious brain on the response of a muscle in the hand of a conscious human subject in response to transcranial magnetic stimulation of the motor cortex showing EMG recordings from muscles in the hand. (From [569]).

The amplitude of the recorded EMG response is seen to increase when the participant in the study "think of the hand," while the amplitude decreases when "thinking of something else" [569]. The response from magnetic stimulation of the cortex is also facilitated by a weak voluntary contraction of the muscles in question, which illustrates the multitude of factors that influences the excitability of α motoneurons.

Segmental control of motion

The neural circuits in the spinal cord can generate commands for many forms of motion. Spinal reflexes play an important role in that respect. The spinal control of motion is modulated by supraspinal input, and by the proprioceptive input. Processing of information in the spinal cord can be modified or modulated through the expression of neuroplasticity.

This means that abnormal motor function may not only be caused by an abnormal input from the descending motor pathways, but also by plastic changes in the spinal cord and changes in proprioceptive feedback. We will discuss these matters in the sections that follow.

Spinal reflexes

Spinal reflexes are important for posture and conscious and unconscious movements. Voluntary control of motion depends to a great extent on modulation of spinal reflexes, from intra- or intersegmental spinal cord neurons and supraspinal sources.

Motor systems of cranial nerves have similar reflexes, but their organization is more diverse than those of the spinal cord. A typical spinal reflex arc consists of a receptor, an afferent pathway (sensory nerve), a reflex center (in the gray matter of the spinal cord), and an efferent pathway that passes the output to the effector organ (striated or smooth muscle or gland).

Some reflexes are simple and involve only one synapse in the spinal cord (monosynaptic stretch reflexes), whereas the reflex center of other (disynaptic and polysynaptic) reflexes involves several synapses. The two most basic spinal reflexes are the stretch reflex, which is a monosynaptic reflex that opposes stretch of a muscle, and the tendon reflex, which is a disynaptic reflex. Other spinal reflexes are more complex and involve supraspinal structures in the brainstem and the cerebral cortex. Spinal reflexes form different "layers" that interact with each other in various ways.

Spinal reflexes are subjected to modulation through the proprioceptive input, from circuits in the spinal cord and supraspinal circuits. The gain in spinal reflexes can be changed by expression of neuroplasticity [86, 287, 727], thus subject to the effect of training and adaptation to injuries and altered demands.

Monosynaptic Stretch Reflex

The monosynaptic stretch reflex is the simplest of the spinal reflexes (Figure D.5). The reflex arc consists of a muscle spindle, the afferent fibers of which travel in peripheral nerves and enters the dorsal horn of the spinal cord in dorsal roots as Ia fibers. In the spinal cord, these fibers travel to the ventral horn, where collaterals connect to the α motoneurons of several agonist muscles.

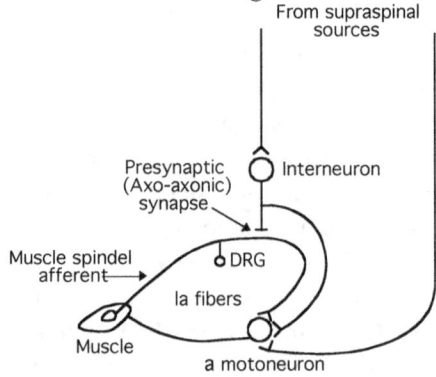

From supraspinal sources

Presynaptic
(Axo-axonic)
synapse

Interneuron

Muscle spindel
afferent

DRG

Ia fibers

Muscle

a motoneuron

Figure D.5. Simplified diagram of the monosynaptic stretch reflex, showing the modulatory input from supraspinal and spinal sources via an interneuron.

The muscle spindles measure the absolute length and rate of length change of muscles. The firing of Ia and group II fibers innervating muscle spindles increases when a muscle is stretched and decreases when it is shortened, such as occurs during normal contraction. In this way, the muscle spindles provide feedback to the spinal cord regarding the length of muscles. When muscle contracts (shortens), the input from its muscle spindles decreases, which decreases the excitatory input to its α motoneurons. This is known as negative feedback because it tends to decrease the contraction. Negative feedback stabilizes control systems.

The H-reflex

Applying a brief force to the patella tendon below the knee and measuring the reflex is a test included in most neurologic examinations. Observing the subsequent stretch of the leg assesses the excitability of α motoneurons. The effect of activation of Ia fibers and group II afferents on α motoneurons can be assessed quantitatively by electrically stimulating a peripheral nerve (containing fibers from muscle spindles) and recording the electromyographic (EMG) responses from the muscle.

This is known as the Hoffman (H) reflex) (Figure D.6). The stimulation used to elicit the H-reflex activates the stretch reflex and thereby provides excitatory input to α motoneurons (Figure D.6).

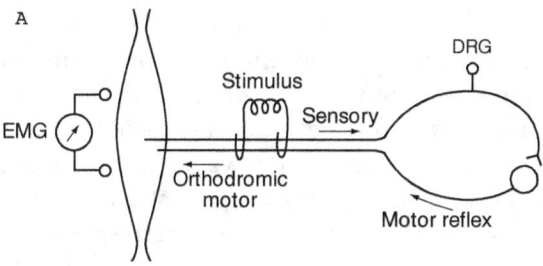

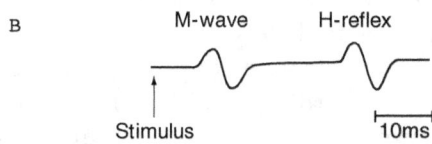

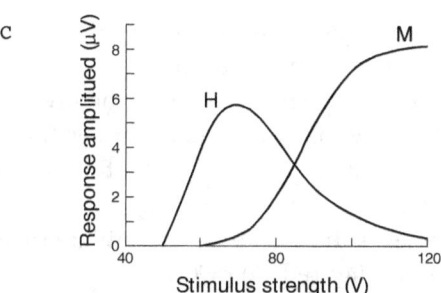

Figure D.6. The Hoffmann reflex.

A. The arrangements for obtaining a Hoffman reflex response.

B: Recording of the direct muscle (M-wave) and the H-reflex from electrodes placed on the muscle.

C: Amplitudes of the M-wave and H-reflex as functions of the stimulus intensity.

The H-response is temporally separated from the M-response and the amplitude of the is proportional to the intensity of a stimulus above a threshold value, but after a point, the relationship becomes the opposite. The amplitude of the direct muscle response (M) continues to increase (Figure D.6) [305, 590]).

At higher stimulus intensities the H-reflex response decreases because the strong stimulation occupies many motor fibers impeding the reflex response from propagating towards the muscle at which the recordings are made (Figure D.6) [590].

A mixed peripheral nerve containing both motor and proprioceptive fibers from muscle spindles is stimulated electrically, eliciting activity that progresses both distally, eliciting a direct muscle contraction (M-wave), and proximally, activating the monosynaptic stretch reflex that causes another and later muscle response (the H-reflex).

Motor reflexes have two components known as the M and H waves. Electrically stimulating the tibialis nerve behind the knee, for example, actually produces two separate responses that can be observed by recording EMG potentials from the soleus muscle. One component, the M-wave, originates from direct activation of the muscle from the stimulation of motor fibers in the nerve. The other component of the response, the H-wave, is from activation of proprioceptive sensory fibers in the nerve eliciting a response from the stretch reflex. When the nerve is stimulated at a location that is close to the muscle it innervates, the M response will occur with a much shorter latency than the H-response, even though they are initiated from the same action (Figure D.6) [590].

The F-response

The F-response, a third kind of response from the target muscle, may also be observed after electrical stimulation of a mixed nerve. This response is a result of firing motoneurons by electrical stimulation of their motor axons. The F-response is used clinically for assessing the excitability of α motoneurons.

Reciprocal spinal reflex

The reciprocal reflex ensures that when one muscle contracts, its reciprocal (or antagonist) muscle relaxes (Figure D.7). Ia neurons that project to a muscle also contact the Ia interneurons that inhibit the α motoneurons of the antagonist's muscles.

The reciprocal reflex is closely related to the monosynaptic stretch reflex because it gets its main input from the Ia afferents from muscle spindles via an interneuron (Figure D.8). Through this reflex, a decrease in the output of muscle spindles causes a decrease in the inhibition of the α motoneurons that innervate antagonist muscles through an Ia inhibitory interneuron.

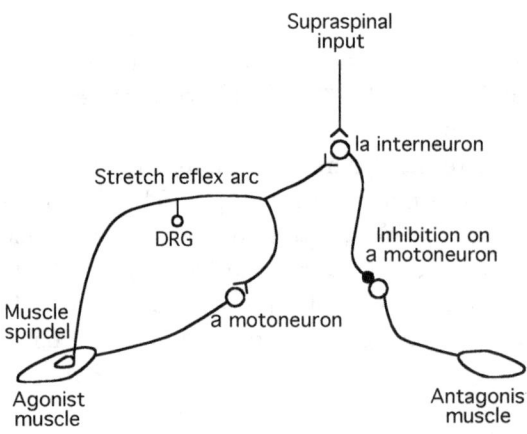

Figure D.7. The reflex arc of the reciprocal spinal reflex. Input from muscle spindles inhibits the antagonist muscle's motoneurons through the Ia interneuron.

Lundberg 1979 [375] demonstrated the importance of Ia inhibitory interneurons in experiments in cats. He and his group showed that the main output of the Ia interneurons is directed to the antagonist muscle's α motoneuron. Axon of the corticospinal and vestibulospinal tracts terminate either directly, or through their propriospinal interneurons, on the Ia interneurons.

This input can modulate the inhibition of the antagonist's muscle when the stretch reflex is activated[365]. The Ia interneuron receives numerous other inputs from the same and other segments of the spinal cord [375, 525] and the inhibition it provides on α motoneurons is therefore complex and can affect motor output across multiple motoneuron pools at multiple spinal levels.

Tendon reflex

The tendon reflex is a disynaptic reflex that receives its afferent input from the Golgi tendon organs via Ib interneurons (Figure D.8). The tendon reflex provides inhibitory input to motoneurons that innervate agonist muscles. Golgi tendon organs that provide the main inputs to Ib interneurons measure the force of muscle contraction.

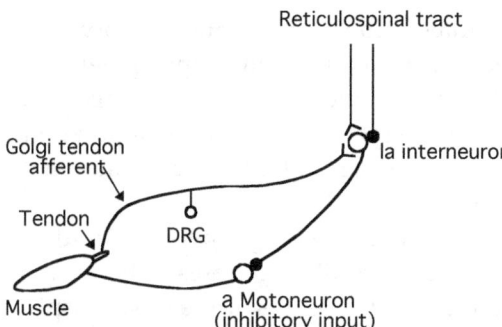

Figure D.8. Tendon reflex.

The output of a muscle's tendon receptors (Golgi organs) inhibits that same muscles α motoneurons through the Ib interneuron. The reflex can be modulated by supraspinal input mainly from the reticulospinal tract. Some descending fibers have an inhibitory influence while some are excitatory.

Since Golgi tendon organs measure the strength of muscle contractions and inhibit α motoneurons accordingly, the tendon reflex provides some protection against overloading muscles. This was earlier regarded to be the main function of the tendon reflex, but more recently it has become apparent that Golgi tendon organs respond over a larger range of muscle tensions[122]. This means that the tendon reflex provides important and continuous feedback to motor systems similar to that of the stretch reflex, which is controlled by the length of a muscle.

The flexor reflex

This has a practical implication for treatment of muscle spasms. Instead of massaging the muscle to relieve spasm that is common, it is more effectives to massage the tendon of the muscle which activates the tendon reflex that has a direct inhibitory effect on the motoneuron.

The flexor reflex, also known as the withdrawal reflex, causes flexor muscles on a limb to contract in response to painful stimuli. For example, it is the flexor reflex that causes the withdrawal of a hand or food from being burned. The flexor reflexes can be elicited by stimulation of several different afferents, known as the FRA (Flexor reflex afferents).

The pathway of the FRA is subject to supraspinal modulation by the dorsal reticulospinal system [86], which descends bilaterally from the pontomedullary reticular formation through the dorsolateral funiculus.

These fibers inhibit first-order interneurons of the FRA reflex pathways. The corticospinal and the rubrospinal pathways facilitate transmission in the FRA reflex [374].

Crossed Extensor Reflex

The crossed extensor reflex is a flexor reflex that is elicited from the opposite side. For example, stepping on a sharp object with one foot cause the other leg to extend to prevent falling.

Renshaw inhibition

Another circuit important to spinal reflexes is the Renshaw (or recurrent) inhibition circuit [86] (Figure D.9). It acts as a negative feedback for the motor systems. This form of feedback adds stability to motor functions.

The Renshaw feedback system consists of the Renshaw cell that acts as an interneuron with input from collaterals of motor nerves. The output of Renshaw cells provides inhibitory input to the same α motoneuron and other agonist motoneurons as well (Figure D.9). Renshaw neurons receive supraspinal input (such as from the corticospinal tract) that can modulate the recurrent inhibition. Renshaw feedback is an important source of negative feedback in motor systems.

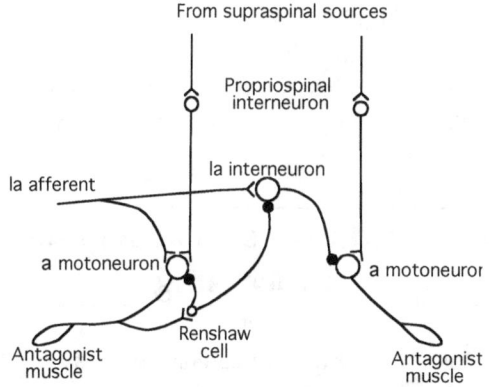

Figure D.9. Renshaw inhibition and the reciprocal reflex.

Inhibitory input from Ia interneurons on the antagonist muscle can be modulated by Renshaw cells. This allows switching from agonist to antagonist, such as from flexor to extensor, and back again as occurs in cyclic movements like stepping.

Renshaw cells also connect to Ia interneurons and can thereby modulate the stretch reflex. Renshaw inhibition has similarities with both the monosynaptic stretch reflex and the tendon reflex in that it provides negative feedback to motor control.

Long reflex arcs

Proprioceptive signals travel in the dorsal column and the spinocerebellar tract from supraspinal sources and form the afferent path of long spinal reflex arcs. The fibers in the dorsal column mainly project to the ventral posterior lateral (VPL) nucleus of the thalamus and these fibers also send collaterals that connect to cells in the corticospinal motor system via thalamocortical and cortico-cortical connections. The medial lemniscus and corticospinal systems are the ascending and descending limbs of these long (spinal) reflexes. These reflexes have much longer latencies than other spinal reflexes.

Long spinal reflexes are affected by many factors such as the degree of wakefulness. Even simple reflexes such as the withdrawal reflex can be modulated by willful actions. For example, it is possible to abort or modify the withdrawal reflex normally elicited by input from skin receptors.

The proprioceptive input from the vestibulospinal (descending) tract to the spinal cord can be modified by training and affected by its use, as is evident from being on a boat. Such changes in function may be described as a form of activation of neuroplasticity, and it can be used in therapy for vestibular disorders.

Inter- and intraspinal segmental processing

Most of the input to cells in the gray matter of the spinal cord originates in other cells in the gray matter of the spinal cord. This complex network of connections between neurons in the spinal cord provides extensive intra- and inter-segmental processing, which is important for the normal function of the motor system.

Local spinal cord connections provide powerful processing of information at the segmental level of the spinal cord, and extensive connections between the segments add to the complexity of the internal processing of information occurring in the spinal cord.

The integration of somatosensory and proprioceptive information with supraspinal motor commands makes the spinal cord a complex system, with wide ranges of computational capabilities regarding voluntary and automatic motor control.

Spinal cord processing involves multiple feedback loops (including reflexes), the gain of which is affected by several sources of supraspinal input as well as proprioceptor input. There are extensive connections between segments of the spinal cord, extending many segments.

The existence of connections between lumbar and cervical segments of the spinal cord is evident, for instance, in the locomotion of quadrupedal animals. Humans have a vestige of this manifestation in the tendency of swinging the arms opposite to leg movements while crawling as infants and walking as adults.

Jendrassik maneuver

Another example that demonstrates the extensive intersegmental connections is the Jendrassik maneuver. That far-away segments can influence excitability is evident from the Jendrassik maneuver that can alter the excitability of lower-extremity stretch reflexes by activating upper limb segments. (The Jendrassik maneuver that is used clinically is a way to increase the excitability of lower extremity stretch reflexes. It is performed by having the person hook the hands together by the flexed fingers and pulling against them with all possible strength).

The medial reticulospinal tract and, to some extent, the vestibulospinal tract mediate facilitatory effects on extensor tone [85], and intersegmental spinal sources provide input to the interneuron as can be shown by the Jendrassik maneuver.

The H-reflex is used to demonstrate the effect of the Jendrassik maneuver. The H-reflex can be up and down-regulated with training, which may enhance the stretch reflex of the lower limb (such as the patellar reflex) by upper limb motor action. This is a clear indication of the interaction between spinal segments, which are far apart.

The role of interneurons

Interneurons are the most common type of cells in the spinal cord. Interneurons are not only an important path to motoneurons from supraspinal motor centers, but these neurons have a much complex role in motor control; most commands from supraspinal sources pass through interneurons. Interneurons receive input not only from descending motor tracts, but also from several types of proprioceptive receptors such as muscle spindles, tendon organs, and joint receptors.

Skin receptors also provide input to interneurons. This provides a means to modulate motor commands that are issued at supraspinal structures. Interneurons send collaterals to many laminas in the dorsal and ventral horns of the spinal cord and extend their connections to several segments.

This means that interneurons are not just relays, but they perform extensive processing of information in their function as links to supraspinal structures and modify motor activity.

This complex role of interneurons was investigated by Lundberg and colleagues who gathered much experimental evidence indicating their complex function in the spinal cord [287]. These investigators also showed that each input alone might not be able to activate interneurons. Some neurons may require input from more than one source to become activated.

Modulation from the brain

The processing that occurs at segmental levels can be modulated by supraspinal input, and by proprioceptive and sensory input from receptors in muscles, tendons, joints, and skin. The spinal proprioceptive interneurons that receive their input from corticospinal neurons, for example, also receive excitatory and inhibitory input from many segmental sources. This input can modulate the descending input to α motoneurons as well as the spinal reflexes [83, 86, 519]. The reciprocal inhibition of the antagonist muscle during stretch reflexes is an example [83].

The organization and function of the inter- and intra-segmental spinal connections have received less attention than the processing that occurs in supraspinal structures. Understanding of these three mechanisms is relatively sparse.

Diagrams of spinal circuitry, such as those for reflexes, appearing in textbooks (including this one), are highly simplified and usually omit intersegmental processing.

The interneurons that relay descending motor information to α motoneurons and interneurons that receive input from peripheral receptors may be involved in the modification of motor control at a pre-motor neuron level [287].

These complex connections make it possible to modulate spinal reflexes from spinal and supraspinal sources. Presynaptic inhibition induced by corticospinal fibers through axo-axonic synapses can control spinal reflexes, including those that involve Ia spindle afferents and large afferents from the skin [573]. Control of spinal reflexes and control of muscle spindles through activation of γ motoneurons are other examples of ways in which the motor cortex can control movement, in addition to their direct activation of α motoneurons, either monosynaptic or via propriospinal interneurons.

This complex control system is normally stable, but pathology can introduce instability that leads to such symptoms as weakness, incoordination, and spasm. The pathologies may alter the processing that occurs at segmental levels of the spinal cord and may change the supraspinal input.

Locomotion and posture

The spinal cord locomotor generator (central pattern generator, CPG) is an example of spinal cord circuits that can generate commands for complex motion without supraspinal input. The CPG can generate the necessary commands for walking and run. These circuits play an important role in locomotion together with spinal reflexes that are under control from the brainstem [152].

Control of locomotion and posture depends on subthalamic, mesencephalic and medullary (locomotor strips) - structures of the brainstem that communicate through the reticulospinal pathway. These structures exert control over the spinal cord CPG that control motion (initiation and speed). The same structures control postural tone and modulate the force that is generated by muscles activated by CPGs.

The weighting of active circuitry in the spinal cord is task specific. For example, when the spinal cord CPGs are turned on during locomotion, Ib neurons are turned off, and there is now synaptic excitation to extensor motoneurons [401].The cerebellum that refines these commands is involved in coordination of movements.

It was earlier believed that the cerebellum was the anatomical site for learning motor skills, but it has later been found that motor skills can be learned without the cerebellum, thus involving other structures, sometimes just the spinal cord.

Gamma motor systems

The spinal neurons that receive their input from corticospinal fibers not only make monosynaptic contact with α motoneurons but also innervate γ motoneurons, which control the length and thereby sensitivity of muscle spindles. The input to the γ motoneuron thereby adjusts the proprioceptive feedback provided by the stretch reflex [83, 86, 519].

In this way, the corticospinal tract not only activates α motoneurons directly by input from the corticospinal tract but also indirectly through Ia afferents from muscle spindles that activate the monosynaptic stretch reflex.

There is evidence that central commands that reach the individual segments of the spinal cords through the corticospinal and rubrospinal tracts exert much of their motor control through their activation of γ motoneurons and thereby activate muscle spindle afferents [184].

There is also evidence for α and γ co-activation.

Startle and freezing reaction

The startle response and the freezing reactions are the results of opposite kinds of commands that are generated in structures in the brainstem. The "freezing" reaction occurs humans and in many animals. It manifests as a temporary blockage of the signal to the skeletal muscles at the brain stem level [132]. This is similar to the blockade that normally occurs during REM (paradoxical) sleep but is elicited by extreme fear.

This arrest of all body motion is an example of an unconscious influence on motor activity. It can occur in some pathological conditions such as Parkinson's disease.

The startle response is nearly the opposite of the freezing reaction. It involves forceful contraction of many skeletal muscles.

Both reactions are influenced by input from the central nucleus of the amygdala [132]. The amygdala is involved in fear reactions, and the cells in its nuclei connect to many structures of the central nervous system. The freezing reaction evidences the amygdala's influence on descending motor pathways via the brainstem nuclei, specifically the PAG [132].

The acoustic startle response is a reflex response that is also related to fear. It occurs most often in response to a strong transient sensory stimulation, but the cause of the response is similar to freezing, namely fear or fright. Startle responses are mediated by circuitry in the brainstem, the main input to which originates in the auditory system. It is mainly elicited by a sharp and loud sound [132]. The acoustic startle response is a short 3-synapse reflex in the brainstem, consisting of the ventral cochlear (VCN) nucleus, the paralemniscal zone of the ventral nucleus of the lateral lemniscus (VLL), and the nucleus reticularis pontis caudalis (RPC).

This reflex can be modulated by activity in other structures, in particular, the amygdala (rostral part of the medial subdivision) [566]. The input from the amygdala is mediated through the N. reticularis pontis caudalis [566]. The startle response can be modified by behavioral interventions, indicating that expression of neuroplasticity

Shivering

Shivering or trembling may occur as a result of either cold or fear. This reaction is yet another example of a non-conscious form of muscle activity. Shivering that occurs because of cooling of the skin is mediated without conscious control, and can occur even though the temperature in the hypothalamus is normal. The increased heat production that is the purpose of shivering occurs in anticipation of a decrease in core temperature [484]. While this is an advantage to the organism because it can restore body temperature by generating heat, the value of shivering that occurs because of fear is questionable.

Muscle tone

Muscle tone is the background contraction of muscles that occur without any voluntary commands. Words like muscle tone and muscle tension are sometimes used synonymously, but some authors [629] define muscle tone only to mean viscoelastic changes in a muscle that occurs in the absence of contractile activity.

There are three different forms of contractile activation of muscles:

(i) electrogenic stiffness caused by activation of motoneurons and neuromuscular endplates (have observable EMG activity);

(ii) electrogenic spasm (pathological and involuntary electrogenic contraction), and

(iii) contracture (occurring within the muscle fibers independent of EMG activity [629] and more a function of tissue properties than activity).

Abnormally increased muscle tone can be caused either by contractile activity mediated by the motor nerve and the motoneurons or by changes in the viscoelastic properties of muscles [629]. Abnormally low muscle tone is known as hypotonus, while abnormally high muscle tone is hypertonia, as may occur in spasticity.

Our understanding of normal muscle tone is, however, incomplete, which hampers our understanding of many pathologic conditions of the motor system.

The resting muscle tone is often assumed to be caused by a low rate of firings of motor nerves, but this assumption seems to rest on a misconception according to Simons and Mense [629]. These investigators described methods to measure muscle tone mechanically, and they credited Walsh [699] for clarifying the misconception that muscle tone was caused by electrical activation of the contractile apparatus of muscles.

Some forms of increased muscle tone are thus not caused by the activity of α motoneurons; instead, the resistance to stretching a muscle is caused by mechanical properties (compliance) of the muscle itself.

The Ia inhibitory interneurons are important for controlling muscle tone. These neurons receive excitatory input from muscle spindles in the agonist muscle, and inhibitory influence from the antagonist muscle spindles in addition to input from supraspinal sources. (Figure D.10).

Some interneurons that have an excitatory influence on inhibitory Ia interneurons receive input from cutaneous receptors (FRA) from both sides [375, 525]. Since the Ia interneurons exert an inhibitory influence on α motoneurons of the agonist muscle, reduced input to these neurons from any of these multiple sources will increase the excitability of α motoneurons, and subsequently, facilitate spinal reflexes and increase the tone of the muscles involved.

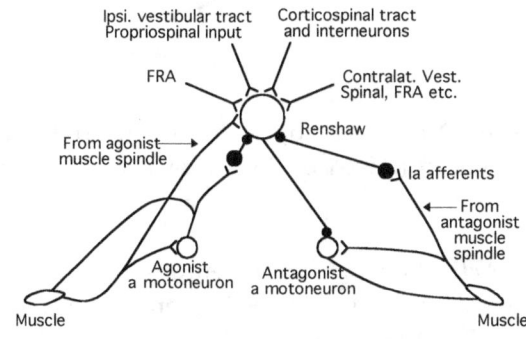

Figure D.10. The input to an Ia inhibitory interneuron (Based on Lundberg, 1979).

The Ib inhibitory interneurons (Figure D.11) receive excitatory input from Golgi tendon organs in the agonist muscle and are inhibitory on agonist α motoneurons [375]. Inhibitory Ib interneurons make multiple connections to α motoneurons of extensor muscles. The Ib interneurons also receive input from supraspinal sources (excitatory input via the corticospinal tract and inhibitory from the reticulospinal tract), and they receive excitatory input from interneurons that receive cutaneous input (FRA). Again, elimination or reduction of such input may increase the excitability of α motoneuron thereby increasing muscle tone [32, 375, 525]. The functions of these circuits are plastic and subject to modifications in their response to demands and response to injuries.

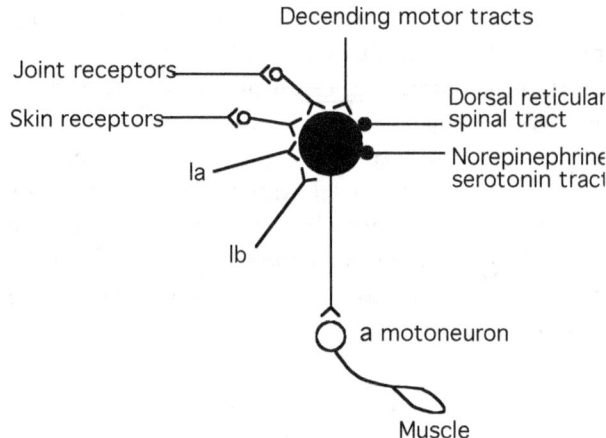

Figure D.11. The input to an Ib (inhibitory) interneuron (Based on Jankowska and Lundberg, 1981).

Activation of γ motoneurons by input from supraspinal sources can influence the tone of skeletal musculature through the stretch reflex.

Brainstem structures are known to exert strong modulatory influence on γ motoneuron (fusimotor) activity. The reticulospinal tract, and especially another tract, the serotonin-norepinephrine tract, exert considerable influence on the excitability of α motoneurons and other neurons within the spinal cord and modulate the excitability of spinal reflexes. These tracts also innervate some γ motoneurons. The tegmental area of the upper brainstem is important in regulating muscle tone in general through the serotonin-norepinephrine descending pathways.

It has also been shown that some drugs used to treat depression, selective serotonin re-uptake inhibitors (SSRI) can unbalance this regulation causing excessive eye movements. These drugs can also increase spasticity that occurs after spinal cord injuries (SCI).

Electrical stimulation of the common peroneal nerve was found to increase the excitability of the motor system. For up to 110 minutes after the cessation of magnetically induced electrical stimulation of the common peroneal nerve, the amplitudes of the motor evoked potentials (MEP) recorded from the tibialis anterior were elevated by an average of 104%. The monosynaptic stretch reflex was not increased, indicating that the effect of peroneal stimulation was not caused by increased excitability of the motoneuron pool.

It was speculated that the anatomical site of increased excitability was the motor cortex [314].

Basal ganglia

Different investigators define the term basal ganglia differently, but the term commonly includes the caudate nucleus, the putamen, and the globus pallidus. Some authors also include the substantia nigra and the subthalamic nucleus (STN) because they are functionally related to the other components [83]. The putamen and the globus pallidus are commonly known as the lentiform nucleus. The caudate nucleus and the putamen have similarities, and these two nuclei are often referred to collectively as the striatum or neostriatum.

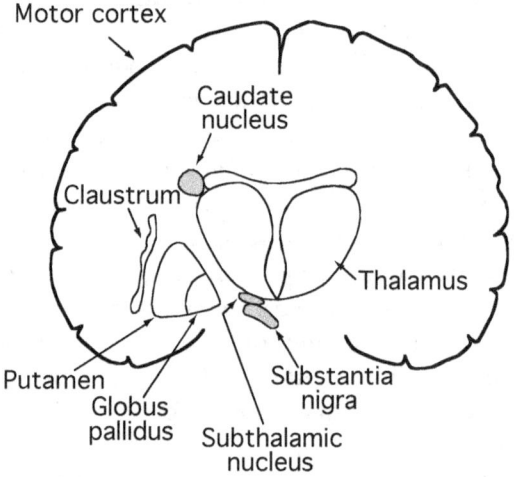

Figure D.12 Anatomical organization of the basal ganglia and the motor thalamus.

The basal ganglia do not issue motor commands, but rather modulate information from the cerebral cortex before sending it back through the motor thalamus (Figure D.13, D.14).

The basal ganglia receive input from cortical motor areas and relay the processed information to the thalamus, which then sends the information back to the motor cortex (Figure D.3). (The basal ganglia also process information from other parts of the cerebral cortex).

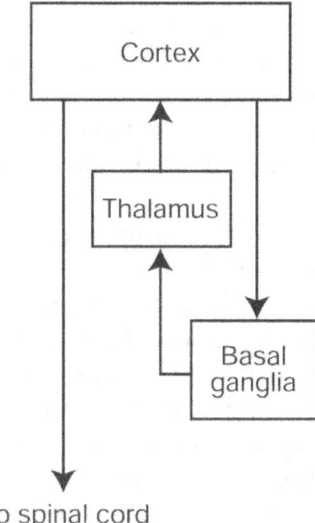

Figure D.13. Connections among the basal ganglia, the thalamus, and the motor cortices.

The basal ganglia are involved in many movement disorders, most characteristically in the more common disorders of PD and HD.

The significant role that the basal ganglia play in PD is responsible for the rapid increase in the interest in these nuclei. It has been demonstrated that various manipulations of these nuclei (surgical lesions, electrical stimulation) can have beneficial effects and can alleviate symptoms movement disorders.

This increased interest has also resulted in a more differentiated view of these ganglia, and several subdivisions of these nuclei are now recognized. Thus, the globus pallidus is commonly divided into an external segment (globus pallidus external part, GPe) and an internal segment (globus pallidus internal part, GPI). Likewise, the substantia nigra is divided into the pars reticulata (SNr) and the pars compacta (SNc) (Figure D.14).

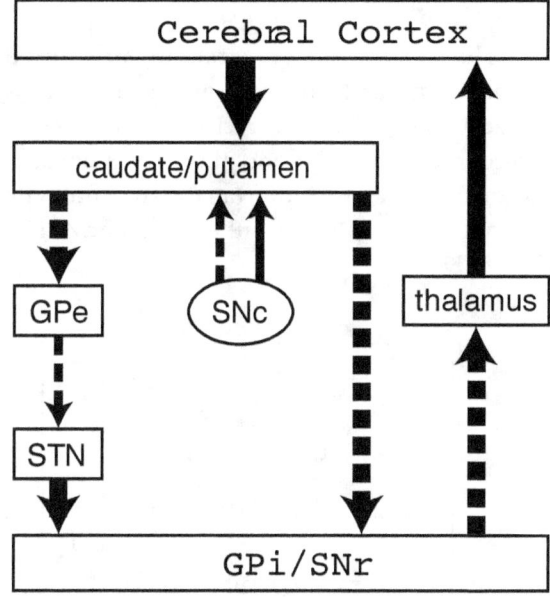

Figure D.14. Simplified schematic of the connections between the cerebral cortex and the nuclei of the basal ganglia and the thalamus. Black arrows show excitation and gray arrows show inhibition.

The functional organization of the basal ganglia is complex and is not completely understood. The function of the basal ganglia must be seen in regards to the interrelationship between components of multiple segregated circuits, including many other structures of the central nervous system [17].

The circuitry of the basal ganglia can be viewed as starting in the motor cortices (M1, PMA, and SMA) and somatosensory cortices (S1) that connect to portions of the putamen, GPe and GPi, the SNr, and the STN, (Figure D.15). The pathway through these nuclei continues through the motor thalamus (ventralis lateralis, pars oralis, VLo, and ventralis anterior, VA and returns the information to the same precentral motor area (MI) from which it originated [17].

The nuclei of the basal ganglia communicate closely with each other and with specific parts of the thalamus that connect to the motor cortices [83].

Direct and indirect routes

The nuclei of the striatum provide direct inhibitory input to the GPi and SNr, forming the "direct" route. The "indirect" route projects to the GPi/SNr via the GPe and the STN. GPi and SNr nuclei thus receive input from the striatum with and without interruption in the GPe and STN [17] (Figure D.15).

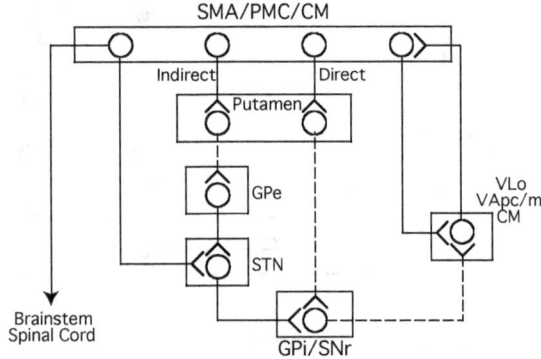

Figure D.15 Schematic of direct and indirect pathways of the basal ganglia. SMA: Supplementary motor area; PMC: Premotor cortex.

The striatum is the main point of entry for incoming information. Input from the cortices converges on the striatum (caudate nucleus and putamen), the centromedian nucleus (CM) of the thalamus and the substantia nigra (Figure D.17). The putamen receives input both from both motor cortex (MI) and somatosensory cortex (SI), but the cortical input to the caudate nucleus mostly originates from association cortices [83] (Figure D.18).

Inhibitory connections dominate the basal ganglia

Except for the connections between the STN and the GPi/SNr which are excitatory, all internal connections between nuclei of the basal ganglia are inhibitory. There is evidence, however, that the output of GPi and SNr provide tonic inhibition on thalamocortical neurons [742]. Whereas the direct dopaminergic nigrostriatal pathway from SNc may modulate the activity in the striatopallidal pathways in two different ways by using two different dopamine receptors. One of these two ways facilitates transmission in the "direct" pathway, while the other inhibits transmission in the "indirect" pathway[15].

The STN has afferent and efferent connections to both the globus pallidus and the substantia nigra and receives input from the motor cortex. The output from the basal ganglia originates mainly from the globus pallidus and the substantia nigra.

Pyramidal and extrapyramidal concepts

The fact that the activity of basal ganglia is intertwined with the descending pathways from the MI (corticospinal tract) (Figure D.17 and D.18) renders the distinction between pyramidal and extrapyramidal tracts invalid from an anatomical and physiological point of view. Nonetheless, that old distinction may retain some relevance for grouping symptoms in disorders of the motor system.

Control of motor activity

Several hypotheses have been presented regarding the role of the basal ganglia in control of motor activity. One hypothesis claims that the basal ganglia are involved in the planning of movements [16]. This hypothesis is supported by the existence of connections to PMA, SMA and prefrontal cortex (PF).

Diseases related to the basal ganglia

The basal ganglia seem to be involved in several important diseases, such as Parkinson's (PD) and Huntington's diseases (HD), and also in some rare diseases, such as Tourette's syndrome, which seem to be caused by pathologies of the basal ganglia.

Much of our understanding of the role of the basal ganglia in motor control has been gained from studies done in people with (PD) and other motor disorders undergoing lesioning or deep brain stimulation (DBS).

The fact that recordings of electrical activity from cells of the target nuclei are essential for making precise lesions or implantation of electrodes for DBS has provided opportunities for studies not previously possible. The methods that are used involve recordings from single nerve cells or small groups of nerve cells using microelectrodes.

This method of recording from deep brain structures in humans with microelectrodes is based on the work by Albe-Fessard and her co-workers [12].

The methods these investigators developed were later used routinely in intraoperative guidance and for basic studies of normal and pathological functions of the motor system [356, 358, 689, 690].

These studies have produced a wealth of information about the pathophysiology of movement disorders, and much information on the normal function of the basal ganglia and various parts of the thalamus have been gained through such studies.

Cerebellum

Like the basal ganglia, the cerebellum is involved in the control of movements but does not initiate movements. Rather, the cerebellum modifies and processes information from other central nervous system structures.

The cerebellum receives extensive input from sensory and proprioceptive sources such as the skin, joints, and muscle spindles through the spinocerebellar tract, and from the vestibular system. Aside from connecting to the basal ganglia and the spinal cord, cells in motor cortices also connect to the cerebellum (Figure D.16). The cerebellum plays an important role in shaping motor commands issued by the MI, but as is the case for the basal ganglia, the cerebellum is not believed to issue commands on its own.

Movement control regions of the cortex send input to the cerebellum through the pontine nuclei. The cerebellum relays information to cortical motor areas, red nucleus, and to the reticular formation of the brainstem (Figure D.17). There are extensive connections between the basal ganglia and the cerebellum.

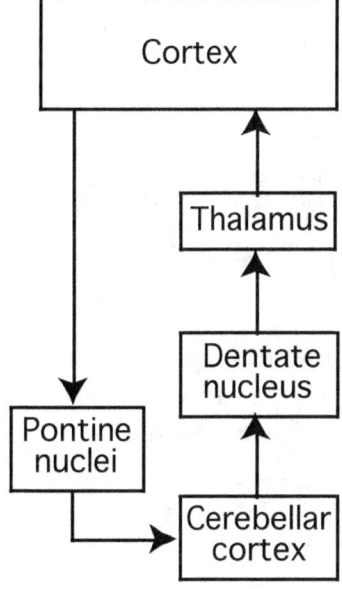

Figure D.16. Some important connections from the motor cortices to the cerebellum (cerebro-cerebellum) (After [83]).

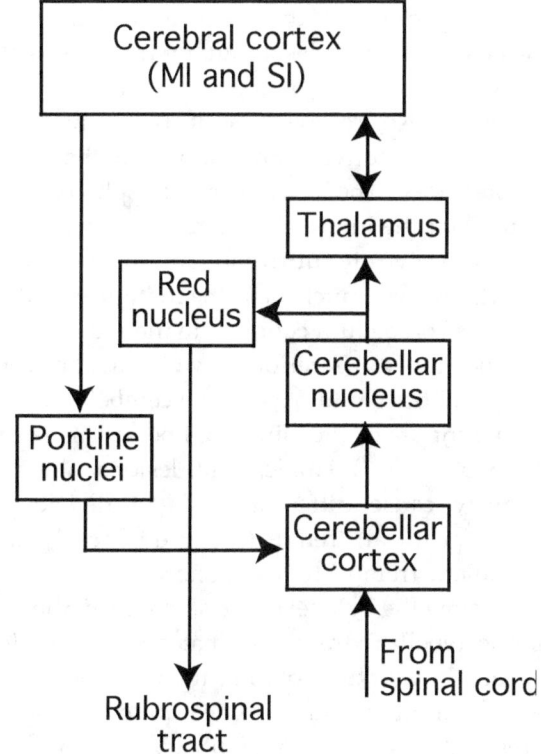

Figure D.17. Connections of the intermediate zone of the cerebellum (After [83]).

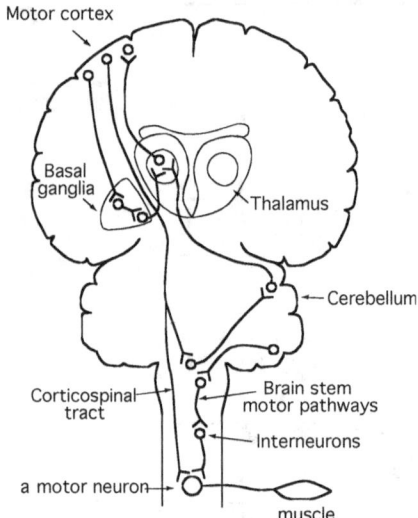

Figure D.18 Anatomical location of major motor pathways.

The pontine nuclei are important relays between the motor and sensory cortices (MI and SI) and the cerebellar cortex. The cerebellar cortex, in turn, provides input to the cerebral cortex via the dentate nucleus of the cerebellum. The dentate nucleus also provides input to the red nucleus, which is the origin of the rubrospinal tract. The thalamus also receives input from the dentate nucleus and conveys that input to the cerebral motor cortex. The cerebellar hemispheres receive input from the inferior olive in the medulla, which in turn receives input from many nuclei including the SC, pretectal nuclei and the red nucleus [83].

The cerebellum connects to the red nucleus, to pontine nuclei (inferior olive) via the central tegmental tract, and back to the cerebellum via the unique inputs of the climbing fibers. This is called the Mollaret's Triangle, and lesions along this pathway cause different kinds of deficits from rubral (postural) tremor (mixture of rest, postural and kinetic tremor) to myoclonus.

Below the T_1 level of the spinal cord, the dorsal spinocerebellar tract originates in the dorsal nucleus of Clarke's column, the neurons of which receive input from muscle spindles and low threshold cutaneous fibers. Above T_1, proprioceptive fibers do not travel in Clarke's column or the dorsal spinocerebellar tract. Instead, such information ascends in the fasciculus cuneatus of the dorsal column, the fibers of which make synaptic contact with cells in the accessory nucleus cuneatus in the lower medulla.

The axons of these cells form the cuneocerebellar tract that joins the dorsal spinocerebellar tract (from the lower body) to reach the restiform body (the larger part of the cerebellar peduncle). The restiform body is an input path to the cerebrum.

The ventral spinocerebellar tract takes a complex route. The fibers originate in cells in the lateral border of the ventral horn of the lumbar spinal cord. These cells receive input from proprioceptive afferent fibers and from collaterals of descending motor pathways. The axons of the spinal border cells cross the midline and ascend as the ventral spinocerebellar tract, through the medulla and pons and enter the cerebellum through the superior cerebellar peduncle.

The fibers cross the midline in the posterior fossa, which implies that this tract innervates predominantly the ipsilateral cerebellum. Afferent fibers from the upper spinal cord also reach cells predominantly in the ipsilateral cerebellum, via the rostral part of the spinocerebellar tract.

The spinocerebellar tract thus provides information to the cerebellum about the motor activity. One part of this tract conveys information from muscle spindles, tendon organs and cutaneous mechanoreceptors to the cerebellum. The other part provides information from spinal cord interneurons.

The reticulospinal and vestibulospinal tracts receive input from the cerebellum and vestibular nuclei, and the cells in the reticular formation provide input to the cerebellum. The number of fibers that connect to the cerebellum is much larger than the number of fibers that provide output from the cerebellum (40:1 in humans [83]).

Diverse functions of the cerebellum

The cerebellum consists of many different parts that have different functions. Earlier, it was assumed that the cerebellum was only involved in the control of movements, but more recently, it has become evident that the cerebellum also plays a role in many other functions, including cognitive functions. It has been hypothesized that the cerebellum is involved in the shifting of attention which as implicated cerebellar dysfunction in developmental disorders characterized by attention shifting deficits such as autism and ADHD [120].

References

1. Aakalu, G., et al., Dynamic visualization of local protein synthesis in hippocampal neurons. Neuron, 2001. 30(2): p. 489-502.

2. Abbott, R., Sensory Rhizotomy for the treatment of childhood spasticity, in Neurophysiology in Neurosurgery, V. Deletis and J.L. Shils, Editors. 2002, Academic Press: Amsterdam. p. 219-230.

3. Ackermans, L., Y. Temel, and V. Visser-Vandewalle, Deep brain stimulation in Tourette's Syndrome. Neurotherapeutics, 2008. 5: p. 339-44.

4. Adkins-Muir, D.L. and T.A. Jones, Cortical electrical stimulation combined with rehabilitative training: Enhanced functional recovery and dendritic plasticity following focal cortical ischemia in rats. Neurol. Res., 2003. 25: p. 780-788.

5. Adlington, P. and J. Warrick, Stellate ganglion block in the management of tinnitus. J. Laryngol. Otol., 1971. 85: p. 159-168.

6. Adour, K.K., J. Wingerd, and H.E. Doty, Prevalence of concurrent diabetes mellitus and idiopathic facial paralysis (Bell's palsy). Diabetes, 1975. 24(5): p. 449-51.

7. Adour, K.K., Mona Lisa syndrome: solving the enigma of the Gioconda smile. Ann. Otol. Rhinol. Laryngol., 1989. 98(3): p. 196-9.

8. Aggarwal, S., Cannabinergic pain medicine: a concise clinical primer and survey of randomized-controlled trial results. Clin J Pain., 2013. 29(2): p. 162-71.

9. Ahissar, E., R. Sosnik, and S. Haidarliu, Transformation from temporal to rate coding in a somatosensory thalamocortical pathway. Nature, 2000. 406(6793): p. 302-6.

10. Aitkin, L.M., The auditory midbrain, structure and function in the central auditory pathway. 1986, Clifton, NJ: Humana Press.

11. Aitkin, L.M., L. Tran, and J. Syka, The responses of neurons in subdivisions of the inferior colliculus of cats to tonal, noise and vocal stimuli. Exp. Brain Res., 1994. 98: p. 53-64.

12. Albe-Fessard, D., et al., Electrophysiological studies of some deep cerebral structures in man. J. Neuro. Sci., 1966. 3: p. 37-51.

13. Alberini, C. and J. LeDoux, Memory reconsolidation. Current Biology, 2013. 23(17): p. 746-50.

14. Alberini, C. and E. Kandel, The Regulation of Transcription in Memory Consolidation. Cold Spring Harb Perspect Biol., 2015. 7(1).

15. Albin, R.L., A.B. Young, and J.B. Penney, The functional anatomy of basal ganglia origin. Trends Neurosci., 1989. 12: p. 366-375.

16. Alexander, G.E. and M.D. Crutcher, Functional architecture of basal ganglia circuits: Neural substrate of parallel processing. Trends Neurosci., 1990(13): p. 266-71.

17. Alexander, G.E., M.D. Crutcher, and M.R. DeLong, Basal ganglia-thalamocortical circuits: Parallel substrates for motor, oculomotor, "prefrontal" and "limbic" functions. Progr. Brain Res., 1990. 85: p. 119-146.

18. Ali, T. and M. Kim, Melatonin ameliorates amyloid beta-induced memory deficits, tau hyperphosphorylation and neurodegeneration via PI3/Akt/GSk3β pathway in the mouse hippocampus. J Pineal Res, 2015. 59(1): p. 47-59.

19. Altschuler, E.L., et al., Rehabilitation of hemiparesis after stroke with a mirror. Lancet., 1999. 353(9169): p. 2035-6.

20. Altschuler, R.A., et al., Rescue and regrowth of sensory nerves following deafferentiation by neurotrophic factors. Ann. N.Y. Acad. Sci., 1999. 884: p. 305-11.

21. Alvarez, J., A. Giuditta, and E. Koenig, Protein synthesis in axons and terminals: significance for maintenance, plasticity and regulation of phenotype. With a critique of slow transport theory. Prog Neurobiol,, 2000. 62: p. 1-62.

22. Amaral, D.G., et al., Anatomical organization of the primate amydaloid complex, in The amygdala, J.P. Aggleton, Editor. 1992, Wiley-Liss: New York. p. 1-66.

23. Amassian, V.E., R.Q. Cracco, and P.J. Maccabee, Focal stimulation of human cerebral cortex with the magnetic coil: a comparison with electrical stimulation. Electroenceph. Clin. Neurophys., 1989. 74: p. 401-416.

24. Amassian, V.E., et al., Suppression of visual perception by magnetic coil stimulation of human occipital cortex. Electroenceph. Clin. Neurophysiol., 1989. 74(6): p. 458-62.

25. Aminoff, M.J., Electromyography in clinical practice. 1998, New York: Churchill Livingstone.

26. Andersen, P., et al., Mapping by microstimulation of overlapping projections from area 4 to motor units of the baboon's hand. Proc. R. Soc. London ser B., 1975. 188: p. 31-60.

27. Andersen, P., P.L. Knight, and M.M. Merzenich, The thalamocortical and corticothalamic connections of AI, AII, and the anterior field (AAF) in the cat: evidence for two largely segregated systems of connections. J. Comp. Neurol., 1980. 194: p. 663-701.

28. Andersen, R.G. and W.L. Meyerhoff, Otologic pathology and tinnitus, in Tinnitus and its management, J.G. Clark and P. Yanick, Editors. 1984, Charles C Thomas Publishers: Springfield, Ill.

29. Apfelbaum, R.I., A comparison of percutaneous radiofrequency trigeminal neurolysis and microvascular decompression of the trigeminal nerve for treatment of tic douloureux. Neurosurgery, 1977(1): p. 16-21.

30. Apkarian, A., J. Hashmi, and M. Baliki, Pain and the brain: specificity and plasticity of the brain in clinical chronic pain. Pain, 2010. 152(3 Suppl): p. 49-64.

31. Aran, J.M. and I. Cazals, Electrical suppression of tinnitus, in Ciba Foundation Symposium 85. 1981, Pitman Books Ltd: London. p. 217-225.

32. Ashby, P. and M. Wiens, Reciprocal inhibition following lesions of the spinal cord in man. J. Physiol., 1989. 414: p. 145-57.

33. Auger, R.G. and J.P. Whisnant, Hemifacial spasm in Rochester and Olmsted County, Minnesota, 1960 to 1984. Arch. Neurol., 1990(47): p. 1233-1234.

34. Bach, S., M.F. Noreng, and N.U. Tjellden, Phantom limb pain in amputees during the first 12 months following limb amputation, after preoperative lumbar epidural blockade. Pain, 1988. 33: p. 297-301.

35. Baguley, D.M., Hyperacusis. J R Soc Med., 2003. 96(12): p. 582-5.

36. Bakin, J.S. and N.M. Weinberger, Induction of a physiological memory in the cerebral cortex by stimulation of the nucleus basalis. Proc. Natl. Acad. Sci. USA, 1996. 93(20): p. 11219-24.

37. Baliki, M., et al., Brain morphological signatures for chronic pain. PLoS One, 2011. 6(10).

38. Baliki, M., et al., Corticostriatal functional connectivity predicts transition to chronic back pain. Nat Neurosci., 2012. 15(8).

39. Baliki, M.N., et al., Chronic pain hurts the brain, disrupting the default-mode network dynamics. J Neurosci., 2008. 28: p. 1398-1403.

40. Baloh, R.W. and V. Honrubia, Clinical neurophysiology of the vestibular system. 1990, Philadelphia: F.A.Davis Company.

41. Bandler, R. and M.T. Shipley, Columnar organization in the midbrain periaqueductal gray: Modules for emotional expression? Trends Neurosci., 1994. 17: p. 379-389.

42. Bano, D., et al., Ageing, neuronal connectivity and brain disorders: an unsolved ripple effect. Mol Neurobiol., 2011. 43(2).

43. Barker, A.T., R. Jalinous, and I.L. Freeston, Non-invasive magnetic stimulation of the human motor cortex. Lancet, 1985: p. 1106-1107.

44. Barker, F.G., et al., Microvascular Decompression for Hemifacial Spasm. J. Neurosurg., 1995. 82: p. 201-210.

45. Barker, F.G., et al., The long-term outcome of microvascular decompression for trigeminal neuralgia. N. Eng. J. Med., 1996. 334: p. 1077-1083.

46. Bartels, S., et al., Noise-induced hearing loss: the effect of melanin in the stria vascularis. Hear. Res., 2001. 154: p. 116-123.

47. Basbaum, A.I. and H.L. Fields, Endogenous pain control systems: brainstem spinal pathways and endorphin circuitry. Ann. Rev. Neurosci., 1984. 7(309-338).

48. Beckes, L., J. Coan, and K. Hasselmo, Familiarity promotes the blurring of self and other in the neural representation of threat. Social Cognitive & Affective Neurosci, 2012. 8: p. 670-7.

49. Beenstock, M., Predicting the stability and growth of acoustic neuromas. Otol. Neurotol., 2002. 23: p. 542-49.

50. Bennett, D.A., et al., Prevalence of parkinsonian signs and associated mortality in a community population of older people. N. Eng. J. Med., 1996. 334: p. 71-76.

51. Bennett, R.M., Fibromyalgia, in Handbook of Pain, P.D. Wall and R. Melzack, Editors. 1999, Churchill Livingstone: Edinburgh. p. 579-601.

52. Benoliel, R. and E. Eliav, Primary headache disorders. Dent Clin North Am., 2013. 57(3): p. 513-39.

53. Benson, D.L., et al., Making memories stick: cell-adhesion molecules in synaptic plasticity. Trends Cell Biol, 2000. 10(11): p. 473-82.

54. Berardelli, A., et al., Pathophysiology of blepharospasm and oromandibular dystonia. Brain, 1985. 108: p. 593-608.

55. Bergmann, C. and M. Sano, Cardiac risk factors and potential treatments in Alzheimer's disease. Neurol Res, 2006. 28(6): p. 595-604.

56. Berthoud, H.R. and W.L. Neuhuber, Functional and chemical anatomy of the afferent vagal system. Autonomic Neurosci., 2000. 85(1-3): p. 1-17.

57. Beurrier, C., et al., High-frequency stimulation produces a transient blockade of voltage-gated currents in subthalamic neurons. J. Neurophys., 2001. 85: p. 1351-1356.

58. Bigal, M.E., et al., Migraine and cardiovascular disease, Possible mechanisms of interaction. Neurology., 2009. 72: p. 1864–1871.

59. Blackburn, S., Hyperbilirubinemia and neonatal jaundice. Neonatal Netw., 1995. 14: p. 15-25.

60. Blackburn-Munro, G. and R.E. Blackburn-Munro, Chronic pain, chronic stress and depression: coincidence or consequence? J Neuroendocrinol, 2001. 13(12): p. 1009-23.

61. Blandini, F., C. Tassorelli, and J.T. Greenamyre, Movement disorders, in Principle of Neural Aging, S.U. Dani, A. Hori, and G.F. Walter, Editors. 1997, Elsevier: Amsterdam.

62. Blask, D., Melatonin, sleep disturbance and cancer risk. Sleep Med Rev, 2009. 13(4): p. 257-64.

63. Blondeau, N.L., RH.;Bourourou, M.; et al, Alpha-Linolenic Acid: An Omega-3 Fatty Acid with Neuroprotective Properties—Ready for Use in the Stroke Clinic? Biomed Res Int, 2015. 2015: p. ID 519830, 8 pages.

64. Bluestone, C.D., Otitis media: A spectrum of diseases, in Pediatric Otology and Neurotology, A.K. Lalwani and K.M. Grundfast, Editors. 1998, Lippincott-Raven: Philadelphia. p. 233-40.

65. Bocca, E., Distorted speech tests, in Sensory-neural hearing processes and disorders, B.A. Graham, Editor. 1965, Little, Brown & Co: Boston.

66. Boeve, B.F., et al., Association of REM sleep behavior disorder and neurodegenerative disease may reflect an underlying synucleinopathy. Movement Disorders, 2001. 16(4): p. 622-30.

67. Boivie, J., Central pain, in Textbook of Pain, P.D. Wall and R. Melzack, Editors. 1999, Churchill Livingstone: Edinburgh. p. 879-914.

68. Bolay, H. and M.A. Moskowitz, Mechanisms of pain modulation in chronic syndromes. Neurology, 2002. 59(5 Suppl. 2): p. S2-7.

69. Bonin von, G. and P. Bailey, The Neocortex of the Macaca mulatia. 1947, Urbana, IL: University of Illinois Press.

70.   Borg, E. and A.R. Møller, Noise and blood pressure: Effects on lifelong exposure in the rat. Acta Physiol. Scand., 1978. 103: p. 340-42.

71.   Borg, E., Noise induced hearing loss in normotensive and spontaneously hypertensive rats. Hear. Res., 1982. 8: p. 117-130.

72.   Borg, E., Noise induced hearing loss in rats with renal hypertension. Hear. Res., 1982. 8: p. 93-99.

73.   Borg-Stein, J. and S.A. Simon, Focused review: myofascial pain. Arch. Phys. Med. Rehab., 2002. 83(3): p. S40-7, S48-9.

74.   Born, D.E. and E.W. Rubel, Afferent influences on brain stem auditory nuclei of the chicken: presynaptic action potentials regulate protein synthesis in nucleu magnocellularis neurons. J. Neurosci., 1988. 8(3): p. 901-919.

75.   Borsel van, J., L.M.G. Curfs, and J.P. Fryns, Hyperacusis in Williams syndrome: A sample survey study. Genetic Counseling, 1997. 8(2): p. 121-126.

76.   Borsook, D.V., R.; Espelding., N.; Borra, R., et al, The Insula: A "Hub of Activity" in Migraine. The neuroscientist, 2016. 22.

77.   Brach, J.S., et al., Facial Neuromuscular Retraining for Oral Synkinesis. Plastic and Reconstructive Surgery, 1997. 99(7): p. 1922-1931.

78.   Brackmann, D.E., C. Shelton, and M.A. Arriaga, Otologic Surgery. Vol. 2nd ed. 2001, Philadelphia: W.B. Saunders Co.

79.   Brandt, T., S. Steddin, and R.B. Daroff, Therapy for benign paroxysmal positioning vertigo, revisted. Neurology, 1994. 44: p. 796-800.

80.   Brattgard, S.O., The importance of adequate stimulation for the chemical composition of retinal ganglion cells during early postnatal develoepment. Acta Radiol. (Stockh.), 1952. Suppl. 96: p. 1-80.

81.   Braun, C.M., et al., Brain modules of hallucination: an analysis of multiple patients with brain lesions. J Psychiatry Neurosci., 2003. 28(6): p. 432-49.

82.   Brodal, P., The central nervous system. 3rd ed. 2004, New York: Oxford Press.

83.   Brodal, P., The Central Nervous System Fourth Edition. 2010, New York: Oxford University Press.

84.   Brown, J.A., et al., Motor cortex stimulation for enhancement of recovery after stroke: Case report. Neurol. Res., 2003. 25: p. 815-818.

85.   Brown, P., Pathophysiology of spasticity. J. Neurol. Neurosurg. Psychiatry, 1994. 57: p. 773-777.

86.   Burke, D., Spasticity as an adaptation to pyramidal tract injury, in Functional Recovery in Neurological Disease, S.G. Waxman, Editor. 1988, Raven Press: New York.

87.   Burns, W. and D.W. Robinson, Hearing and noise in Industry. 1970, London: Her Majesty's Stationery Office.

88.   Burstein, R., M.F. Cutrer, and D. Yarnitsky, The development of cutaneous allodynia during a migraine attack clinical evidence for the sequential recruitment of spinal and supraspinal nociceptive neurons in migraine. Brain, 2000. 123(8): p. 1703-9.

89.   Busch, V., et al., The effect of transcutaneous vagus nerve stimulation on pain perception--an experimental study. Brain Stimul., 2013. 6(2): p. 202-9.

90.   Bushnell, M.C., Ceko M, and L. LA., Cognitive and emotional control of pain and its disruption in chronic pain. Nat Rev Neurosci, 2013. 14(7): p. 502-11.

91.   Buzsaki, G. and A. Draguhn, Neuronal oscillations in cortical networks. Science, 2004. 304: p. 1926-29.

92.   Cacace, A.T., et al., Anomalous cross-modal plasticity following posterior fossa surgery: Some speculations on gaze-evoked tinnitus. Hear. Res., 1994. 81: p. 22-32.

93.   Cacace, A.T., et al., Cutaneous-evoked tinnitus. II: Review of neuroanatomical, physiological and functional imaging studies. Audiol. Neurotol., 1999. 4(5): p. 258-268.

94.   Cacace, A.T., et al., Cutaneous-evoked tinnitus. I: Phenomenology, psychophysics and functional imaging. Audiol. Neurotol, 1999. 4(5): p. 247-257.

95.   Cacace, A.T., Expanding the biological basis of tinnitus: crossmodal origins and the role of neuroplasticity. Hear. Res., 2003. 175: p. 112-132.

96.   Cai, Z.G., et al., Efficacy of functional training of the facial muscles for treatment of incomplete peripheral facial nerve injury. Chin J Dent Res, 2010. 13(1): p. 37-43.

97.   Calford, M.B. and L.M. Aitkin, Ascending projections to the medial geniculate body of the cat: Evidence for multiple, parallel auditory pathways through the thalamus. J. Neurosci., 1983. 3(2): p. 365-380.

98.   Canavero, S., et al., Low-rate repetitive TMS allays central pain. Neurol. Res., 2003. 25: p. 151-152.

99.   Canlon, B., E. Borg, and A. Flock, Protection against noise trauma by pre-exposure to a low level acoustic stimulus. Hear. Res., 1988. 34: p. 197-200.

100.   Cant, N.B., Structural developemnt of the mammalien auditory pathways, in Development of the auditory system, E.W. Rubel, A.N. Popper, and R.R. Fay, Editors. 1998, Springer: New York. p. 315-413.

101.   Caspary, D.M., et al., Immunocytochemical and neurochemical evidence for age-related loss of GABA in the inferior colliculus: Implications for neural presbycusis. J. Neurosci., 1990. 10: p. 2363-2372.

102.   Caspary, D.M., J.C. Milbrandt, and R.H. Helfert, Central auditory aging: GABA changes in the inferior colliculus. Exp. Gerontol., 1995. 30: p. 349-360.

103.   Caspary, D.M., et al., Age-related changes in GABA$_A$ Receptor subunit composition and function in rat auditory system. Neuroscience, 1999. 93(1): p. 307-312.

104.   Cazals, Y., M. Negrevergne, and J.M. Aran, Electrical stimulation of the cochlea in man: Hearing induction and tinnitus suppression. J. Am. Audiol. Soc., 1978. 3: p. 209-213.

105.   Cervero, F., Sensory innervation of the viscera: peripheral basis of visceral pain. Physiol. Rev., 1994. 74: p. 95-138.

106.   Chan, B.L., et al., Mirror therapy for phantom limb pain. N Engl J Med., 2007. 357(21): p. 2206-7.

107. Chan, S.L. and M.M. Mattson, Caspase and calpain substrates: roles in synaptic plasticity and cell death. J. Neurosci. Res., 1999. 58(1): p. 167-90.

108. Chandler, M.J., et al., Effects of vagal afferent stimulation on cervical spinothalamic tract neurons in monkeys. Pain, 1991. 44: p. 81-87.

109. Chapman, C.V., CJ., The Transition of Acute Postoperative Pain to Chronic Pain: An Integrative Overview of Research on Mechanisms. The Journal of Pain, 2016.

110. Charabi, S., et al., Acoustic neuroma/vestibular schwannoma growth: past, present and future. Acta Otolaryngol. (Stockh), 1998. 118: p. 327-32.

111. Chen, S.X., et al., Subtype-specific plasticity of inhibitory circuits in motor cortex during motor learning. Nat Neurosci,, 2015. 18: p. 1109-1115.

112. Citri, A. and R. Malenka, Synaptic Plasticity: Multiple Forms, Functions, and Mechanisms. Neuropsychopharmacology, 2008. 33: p. 18-41.

113. Cleare, A., et al., Chronic fatigue syndrome. BMJ Clin Evid, 2015. Sep 28.

114. Coad, M.L., et al., Characteristics of patients with gaze-evoked tinnitus. Otol. Neurotol., 2001. 22: p. 650-4.

115. Coderre, T.J., et al., Contribution of central neuroplasticity to pathological pain: Review of clinical and experimental evidence. Pain, 1993. 52: p. 259-285.

116. Cole, J., et al., Exploratory findings with virtual reality for phantom limb pain; from stump motion to agency and analgesia. Disabil Rehabil., 2009. 31(10): p. 846-54.

117. Colletti, V., et al., Hearing habilitation with auditory brainstem implantation in two children with cochlear nerve aplasia. Int. J. Pediatric Otorhinolaryngol., 2001. 60(2): p. 99-111.

118. Conlon, B.J. and D.W. Smith, Attenuation of neomycin ototoxicity by iron chelation. Larygoscope, 1998. 108: p. 284-7.

119. Cooper, I.S., Ligation of the anterior choroidal artery for involuntary movements in parkinsonism. Psychiatry, 1953. 27: p. 317-319.

120. Courchesne, E., et al., Impairment in shifting attention in autistic and cerebellar patients. Behav. Neurosci., 1994. 108: p. 848-865.

121. Cousins, M.J. and P.O. Bridenbbaugh, Neural blockade in clinical anesthesia and management of pain. 3rd ed. 1998, Philadelphia: Lippingcott-Raven.

122. Crago, A., J.C. Houk, and W.Z. Rymer, Sampling of total muscle force by tendon organs. J. Neurophys., 1982. 47: p. 1069-1083.

123. Craig, A., How do you feel? Interoception: the sense of the physiological condition of the body. Nat Rev Neurosci., 2002. 3(8): p. 655-66.

124. Cramer, S.C., et al., Mapping individual brains to guide restorative therapy after stroke: Rationale and pilot studies. Neurol Res, 2003(25): p. 811-814.

125. Crofford, L.J., Pain management in fibromyalgia. Curr Opin Rheumatol, 2008. 20(3): p. 246-50.

126. Crowley, W.R., J.F. Rodriguez-Sierra, and B.R. Komisaruk, Analgesia induced by vagina stimulation in rats is apparently independent of a morphine-sensitive process. Psychopharmacology, 1977. 54(3): p. 223-5.

127. Culp, W.J., J. Ochoa, and H.E. Torebjoerk, Ectopic impulse generation in myelinated sensory nerve fibers in man, in Abnormal nerves and muscles as impulse generators, W.J. Culp and J. Ochoa, Editors. 1982, Oxford University Press: New York. p. 490-512.

128. Cushing, H., The major trigeminal neuralgias and their surgical treatment based on experience with 332 gasserian operations. Am. J. Med. Sci., 1920(160): p. 158-184.

129. Dahlöf, C.G.H., Management of primary headaches: Current and future aspects, in Pain 2002 - An updated review: Refresher course syllabus, M.A. Giamberardino, Editor. 2002, IASP Press: Seattle.

130. Damasio, A. and G. Carvalho, The nature of feelings: evolutionary and neurobiological origins. Nat Rev Neurosci., 2013. 14(2): p. 143-52.

131. Dancer, A.L., et al., Noise induced hearing loss. 1990, St. Louis: Mosby Year Book.

132. Davis, M., The role of the amygdala in fear and anxiety. Ann. Rev. Neurosci, 1992. 15: p. 353-375.

133. de Jong, P., Age-related macular degeneration. N Engl J Med., 2006. 355(14): p. 1474-85.

134. De Ridder, D., et al., Magnetic and electrical stimulation of the auditory cortex for intractable tinnitus. J. Neurosurg., 2004. 100(3): p. 560-4.

135. De Ridder, D., et al., Somatosensory cortex stimulation for deafferentation pain. Acta Neurochir, 2007. 97(Suppl. Pt. 2): p. 67-74.

136. De Ridder, D. and S. Vanneste, Auditory cortex stimulation for tinnitus, in Textbook of Tinnitus, A.R. Møller, et al., Editors. 2010, Springer: New York. p. 717-726.

137. De Ridder, D., et al., Microvascular decompression for tinnitus: significant improvement for tinnitus intensity without improvement for distress. A 4-year limit. Neurosurgery. , 2010. 66(4): p. 656-60.

138. De Ridder, D., et al., Phantom percepts: tinnitus and pain as persisting aversive memory networks. Proc Natl Acad Sci U S A, 2011. 108(20): p. 8075-80.

139. De Ridder, D., et al., Phantom percepts: tinnitus and pain as persisting aversive memory networks. Proc Natl Acad Sci U S A. , 2011. 108(20): p. 8075-80.

140. De Ridder, D., et al., An integrative model of auditory phantom perception: tinnitus as a unified percept of interacting separable subnetworks. Neurosci Biobehav Rev., 2014. 44: p. 16-32.

141. De Ridder D, V.S., Engineer ND, Kilgard MP., Safety and efficacy of vagus nerve stimulation paired with tones for the treatment of tinnitus: a case series. Neuromodulation, 2014. 17(2): p. 170-9.

142. DeCandia, M., L. Provini, and H. Taborikova, Mechanisms of the reflex discharge depression in spinal motoneurone during repetitive orthodromic stimulation. Brain Res., 1967. 4: p. 284-291.

143. Dehmel, S., Y.L. Cui, and S.E. Shore, Cross-modal interactions of auditory and somatic inputs in the brainstem and midbrain and their imbalance in tinnitus and deafness. Am J Audiol, 2008. 17(2): p. S193-209.

144. Deletis, V., Intraoperative neurophysiology and methodologies used to monitor the functional integrity of the motor system, in Neurophysiology in Neurosurgery, V. Deletis and J.L. Shils, Editors. 2002, Academic Press: Amsterdam. p. 25-51.

145. Delwaide, P.J. and E. Oliver, Short latency autogenic inhibition (Ib inhibition) in human spasticity. J. Neurol. Neurosurg. Psych., 1988. 51: p. 1548-50.

146. Densert, B. and K. Sass, Control of symptoms in patients with Ménière's disease using middle ear pressure applications: Two years follow-up. Acta Otolaryng. (Stockh.), 2001. 121: p. 616-621.

147. Densert, O., Adrenergic innervation in the rabbit cochlea. Acta Otolaryngol. (Stockh.), 1974. 78: p. 345-356.

148. Dergacheva, O., et al., The Lateral Paragigantocellular Nucleus Modulates Parasympathetic Cardiac Neurons: A Mechanism for Rapid Eye Movement Sleep-Dependent Changes in Heart Rate. J Neurophysiol., 2010. 104: p. 685-694.

149. Devor, M., The pathophysiology of damaged peripheral nerves, in Textbook of pain, P.D. Wall and R. Melzack, Editors. 1994, Churchill Livingstone: Edinburgh. p. 79-100.

150. Devor, M. and Z. Seltzer, Pathophysiology of damaged nerves in relation to chronic pain, in Textbook of Pain, P.D. Wall and R. Melzack, Editors. 1999, Churchill Livingstone: Edinburgh. p. 129-164.

151. Diamond, M.E. and M. Armstrong-James, The role of parallel sensory pathways and cortical columns in learning. Concepts Neurosci., 1992. 3: p. 55-78.

152. Dietz, V., Spinal cord pattern generators for locomotion. Clin. Neurophysiol., 2003. 114(8): p. 1379-89.

153. Dimitrijevic, M.R., Model for the study of plasticity of the human nervous system: features of residual spinal cord motor activity resulting from established post-traumatic injury, in Plasticity of the neuromuscular system (Chiba Foundation Symposium 138). 1988, Wiley: Chichester. p. 227-239.

154. Dinse, H.R., et al., Optical imaging of cat auditory cortex cochleotopic selectivity evoked by acute electrical stimualtion of a multi-channel cochlear implant. Eur. J. Neurosci, 1997. 9(9): p. 113-9.

155. Diorio, J. and M. Meaney, Maternal programming of defensive responses through sustained effects on gene expression. J Psychiatry Neurosci, 2007. 32(4): p. 275-84.

156. Dobie, R. and U. Fisch, Primary and revision surgery (selective neurectomy) for facial hyperkinesis. Arch. Otolaryngol. Head Neck Surg., 1986(112): p. 154-163.

157. Donoghue, J.P., S. Suner, and J.N. Sanes, Dynamic organization of primary motor cortex output to target muscles in adult rats. II. Rapid reorganization following motor nerve lesions. Exp. Brain Res., 1990. 79(3): p. 492-503.

158. Doubell, T.P., R.J. Mannion, and C.J. Woolf, The dorsal horn: state-dependent sensory processing, plasticity and the generation of pain, in Handbook of Pain, P.D. Wall and R. Melzack, Editors. 1999, Churchill Livingstone: Edinburgh. p. 165-181.

159. Dum, R. and P. Strick, The origin of corticospinal projections from the premotor areas in the frontal lobe. J Neurosci., 1991. 11: p. 667-89.

160. Ebert, D.H., Activity-dependent neuronal signalling and autism spectrum disorder. Nature, 2013. 493: p. 327-37.

161. Eccles, J.C., Plasticity at its simplest level, in Centennial lectures of E.E. Squibb & Son. 1959, Putnam & Sons: New York. p. 217-244.

162. Edeline, J.M., The thalamo-cortical auditory receptive fields: regulation by the states of vigilance, learning and the neuromodulatory system. Exp. Brain Res., 2003. 153(4): p. 554-72.

163. Eggermont, J. and P. Tass, Maladaptive neural synchrony in tinnitus: origin and restoration. Front Neurol., 2015. Feb 17;6:29.

164. Eggermont, J.J., On the pathophysiology of tinnitus: A review and a peripheral model. Hear. Res., 1990. 48: p. 111-124.

165. Elbert, T., et al., Increased cortical representation of the fingers of the left hand in string players. Science, 1995. 270(5234): p. 305-7.

166. Engel, A.K. and G.W. Kreutzberg, Neuronal surface changes in the dorsal vagal motor nucleus of the guinea pig in response to axotomy. J. Comp. Neurol., 1988. 275: p. 181-200.

167. Engert, F. and T. Bonhoeffer, Dendritic spine changes associated with hippocampal long-term synaptic plasticity. Nature., 1999. 399(6731): p. 66-70.

168. Engineer, N.D., et al., Reversing pathological neural activity using targeted plasticity. Nature, 2011. 470(7332): p. 101-4.

169. Engineer, N.D., Møller, A.R., Kilgard, M.P., Directing neural plasticity to understand and treat tinnitus. Hearing Research, 2013. 295: p. 58-66.

170. Englot, D.J., E.F. Chang, and K.I. Auguste, Vagus nerve stimulation for epilepsy: a meta-analysis of efficacy and predictors of response. J Neurosurg., 2011. 115(6): p. 1248-55.

171. Eroglu, C. and B.A. Barres, Regulation of synaptic connectivity by glia. Nature, 2010. 468(7321): p. 223-31.

172. Esslen, E., Der Spasmus facialis -- eine Parabiosserscheinung: Elektrophysiologische Untersuchungen zum Enstehungsmechanismus des Facialisspasmus. Dtsch. Z. Nervenheil., 1957. 176: p. 149-172.

173. Esteban, A. and P. Molina-Negro, Primary hemifacial spasm: a neurophysiological study. J. Neurol. Neurosurg. Psych., 1986. 49: p. 58-63.

174. Eyo, U.B. and M.E. Dailey, Microglia: key elements in neural development, plasticity, and pathology. Neuroimmmune Pharmacology, 2013. 8(3): p. 494-509.

175. Falck, B., et al., Fluorescence of catcholamines and related compound condensed with formaldehyde. Brain Res. Bull., 1982. 9: p. 1-6.

176. Farmer, M.A., M.N. Baliki, and A.V. Apkarian, A dynamic Network perspective of chronic pain. Neurosci Lett, 2012. 520(2): p. 197-203.

177. Fasano, V.A., G. Broggi, and S. Zeme, Intraoperative electrical stimulation for functional posterior rhizotomy. Scand. J. Rehab. Med., 1988. 17: p. 149-54.

178. Ferguson, J.H., Hemifacial spasm and the facial nucleus. Ann. Neurol., 1978. 4: p. 97 103.

179. Fernandes, D. and A. Carvalho, Mechanisms of homeostatic plasticity in the excitatory synapse. J Neurochem., 2016. 139(6): p. 973-996.

180. Ferry, B., B. Roozendaal, and J.L. McGaugh, Role of norepinephrine in mediating stress hormone regulation of long term memory storage: a critical involvement of the amygdala. Biol. Psychiatry, 1999. 46(9): p. 1142-1152.

181. Fetz, E.E., K. Toyama, and W. Smith, Synaptic interaction between cortical neurons, in Cerebral cortex, E.G. Jones and A. Peters, Editors. 1990, Plenum: New York. p. 1-47.

182. Fields, H.L. and A.I. Basbaum, Central nervous system mechanism of pain modulation, in Textbook of Pain, P.D. Wall and R. Melzack, Editors. 1999, Churchill Livingstone: Edinburgh. p. 309-329.

183. Fitzgerald, D.C. and A.S. Mark, Sudden hearing loss: frequency of abnormal findings on contrast-enhanced MR studies. Am J Neuroradiol., 1998. 19(8): p. 1433-6.

184. Flament, D., P.A. Fortier, and E.E. Fetz, Response patterns and post-spike effects of peripheral afferents in dorsal root ganglia of behaving monkeys. J.Neurophysiol., 1992. 67: p. 875-889.

185. Flor, H., et al., Phantom-limb pain as a perceptual correlate of cortical reorganization following arm amputation. Nature, 1995. 375(6531): p. 482-4.

186. Forge, A. and J. Schacht, Aminoglycoside antibiotics. Audiol. Neurotol., 2000. 5: p. 3-22.

187. Fowler, E.P., The illusion of loudness of tinnitus-its etiology and treatment. Ann. Otol. Laryngol., 1942. 52: p. 275-285.

188. Freckmann, N., et al., Treatment of neurogenic torticollis by microvascular lysis of the accessory nerve roots: Indication, technique, and first results. Acta Neurochir. (Wien), 1981(59): p. 167-175.

189. French, J.D., M. Verzeano, and H.W. Magoun, An extralemniscal sensory system of the brain. AMA Arch. Neurol. Psychiat.,, 1953. 69: p. 505-519.

190. Friston, K., Functional and Effective Connectivity: A Review. Brain Connectivity, 2011. 1.

191. Frith, U. and F. Happé, Autism: beyond "theory of mind. Cognition, 1994. 50(1-3): p. 115-32.

192. Froehling, D.A., et al., Benign positional vertigo: incidence and prognosis in a population-based study in Olmsted County, Minnesota. Mayo Clinic Proceedings, 1991. 66(6): p. 596-601.

193. Fromm, G., Medical treatment of patients with trigeminal neuralgia, in Fromm G.H and Sessle B.J. Trigeminal Neuralgia. 1991, Butterworth-Heinemann: Boston. p. 133-144.

194. Fromm, G.H., et al., Role of inhibitory mechanisms in trigeminal neuralgia. Neurology, 1981. 31: p. 683-687.

195. Fromm, G.H., Pathophysiology of trigeminal neuralgia, in Trigeminal Neuralgia, G.H. Fromm and B.J. Sessle, Editors. 1991, Butterworth-Heinemann: Boston. p. 105-130.

196. Fromm, G.H. and B.J. Sessle, Trigeminal Neuralgia. 1991, Boston: Butterworth-Heinemann.

197. Fu, K.M., et al., Auditory cortical neurons respond to somatosensory stimulation. J. Neurosci., 2003. 23(20): p. 7510-5.

198. Gajewski, P.D., et al., The Met-allele of the BDNF Val66Met polymorphism enhances task switching in elderly. Neurobiol Aging, 2011. 32: p. e2327-2319.

199. Galambos, R., R. Myers, and G. Sheatz, Extralemniscal activation of auditory cortex in cats. Am. J. Physiol., 1961. 200: p. 23-28.

200. Gallowitsch-Puerta, M. and V.A. Pavlov, Neuro-immune interactions via the cholinergic anti-inflammatory pathway. Life Sci. , 2007. 80(24-25): p. 2325-9.

201. Gardner, W.J. and M. Miklos, Response of trigeminal neuralgia to "decompression" of sensory root. JAMA, 1959(170): p. 1773-1776.

202. Gardner, W.J., Concerning the mechanism of trigeminal neuralgia and hemifacial spasm. J. Neurosurg., 1962(19): p. 947-958.

203. Gardner, W.J. and G.A. Sava, Hemifacial spasm -- a reversible pathophysiologic state. J. Neurosurg., 1962(19): p. 240-247.

204. Gardner, W.J., Crosstalk -- The paradoxical transmission of a nerve impulse. Arch. Neurol., 1966. 14: p. 149-156.

205. Gates, G.A., N.N. Couropmitree, and R.H. Myers, Genetic associations in age-related hearing thresholds. Arch. Otolaryngol. Head &Neck Surg., 1999. 125(6): p. 654-9.

206. Gebhart, G.F. and A. Randich, Vagal modulation of nociception. Am. Pain Soc. J., 1992. 1: p. 26-32.

207. Geha, P., et al., The brain in chronic CRPS pain: abnormal gray-white matter interactions in emotional and autonomic regions. Neuron., 2008. 60(4): p. 570-81.

208. Gejrot, T., Intravenous xylocaine in the treatment of attacks of Ménière's disease. Acta Otolaryngol. (Stockh), 1963. Suppl 188: p. 190-195.

209. Gerhart, K.D., R.P. Yezierski, and G.J. Giesler, Inhibitory receptive fields of primate spinothalamic tract cells. J. Neurophys, 1981. 46: p. 1309-25.

210. Gerken, G.M., Temporal summation of pulsate brain stimulation in normal and deafened cats. J. Acoust. Soc. Am., 1979. 66: p. 728-734.

211. Gerken, G.M., S.S. Saunders, and R.E. Paul, Hypersensitivity to electrical stimulation of auditory nuclei follows hearing loss in cats. Hear. Res., 1984. 13: p. 249-260.

212. Gerken, G.M., J.M. Solecki, and F.A. Boettcher, Temporal integration of electrical stimulation of auditory nuclei in normal hearing and hearing-impaired cat. Hear. Res., 1991. 53: p. 101-112.

213. Gerken, G.M., P.S. Hesse, and J.J. Wiorkowski, Auditory evoked responses in control subjects and in patients with problem tinnitus. Hear. Res., 2001. 157: p. 52-64.

214. Giardino, L., et al., Plasticity of GABAᴀ system during aging: focus on vestibular compensation and possible pharmacological intervention. Brain Res., 2002. 929: p. 76-86.

215. Glasgold, A. and F. Altman, The effect of stapes surgery on tinnitus in otosclerosis. Laryngoscope, 1966. 76: p. 1524-1532.

216. Glasscock, M.C., B.A. Thedinger, and P.A. Cueva, An analysis of the retrolabyrinthine vs the retrosigmoid vestibular nerve section. Otolaryngol. Head Neck Surg., 1991. 104: p. 88-95.

217. Goda, Y. and G.W. Davis, Mechanisms of synapse assembly and disassembly. Neuron, 2003. 40(2): p. 243-64.

218. Goddard, G.V., Amygdaloid stimulation and learning in the rat. J. Comp. Physiol. Psychol., 1964. 58: p. 23-30.

219. Goodale, M.A. and A.D. Milner, Separate pathways for perception and action. Trends Neurosci., 1992. 15(1): p. 20-25.

220. Goodin, B., T. Ness, and M. Robbins, Oxytocin - a multifunctional analgesic for chronic deep tissue pain. Curr Pharm Des, 2015. 21(7): p. 906-13.

221. Goodwin, P.E. and P.M. Johnson, The loudness of tinnitus. Acta Otolaryngol. (Stockh), 1980. 90: p. 353-359.

222. Gouda, J.J. and J.A. Brown, Atypical facial pain and other pain syndromes. Neurosurgery Clinics of North America, 1997. 8(1): p. 87-100.

223. Granit, R., L. Leksell, and C.R. Skoglund, Fibre interaction in injured or compressed region of nerve. Brain, 1944(67): p. 125-140.

224. Graven-Nielsen, T. and S. Mense, The peripheral apparatus of muscle pain: evidence from animal and human studies. Clin. J. Pain., 2001. 17(1): p. 2-10.

225. Graybiel, A.M., The thalamocortical projection of the so-called posterior nuclear group: A study with anterograde degeneration methods in the cat. Brain. Res., 1973. 49: p. 229-244.

226. Grevert, P., L.H. Albert, and A. Goldstein, Partial antagonism of placebo analgesia by naloxone. Pain, 1983. 16: p. 129-143.

227. Grosser, T.W., CJ.; FitzGerald, GA., Time for nonaddictive relief of pain. Science, 2017. 355(6329): p. 1026-1027.

228. Grouios, G., Phantom smelling. Percept Mot Skills., 2002. 94(3): p. 841-50.

229. Grundy, B., Evoked potentials monitoring, in Monitoring in Anesthesia and Critical Care Medicine., C. Blitt, Editor. 1985, Churchill-Livingstone: New York. p. 345-411.

230. Guo, L., et al., Dynamic rewiring of neural circuits in the motor cortex in mouse models of Parkinson's disease. Nat Neurosci,, 2015. 18: p. 1299-1309.

231. Gupta, R. and O. Steward, Chronic nerve compression induces concurrent apoptosis and proliferation of Schwann cells. J. Comp. Neurol., 2003. 461(2): p. 174-86.

232. Gybels, J.M. and R.R. Tasker, Central neurosurgery, in Textbook of Pain, P.D. Wall and R. Melzack, Editors. 1999, Churchill Levingstone: Edinburgh. p. 1307-1339.

233. Hall, E.J., et al., Non-invasive brain stimulation reveals reorganized cortical outputs in amputees. Neurosci. Lett., 1990. 116: p. 379-386.

234. Halpern, M., The organization and function of the vomeronasal system. Ann. Rev. Neurosci., 1987. 10: p. 325-62.

235. Halstead, L.S. and S.W.J. Seager, The effects of rectal probe electrostimulation on spinal cord injury spasticity. Paraplegia, 1991. 29: p. 43-47.

236. Halstead, L.S., et al., Relief of spasticity in SCI men and women using rctal probe electrostimulation. Paraplegia, 1993. 31: p. 715-721.

237. Hamernik, R.P., D. Henderson, and R.J. Salvi, New Perspectives on Noise-Induced Hearing Loss. 1982, New York: Raven Press.

238. Han, S.C. and P. Harrison, Myofascial pain syndrome and trigger-point management. Regional Anesthesia, 1997. 95(2): p. 89-101.

239. Happel, L. and D. Kline, Intraoperative Neurophysiology of the Peripheral Nervous System, in Neurophysiology in Neurosurgery, V. Deletis and J.L. Shils, Editors. 2002, Academic Press: Amsterdam. p. 169-195.

240. Harlow, H.F. and R.R. Zimmermann, Affectional responses in the infant monkey; orphaned baby monkeys develop a strong and persistent attachment to inanimate surrogate mothers. Science, 1959. 130: p. 421-32.

241. Harrison, J.M. and M.E. Howe, Anatomy of the descending auditory system in auditory system., in Handbook of sensory physiology, W.D. Keidel and W.D. Neff, Editors. 1974, Springer Verlag: Berlin. p. 363-388.

242. Harrison, N., Inflammation and mental illness. J Neurol Neurosurg Psychiatry, 2013. 84(9).

243. Hartmann, R., et al., Response of the primary auditory cortex to electrical stimulation of the auditory nerve in the congenitally deaf white cat. Hear Res., 1997. 112: p. 115-33.

244. Hartong, D., E. Berson, and T. Dryja, Retinitis pigmentosa. Lancet, 2006. 368(9549): p. 1795-809.

245. Harvey, J., Peptin regulation of neuronal morphology and hippocampal synaptic function. Froniers in Snaptic Neuroscience, 2013. 5(3): p. 1-12.

246. Hashmi, A.M., Z. Butt, and M. Umair, Is depression an inflammatory condition? A review of available evidence. J. Pak Med Assoc, 2013. 63(7): p. 899-906.

247. Hashmi, J., et al., Shape shifting pain: chronification of back pain shifts brain representation from nociceptive to emotional circuits. Brain, 2013. 136(9): p. 2751-68.

248. Hassenbusch, S.J., P.K. Pillay, and G.H. Barnett, Radiofrequency cingulotomy for intractable cancer pain using stereotaxis guided by magnetic resonance imaging. Neurosurg., 1990. 27(2): p. 220-3.

249. Hawkins, J.E., Auditory physiologic history: A surface view., in Physiology of the ear, A.F. Jahn and J. Santos-Sacchi, Editors. 1988, Raven Press: New York.

250. Hebb, D.O., The organization of behavior. 1949, New York: Wiley.

251. Heid, S., et al., Afferent projection patterns in the auditory brainstem in normal and congenitally deaf white cats. Hear. Res., 1997. 110: p. 191-199.

252. Henkin, R.I., L.M. Levy, and C.S. Lin, Taste and smell phantoms revealed by brain functional MRI (fMRI). J. Comput. Assist. Tomogr., 2000. 24(1): p. 106-23.

253. Hensch, T., Critical period mechanisms in developing visual cortex. Curr Top Dev Biol., 2005. 69: p. 215-37.

254. Herbert, H. and C.B. Saper, Organization of medullary adrenergic and noradrenergic projections to periaqueductal gray matter in the rat. J. Comp. Neurol., 1992. 315: p. 34-52.

255. Herweg, N.A., et al., Oscillations Bind the Hippocampus, Prefrontal Cortex, and Striatum during Recollection:Evidence from Simultaneous EEG-fMRI. The Journal of neuroscience, 2016. 36: p. 3579-3587.

256. Hilbig, H., et al., In contrast to neuronal NOS-I, the inducible NOS-II expression in aging brains is modifled by enriched environmental conditions. Experimental & Toxicologic Pathology, 2002. 53(6): p. 427-31.

257. Hill, J.L., et al., Loss of promoter IV-driven BDNF expression impacts oscillatory activity during sleep, sensory information processing and fear regulation. Transl Psychiatry, 2016. 6: p. e873.

258. Hillig, K. and P. Mahlberg, A chemotaxonomic analysis of cannabiod variations in cannabis (cannabaceae). Am. J. Botany, 2004. 91(6): p. 966-75.

259. Hirato, M., et al., Pathophysiology of central (thalamic) pain: combined change of sensory thalamus with cerebral cortex around central sulcus. Stereotact. Funct. Neurosurg., 1994. 62(1-4): p. 300-3.

260. Hitzelberger, W.E. and R.M. Witten, Abnormal myelograms in asymptomatic patients. J. Neurosurg., 1968. 28: p. 204-6.

261. Hofman, M., Evolution of the human brain: when bigger is better. Front Neuroanat., 2014. 8: p. 15.

262. Hoheisel, U., G. Beylich, and S. Mense, Effects of an acute muscle nerve section on excitability of dorsal horn neurons in the rat. Pain, 1995. 60(22): p. 151-158.

263. Hoistad, D.L., et al., Update on conservative management of acoustic neuroma. Otol. Neurotol., 2001. 22: p. 682-685.

264. Hong, C.Z. and D.G. Simons, Pathophysiologic and electrophysiologic mechanisms of myofascial trigger points. Arch Phys. Med. Rehab., 1998. 79(7): p. 863-72.

265. Horng, S.H. and M. Sur, Visual activity and cortical rewiring: Activity-dependent plasticity of cortical networks, in Reprogramming the brain, Progress in Brain Research, A.R. Møller, Editor. 2006, Elsevier: Amsterdam. p. 3-11.

266. Hosp, J.A., et al., Dopaminergic projections from midbrain to primary motor cortex mediate motor skill learning. J Neurosci,, 2011. 31: p. 2481-2487.

267. Hotta, T. and K. Kameda, Interactions between somatic and visual or auditory responses in the thalamus of the cat. Exp. Neurol., 1963. 8: p. 1-13.

268. Howe, J.E., J.D. Loeser, and J.H. Calvin, Mechanosensitivity of dorsal root ganglia and chronically injured axons: a physiologic basis for radically pain of nerve root compression. Pain, 1977. 3: p. 25-41.

269. Howe, J.F., W.H. Calvin, and J.D. Loeser, Impulses reflected from dorsal root ganglia and from focal nerve injuries. Brain Res., 1976: p. 116-144.

270. Howland, R., Vagus Nerve Stimulation. Curr Behav Neurosci Rep, 2014. 1(2): p. 64-73.

271. Hubbard, D.R. and G.M. Berkoff, Myofascial trigger points show spontaneous needle EMG activity. Spine, 1993. 18(13): p. 1803-7.

272. Hughes, G.B., et al., Sudden sensorineural hearing loss. Otolaryngol Clin North Am., 1996. 29(3): p. 393-405.

273. Hunt, S.P. and C.E. Urch, Pain, Opiates and Addiction, in Wall and Melzack's Textbook of Pain, S.B. McMahon and M. Koltzenburg, Editors. 2006, Elsevier: Amsterdam. p. 349-359.

274. Hunter, J.P., J. Katz, and K.D. Davis, The effect of tactile and visual sensory inputs on phantom limb awareness. Brain, 2003. 126(3): p. 579-89.

275. Huynh, L. and S. Fields, Alprazolam for tinnitus. Ann Pharmacother, 1995. 29(3): p. 311-2.

276. Hyson, R.L. and E.W. Rubel, Activity-dependent regulation of a ribosomal RNA epitope in the chick cochlear nucleus. Brain Res., 1995. 672(1-2): p. 196-204.

277. Illing, R.B., Activity-dependent plasticity in the adult auditory brainstem. Audiol. Neuro-Otol., 2001. 6(6): p. 319-345.

278. Irvine, D.R. and R. Rajan, Injury- and use-related plasticity in the primary sensory cortex of adult mammals: possible relationship to perceptual learning. Clin. Exp. Pharmacol. Physiol., 1996. 23(10-11): p. 939-947.

279. Irving, A. and J. Harvey, Leptin regulation of hippocampal synaptic function in health and disease. Philos Trans R Soc Lond B Biol Sci., 2013. 369(1633).

280. Ishiyama, A., K.M. Jacobson, and R.W. Baloh, Migraine and benign positional vertigo. Ann. Otol. Rhinol. Laryngol., 2000. 109: p. 377-80.

281. Itagaki, S., S. Saito, and O. Nakai, Electrophysiological study on hemifacial spasm - usefulness in etiological diagnosis and pathophysiological mechanism. Brain Nerve (Tokyo), 1989. 41: p. 1005 1011.

282. Itoh, K., et al., Direct projections from dorsal column nuclei and the spinal trigeminal nuclei to the cochlear nuclei in the cat. Brain Res., 1987. 400: p. 145-150.

283. Jacobs, K.M. and J.P. Donoghue, Reshaping the cortical motor map by unmasking latent intracortical connections. Science, 1991. 251: p. 944-947.

284. Jänig, W., et al., The role of vagal visceral afferents in the control of nociception. Prog Brain Res., 2000. 122: p. 273-87.

285. Jankovic, J., Tics in other neurological disorders, in Handbook of Tourette's Syndrome and Related Tic and Behavioral Disorders, R. Kurlan, Editor. 1993, Marcel Dekker: New York. p. 167-182.

286. Jankowska, E. and W.J. Roberts, Synaptic actions of single interneurons mediating reciprocal Ia inhibition to motoneurons. J. Physiol., 1972. 222: p. 623-642.

287. Jankowska, E. and A. Lundberg, Interneurons in the spinal cord. Trends Neurosci., 1981. 4: p. 230-233.

288. Jannetta, P.J., Microsurgical exploration and decompression of the facial nerve in hemifacial spasm. Curr. Top. Surg. Res., 1970(2): p. 217-222.

289. Jannetta, P.J., Observations on the etiology of trigeminal neuralgia, hemifacial spasm, acoustic nerve dysfunction and glossopharyngeal neuralgia. Definitive microsurgical treatment and results in 117 patients. Neurochirurgia (Stuttg), 1977. 20: p. 145-154.

290. Jannetta, P.J., Hemifacial spasm caused by a venule: Case report. Neurosurgery, 1984. 14: p. 89-92.

291. Jannetta, P.J., M.B. Møller, and A.R. Møller, Disabling positional vertigo. New Engl. J. Med., 1984(310): p. 1700-1705.

292. Jastreboff, P.J., Phantom auditory perception (tinnitus): Mechanisms of generation and perception. Neurosci. Res., 1990. 8: p. 221-254.

293. Jastreboff, P.J. and M.M. Jastreboff, Tinnitus Retraining Therapy (TRT) as a method for treatment of tinnitus and hyperacusis patients. J. Am. Acad. Audiol., 2000. 11(3): p. 162-77.

294. Jastreboff, P.J., Tinnitus Retraining Therapy, in Textbook of Tinnitus, A.R. Møller, et al., Editors. 2010, Springer: New York. p. 575-596.

295. Jenkins, W.M., et al., Functional reorganization of primary somatosensory cortex in adult owl monkeys after behaviorally controlled tactile stimulation. J. Neurophysiol., 1990. 63(1): p. 82-104.

296. Jensen, R., Peripheral and central mechanisms in tension-type headache: an update. Cephalalgia, 2003. 23(Suppl. 1): p. 49-52.

297. Jiang, L., H. Xu, and C. Yu, Brain connectivity plasticity in the motor network after ischemic stroke. Neural Plast, 2013: p. 1-11.

298. Joachims, H.Z., et al., Antioxidants in treatment of idiopathic sudden hearing loss. Otol. Neurotol., 2003. 24: p. 572-5.

299. Johnson, L.R., L.E. Westrum, and M.A. Henry, Anatomic organization of the trigeminal system and the effects of deafferentation, in Trigeminal neuralgia, G.H. Fromm and B.J. Sessle, Editors. 1991, Butterworth-Heinemann: Boston. p. 27-69.

300. Johnson, M.H., Development of human brain functions. Biol Psychiatry, 2003. 54(12): p. 1312-6.

301. Johnson, R.M., R. Brummett, and A. Schleuning, Use of Alprazolam for relief of tinnitus. Arch. Otolaryngol. Head & Neck Surg., 1993. 119: p. 842 845.

302. Johnsson, L.G. and H.L. Hawkins, Sensory and neural degeneration with aging, as seen in microdissections of the human inner ear. Ann. Otol. Rhinol. Laryngol., 1972. 81: p. 179-193.

303. Johnston, M.V., Clinical disorders of brain plasticity. Brain Dev., 2004. 26(2): p. 73-80.

304. Jones, T.A., et al., Importance of behavioral manipulations and measures in rat models of brain damage and brain repair. Ilar Journal, 2003. 44(2): p. 144-52.

305. Joodaki, M.R., G.R. Olyaei, and H. Bagheri, The effects of electrical nerve stimulation of the lower extremity on H-reflex and F-wave parameters. Electromyography Clin. Neurophysiol., 2001. 41(1): p. 23-8.

306. Kakigi, R., et al., Cerebral responses following stimulation of unmyelinated C-fibers in humans: eletro- and magneto-encephalographic study. Neurosci. Res., 2003.

307. Kaltenbach, J.A. and C.E. Afman, Hyperactivity in the dorsal cochlear nucleus after intense sound exposure and its resemblance to tone-evoked activity: a physiological model for tinnitus. Hear. Res., 2000. 140: p. 165-72.

308. Kanold, P.O., et al., Co-regulation of ocular dominance plasticity and NMDA receptor subunit expression in glutamic acid decarboxylase-65 knockout mice. J Physiol,, 2009. 587: p. 2857-2867.

309. Katagiri, H., M. Fagiolini, and T. Hensch, Optimization of somatic inhibition at critical period onset in mouse visual cortex. Neuron, 2007. 53(6): p. 805-12.

310. Katayama, Y., T. Tsubokawa, and T. Yamamoto, Chronic motor cortex stimulation for central deafferentation pain: experience with bulbar pain secondary to Wallenberg syndrome. Stereotact. Funct. Neurosurg. , 1995. 34: p. 42-48.

311. Katusic, S., et al., Incidence and clinical features of trigeminal neuralgia, Rochester, Minnesota 1945-1984. Ann Neurol, 1990(27): p. 89-95.

312. Keay, K., A, and R. Bandler, Parallel circuits mediating distinct emotional coping reactions to different types of stress. Neurosci Biobehav Rev, 2001. 25(7-8): p. 669-78.

313. Kelly, D., T. O'Dowd, and U. Reulbach, Use of folic acid supplements and risk of cleft lip and palate in infants: a population-based cohort study. Br J Gen Pract., 2012. 62(600): p.:e466-72.

314. Khaslavskaia, S., M. Ladouceur, and T. Sinkjaer, Increase in tibialis anterior motor cortex excitability following repetitive electrical stimulation of the common peroneal nerve. Exp. Brain Res., 2002. 143(3): p. 309-315.

315. Khodaparast, N., et al., Vagus nerve stimulation delivered during motor rehabilitation improves recovery in a rat model of stroke. Neurorehabil Neural Repair, 2014. 28(7): p. 698-706.

316. Kilgard, M.P. and M.M. Merzenich, Cortical map reorganization enabled by nucleus basalis activity. Science, 1998. 279: p. 1714-1718.

317. Kilgard, M.P. and M.M. Merzenich, Plasticity of temporal information processing in the primary auditory cortex. Nature Neurosci., 1998. 1: p. 727-731.

318. Kim, S. and L. Strathearn, Oxytocin and Maternal Brain Plasticity. New Dir Child Adolesc Dev., 2016. 2016(153): p.:59-72.

319. Kimura, J., A method for estimating the refractory period of motor fibers in the human peripheral nerve. J. Neurol. Sci., 1976. 28: p. 485-90.

320. Kirchner, A., et al., Left vagus nerve stimulation suppresses experimentally induced pain. Neurology, 2000. 55(8): p. 1167-71.

321. Kitagawa, H. and A.R. Møller, Conduction pathways and generators of magnetic evoked spinal cord potentials: a study in monkeys. Electroenceph. Clin. Neurophys., 1994. 93: p. 57-67.

322. Kleim, J.A., et al., BDNF val66met polymorphism is associated with modified experience-dependent plasticity in human motor cortex. Nat Neurosci,, 2006. 9: p. 735-737.

323. Kleinjung, T., et al., Long-term effects of repetitive transcranial magnetic stimulation (rTMS) in patients with chronic tinnitus. Otolaryngol Head Neck Surg, 2005. 132(4): p. 566-9.

324. Klinke, R., et al., Plastic changes in the auditory cortex of congenitally deaf cats following cochlear implantation. Audiol. Neurootol., 2001. 6: p. 203-206.

325. Klumpers, L., et al., Novel Δ(9) -tetrahydrocannabinol formulation Namisol® has beneficial pharmacokinetics and promising pharmacodynamic effects. Br J Clin Pharmacol. , 2012. 74(1).

326. Kohama, I., K. Ishikawa, and J.D. Kocsis, Synaptic reorganization in the substantia gelatinosa after peripheral nerve neuroma formation: aberrant innervation of lamina II neurons by beta afferents. J. Neurosci., 2000. 20: p. 1538-1549.

327. Komisaruk, B.R., C.A. Gerdes, and B. Whipple, 'Complete' spinal cord injury does not block perceptual responses to genital self-stimulation in women. Arch. Neurol., 1997. 54(12): p. 1513-20.

328. Kommerell, G., et al., Oculomotor palsy with cyclic spasms: Electromyographic and electron microscopic evidence of chronic peripheral neuronal involvement. Neuro-Ophthalmol., 1988. 8: p. 9-21.

329. Kondo, A., et al., Microvascular decompression of cranial nerves, particularly of the seventh cranial nerve. Neurol. Med. Chir. (Tokyo), 1980. 20: p. 739-751.

330. Kondo, A., Morota, N, Date, H, Yoshifuji, K, Morishima, T, Miyazato, M, Shirane, R, Sakai, H, Pooh, KH, Watanabe, T, Awareness of folic acid use increases its consumption, and reduces the risk of spina bifida. Br J Nutr., 2015. 114(1): p. 84-90.

331. Kondziolka, D., L.D. Lunsford, and J.C. Flickinger, Stereotactic radiosurgery for the treatment of trigeminal neuralgia. Clin. J. Pain, 2002. 18(1): p. 42-47.

332. Korsan-Bengtsen, M. and (aka MB Møller), Distorted Speech Audiometry. Acta Otolaryng. (Stockholm), 1973. Suppl. 310.

333. Kral, A., et al., Congenital auditory deprivation reduces synaptic activity within the auditory cortex in layer specific manner. Cerebral Cortex, 2000. 10: p. 714-726.

334. Kral, A., Auditory critical periods: A review from system's perspective. Neuroscience Letters, 2013. 247: p. 117-33.

335. Kraus, K.S. and B. Canlon, Neuronal connectivity and interactions between the auditory and limbic systems. Effects of noise and tinnitus. Hear Res, 2012. 288: p. 34-46.

336. Kreutzberg, G.W., Neurobiology of regeneration and degeneration the facial nerve, in The facial nerve, M. May, Editor. 1986, Thieme: New York.

337. Kruit, M.C., et al., Migraine as a risk factor for subclinical brain lesions. JAMA, 2004. 291(4): p. 427-34.

338. Kugelberg, E., "Injury activity" and "trigger zones" in human nerves. Brain, 1946(69): p. 310-324.

339. Kugelberg, E., Activation of human nerves by ischemia. Arch. Neurol. Psychiat., 1948. 60: p. 140-152.

340. Kuypers, H.G.J.M., Anatomy of the descending pathways, in Handbook of physiology-the nervous system, J.M. Brookhart and V.B. Mountcastle, Editors. 1981, American Physiological Society: Bethesda, MD. p. 597-666.

341. Kwiat, G.C. and A.I. Basbaum, The origin of brainstem noradrenergic and serotonergic projections to the spinal cord dorsal horn in the rat. Somatosensory and Motor Res., 1992. 9: p. 157-173.

342. LaBerge, D. and M.S. Buchsbaum, Positron emission tomographic measurements of pulvinar activity during an attention task. J Neurosci., 1990. 10(2): p. 613-9.

343. Laha, R.K. and P.J. Jannetta, Glossopharyngeal Neuralgia. J. Neurosurg., 1977(47): p. 316-320.

344. Lamm, K., H. Lamm, and W. Arnold, Effect of hyperbaric oxygen therapy in comparison to conventional or placebo therapy or no treatment in idiopathic sudden hearing loss, acoustic trauma, noise-induced hearing loss and tinnitus. A literature survey. Adv. Otorhinolaryngol., 1998. 54: p. 86-99.

345. Lampl, Y., et al., Minocycline treatment in acute stroke: an open-label, evaluator-blinded study. Neurology., 2007 69(14): p. 1404-10.

346. Landgren, S. and H. Silfvenius, Nucleus Z , the medullary relay in the projection path to the cerebral cortex of group i muscle afferents from the cat's hind limb. J. Physiol. (Lond), 1971. 218: p. 551-71.

347. Langers, D.R.M., E. Kleine, and P. van Dijk, Tinnitus does not require macroscopic tonotopic map reorganization. Frontiers in System Neuroscience, 2012. 6.

348. Langguth, B., T. Kleinjung, and M. Landgrebe, Severe tinnitus and depressive symptoms: a complex interaction. Otolaryngol Head Neck Surg., 2011. 145(3).

349. Langguth, B., et al., Tinnitus and depression. World J Biol Psychiatry, 2011. 12(7): p. 489-500.

350. Laurikainen, E.A., et al., Stellate ganglion drives sympathetic regulation of cochlear blood flow. Hear. Res., 1993. 64: p. 199-204.

351. Layzer, R.B., Muscle Pain, Cramps, and Fatigue, in Myology, 2nd ed, A.G. Engel and C. Franzini-Armstrong, Editors. 1994, McGraw-Hill: New York. p. 1754–1768.

352. LeDoux, J.E., A. Sakaguchi, and D.J. Reis, Subcortical efferent projections of the medial geniculate mediate emotional responses conditioned by acoustic stimuli. J. Neurosci., 1984. 4: p. 683-698.

353. LeDoux, J.E., Brain mechanisms of emotion and emotional learning. Curr. Opin. Neurobiol., 1992. 2: p. 191-197.

354. Leistedt, S.J. and P. Linkowski, Brain, networks, depression, and more. Eur Neuropsychopharmacol, 2013. 23(1): p. 55-62.

355. Lenarz, T., Treatment of tinnitus with lidocaine and tocainide. Scand. Audiol. (Stockh), 1986. 26: p. 49-51.

356. Lenz, F.A., et al., Methods for microstimulation and recording of single neurons and evoked potentials in the human central nervous system. J. Neurosurg.. 1988. 68(4): p. 630-4.

357. Lenz, F.A., et al., Reorganization of sensory modalities evoked by microstimulation in region of the thalamic principal sensory nucleus in patients with pain due to nervous system injury. J. Comp. Neurol., 1998. 399(1): p. 125-38.

358. Lenz, F.A., et al., Thalamic single neuron activity in patients with dystonia: dystonia-related activity and somatic sensory reorganization. J. Neurophysiol., 1999. 82(5): p. 2372-92.

359. Lepeta, K., et al., Synaptopathies: synaptic dysfunction in neurological disorders - A review from students to students. J Neurochem., 2016. 138: p. 785-805.

360. Lessell, S. and M.M. Cohen, Phosphenes induced by sound. Neurology, 1979. 29(11): p. 1524-6.

361. Levine, J.D., N.C. Gordon, and H.L. Fields, The mechanism of placebo analgesia. Lancet, 1978: p. 654-657.

362. Levine, R.A., Somatic (craniocervical) tinnitus and the dorsal cochlear nucleus hypothesis. Am. J. Otolaryngol., 1999. 20(6): p. 351-62.

363. Liang, C., et al., New hypothesis of chronic back pain: low pH promotes nerve ingrowth into damaged intervertebral disks. Acta Anaesthesiol Scand., 2013. 57(3): p. 271-7.

364. Lidén, G., Audiology. 1985, Stockholm: Almquist & Wiksell.

365. Lindstrom, S., Recurrent control from motor axon collaterals on Ia inhibitory pathways in the spinal cord of the cat. Acta Physiol. Scand. Suppl., 1973. 392: p. 1-43.

366. Liu, H., C.R. Mantyh, and A.I. Basbaum, NMDA-receptor regulation of substance-P release from primary nociceptors. Nature, 1997. 386: p. 721-724.

367. Llinas, R.R., et al., Thalamocortical dysrhythmia: A neurological and neuropsychiatric syndrome characterized by magnetoencephalography. Proc Natl Acad Sci, 1999. 96(26): p. 15222-7.

368. Lockwood, A., et al., The functional neuroanatomy of tinnitus. Evidence for limbic system links and neural plasticity. Neurology, 1998. 50: p. 114-120.

369. Long, D.M., Chronic back pain, in Handbook of Pain, P.D. Wall and R. Melzack, Editors. 1999, Churchill Livingstone: Edinburgh. p. 539-538.

370. Lovely, T.J. and P.J. Jannetta, Surgical treatment of geniculate neuralgia. Am. J. Otol., 1997. 18(4): p. 512-7.

371. Lu, B., Pro-region of neurotrophines: role in synaptic modulation. Neuron, 2003. 39(5): p. 735-8.

372. Lu, B., et al., BDNF-based synaptic repair as a disease-modifying strategy for neurodegenerative diseases. Nat Rev Neurosci, 2013. 14(6): p. 401-16.

373. Luft, A.R., et al., Motor skill learning depends on protein synthesis in motor cortex after training. J Neurosci, 2004. 24: p. 6515-6520.

374. Lundberg, A. and P. Voorhoeve, Effects from pyramidal tract on spinal reflex arcs. Acta Physiol. Scand., 1962. 56: p. 201-219.

375. Lundberg, A., Multisensory control of spinal reflex pathways. Prog. Brain Res., 1979. 50: p. 11-28.

376. Ma, L., et al., Lutein and zeaxanthin intake and the risk of age-related macular degeneration: a systematic review and meta-analysis. Br J Nutr., 2012. 107(3): p. 350-9.

377. Magnan, J., B. Lafont, and C. Rameh, Long Term Follow Up of Microvascular Decompression for Tinnitus, in Textbook of Tinnitus, A.R. Møller, et al., Editors. 2010, Springer: New York. p. 669-680.

378. Maison, S.F. and M.C. Liberman, Predicting vulnerability to acoustic injury with a non-invasive assay of olivocochlear reflex strength. J. Neurosci., 2000. 20: p. 4701-4707.

379. Maletic, V., Raison, CL, Neurobiology of depression, fibromyalgia and neuropathic pain. Front Biosci, 2009. 14: p. 5291-5338.

380. Malmberg, A.B., Central changes, in Pain in Peripheral Nerve diseases. Pain Headache, C. Sommer, Editor. 2001, Karger: Basel. p. 149-167.

381. Mansour, A., et al., Brain white matter structural properties predict transition to chronic pain. Pain, 2013. 154(10): p. 2160-8.

382. Mansour, A., et al., Brain white matter structural properties predict transition to chronic pain. Pain, 2013. 154(10): p. 2160-8.

383. Mansour, A., et al., Chronic pain: The role of learning and brain plasticity. Restor Neurol Neurosci, 2013.

384. Marchand, F., M. Perretti, and S.B. McMahon, Role of the immune system in chronic pain. Nat. Rev. Neurosci. , 2005. 6(7): p. 521–32.

385. Marczynski, T.J., J. Artwohl, and B. Marczynska, Chronic administration of flumazenil increases life span and protects rats from age-related loss of cognitive functions: a benzodiazepine/GABAergic hypothesis of brain aging. Neurobiology of Aging, 1994. 15(1): p. 69-84.

386. Margolis, R.L., D.M. Chuang, and R.l.M. Post, Programmed cell death: implications for neuropsychiatric disorders. Biol. Psychiatry., 1994. 35(12): p. 946-56.

387. Marlin, B., Froemke, RC, Oxytocin modulation of neural circuits for social behavior. Dev Neurobiol, 2017. 77(2): p. 69-189.

388. Maroon, J., C. and J.W. Bost, Omega-3 fatty acids (fish oil) as an anti-inflammatory: an alternative to nonsteroidal anti-inflammatory drugs for discogenic pain. Surg Neurol., 2006. 65(4): p. 326-31.

389. Martich-Kriss, V., S.S. Kollias, and W.S. Ball Jr., MR findings in kernicterus. Am. J. Neuroradiol., 1995. 16: p. 819-21.

390. Martin, K. and E. Kandel, Cell adhesion molecules, CREB, and the formation of new synaptic connections. Neuron, 1996. 17(4): p. 567-70.

391. Martinez de Villarreal, L.E., et al., Weekly Administration of Folic Acid and Epidemiology of Neural Tube Defects. Matern Child Health J, 2006. 10(5): p. 397-401.

392. Mathews, E.S. and S.J. Scrivani, Percutaneous stereotactic radiofrequency thermal rhizotomy for the treatment of trigeminal neuralgia. Mount Sinai J. Med., 2000. 67(4): p. 288-99.

393. Mattox, D.E. and F.B. Simmons, Natural history of sudden hearing loss. Otolaryngol. Head Neck Surg., 1977. 88: p. 111-3.

394. Mäurer, M. and K. Reiners, Mononeuropathies, in Pain in Peripheral Nerve diseases. Pain Headache, C. Sommer, Editor. 2001, Karger: Basel. p. 37-52.

395. Maxwell, A.P., S.M. Mason, and G.M. O'Donoghue, Cochlear nerve aplasia: its importance in cochlear implantation. Am. J. Otol., 1999. 20(3): p. 335-337.

396. Mayford, M., S. Siegelbaum, and E. Kandel, Synapses and Memory Storage. Cold Spring Harb Perspect Biol., 2012. 4(6).

397. Mazelova, J., J. Popelar, and J. Syka, Auditory function in presbycusis: peripheral vs. central changes. Exp Gerontol, 2003. 38.: p. 87-94.

398. McCabe, B., Management of hyperfunction of the facial nerve. Ann. Otol. Rhin. Laryng., 1970(79): p. 252-258.

399. McCabe, C.S., et al., Phantoms in rheumatology. Novartis Found Symp., 2004. 260: p. 154-74.

400. McCormick, M.S. and J.N. Thomas, Mexiletine in the relief of tinnitus: a report on a sequential double-blind crossover trial. Clin. Otolaryngol. Allied Sci., 1981. 6(4): p. 255-8.

401. McCrea, D.A., Spinal circuitry of sensorimotor control of locomotion. J. Physiol., 2001. 533(1): p. 41-50.

402. McDonald, A.J., Cortical pathways to the mammalian amygdala. Progr. Neurobiol., 1998. 55(3): p. 257-332.

403. McHughen, S.A. and S.C. Cramer, The BDNF val(66)met polymorphism is not related to motor function or short-term cortical plasticity in elderly subjects. Brain Res, 2013. 1495: p. 1-10.

404. McIntyre, C.K., J.L. McGaugh, and C.L. Williams, Interacting brain systems modulate memory consolidation. Neurosci Biobehav Rev., 2011.

405. McKay, B., M. Oh, and J. Disterhoft, Learning increases intrinsic excitability of hippocampal interneurons. J Neurosci., 2013. 33(13): p. 5499–5506.

406. McNicol, E., Midbari A, and E. E., Opioids for neuropathic pain. Cochrane Database Syst Rev. , 2013. 8(Aug 29).

407. McQuay, H., Do preemptive treatments provide better pain control?, in Progr. Pain Res. Management, G.F. Gebhart, D.L. Hammond, and T. Jensen, Editors. 1994, IASP Press: Seattle, WA. p. 709-723.

408. Meaney, M.J., Maternal care, gene expression, and the transmission of individual differences in stress reactivity across generations. Annu Rev Neurosci, 2001. 24: p. 1161-1192.

409. Melding, P.S., R.J. Goodey, and P.R. Thorne, The use of lignocaine in the diagnosis and treatment of tinnitus. J. Laryngol. Otol., 1978. 92: p. 115-121.

410. Melzack, R. and P.D. Wall, Pain mechanisms: A new theory. Science, 1965. 150: p. 971-979.

411. Melzack, R., Phantom limbs. Sci. Am., 1992. 266: p. 120-126.

412. Mense, S. and M. H., Bradykinin-induced modulation of the response behaviour of different types of feline group III and IV muscle receptors. J. Physiol., 1988. 398: p. 49-63.

413. Merskey, H. and N. Bogduk, Classification of chronic pain. 1994, IASP Press: Seattle. p. 1-222.

414. Merton, P.A. and H.B. Morton, Electrical stimulation of human motor and visual cortex through the scalp. J. Physiol., 1980. 305: p. 9-10P.

415. Merzenich, M.M., et al., Topographic reorganization of somatosensory cortical areas 3b and 1 in adult monkeys following restricted deafferentiation. Neuroscience, 1983. 8(1): p. 3-55.

416. Meschia, J., et al., Guidelines for the primary prevention of stroke: a statement for healthcare professionals from the American Heart Association/American Stroke Association. Stroke, 2014 45(12): p. 3754-832.

417. Meyer, K., Another Remembered Present. Science, 2012. 335: p. 415-6.

418. Meyerson, B.A., et al., Motor cortex stimulation as treatment of trigeminal neuropathic pain. Acta Neurochir. - Supplementum, 1993. 58: p. 105-3.

419. Meyerson, B.A. and B. Linderoth, Mechanism of spinal cord stimulation in neuropathic pain. Neurol. Res., 2000. 22: p. 285-292.

420. Miller, J.M., C.S. Watson, and W.P. Covell, Deafening effects of noise on the cat. Acta Oto Laryng. Suppl. 176, 1963: p. 1-91.

421. Mishkin, M., L.G. Ungerleider, and K.A. Macko, Object vision and spatial vision: Two cortical pathways. Trends Neurosci., 1983. 6: p. 415-417.

422. Mitsi, V.a.Z., V., Modulation of pain, nociception, and analgesia by the brain reward center. Neuroscience, 2016.

423. Møller, A., Hearing: Its Physiology and Pathophysiology. 2000, San Diego: Academic Press.

424. Møller, A., Pathogenesis and Treatment of Hemifacial Spasm, in Microvascular Decompression Surgery, S.-T. Li, et al., Editors. 2016, Springer. p. 35-49.

425. Møller, A.R., Pathophysiology of tinnitus. Ann. Otol. Rhinol. Laryngol., 1984. 93: p. 39-44.

426. Møller, A.R. and P.J. Jannetta, On the origin of synkinesis in hemifacial spasm: Results of intracranial recordings. J. Neurosurg., 1984. 61: p. 569-576.

427. Møller, A.R. and P.J. Jannetta, Microvascular decompression in hemifacial spasm: Intraoperative electrophysiological observations. Neurosurgery, 1985. 16: p. 612-618.

428. Møller, A.R. and P.J. Jannetta, Hemifacial spasm: Results of electrophysiologic recording during microvascular decompression operations. Neurology, 1985. 35: p. 969-974.

429. Møller, A.R. and P.J. Jannetta, Physiological abnormalities in hemifacial spasm studied during microvascular decompression operations. Exp. Neurol., 1986. 93: p. 584 600.

430. Møller, A.R. and P.J. Jannetta, Blink reflex in patients with hemifacial spasm: Observations during microvascular decompression operations. J. Neurol. Sci., 1986. 72: p. 171-182.

431. Møller, A.R., Hemifacial spasm: Ephaptic transmission or hyperexcitability of the facial motor nucleus? Exp. Neurol., 1987. 98: p. 110-119.

432. Møller, A.R., Electrophysiological monitoring of cranial nerves in operations in the skull base, in Tumors of the Cranial Base: Diagnosis and Treatment, L.N. Sekhar and V.L. Schramm Jr, Editors. 1987, Futura Publishing Co: Mt. Kisco, New York. p. 123-132.

433. Møller, A.R. and P.J. Jannetta, Monitoring facial EMG during microvascular decompression operations for hemifacial spasm. J. Neurosurg., 1987. 66: p. 681-685.

434. Møller, A.R. and M.B. Møller, Does intraoperative monitoring of auditory evoked potentials reduce incidence of hearing loss as a complication of microvascular decompression of cranial nerves? Neurosurgery, 1989. 24: p. 257-263.

435. Møller, A.R., Interaction between the blink reflex and the abnormal muscle response in patients with hemifacial spasm: Results of intraoperative recordings. J. Neurol. Sci., 1991. 101: p. 114-123.

436. Møller, A.R., The cranial nerve vascular compression syndrome: I. A review of treatment. Acta Neurochir. (Wien), 1991. 113: p. 18-23.

437. Møller, A.R., et al., Compound action potentials recorded from the exposed eighth nerve in patients with intractable tinnitus. Laryngoscope, 1992. 102: p. 187-197.

438. Møller, A.R., M.B. Møller, and M. Yokota, Some forms of tinnitus may involve the extralemniscal auditory pathway. Laryngoscope, 1992. 102: p. 1165-1171.

439. Møller, A.R., Cranial nerve dysfunction syndromes: Pathophysiology of microvascular compression., in Neurosurgical Topics Book 13, 'Surgery of Cranial Nerves of the Posterior Fossa,' Chapter 2, D.L. Barrow, Editor. 1993, American Association of Neurological Surgeons: Park Ridge. IL. p. 105-129.

440. Møller, A.R., Intraoperative neurophysiologic monitoring. 1995, Luxembourg: Harwood Academic Publishers.

441. Møller, A.R., Pathophysiology of hemifacial spasm, in Hemifacial spasm: A Multidisciplinary Approach, M. Sindou, Y. Keravel, and A.R. Møller, Editors. 1997, Springer. p. 51-62.

442. Møller, A.R. and T. Pinkerton, Temporal integration of pain from electrical stimulation of the skin. Neurol. Res, 1997. 19: p. 481-488.

443. Møller, A.R., Vascular compression of cranial nerves. I: History of the microvascular decompression operation. Neurol. Res., 1998. 20: p. 727-731.

444. Møller, A.R., Similarities between severe tinnitus and chronic pain. J. Amer. Acad. Audiol., 2000. 11: p. 115-124.

445. Møller, A.R., Diagnosis of acoustic tumors. Am. J. Otol., 2000. 21: p. 151-152.

446. Møller, A.R. and P. Rollins, The non-classical auditory system is active in children but not in adults. Neurosci. Lett., 2002. 319: p. 41-44.

447. Møller, A.R., J.K. Kern, and B. Grannemann, Are the non-classical auditory pathways involved in autism and PDD? Neurol Res, 2005. 27: p. 625-629.

448. Møller, A.R., Neural plasticity and disorders of the nervous system. 2006, Cambridge: Cambridge University Press

449. Møller, A.R., Neurophysiologic abnormalities in autism, in New Autism Research Developments, B.S. Mesmere, Editor. 2007, Nova Science Publishers: New York. p. 137-158.

450. Møller, A.R., Neural Plasticity: For Good and Bad. Progress of Theoretical Physics, 2008. Supplement No 173: p. 48-65.

451. Møller, A.R., Similarities between tinnitus and pain in Textbook of Tinnitus, A.R. Møller, et al., Editors. 2010, Springer: New York. p. 113-120.

452. Møller, A.R., Misophonia, phonophobia and "exploding head" syndrome, in Textbook of Tinnitus, A.R. Møller, et al., Editors. 2010, Springer: New York. p. 25-27.

453. Møller, A.R., Different forms of tinnitus, in Textbook of Tinnitus, A.R. Møller, et al., Editors. 2010, Springer: New York. p. 9-12.

454. Møller, A.R., The role of neural plasticity in tinnitus, in Textbook of Tinnitus, A.R. Møller, et al., Editors. 2010, Springer: New York. p. 99-102.

455. Møller, A.R., The role of auditory deprivation, in Textbook of Tinnitus, A.R. Møller, et al., Editors. 2010, Springer: New York. p. 95-98.

456. Møller, A.R., Epidemiology of tinnitus in adults, in Textbook of Tinnitus, A.R. Møller, et al., Editors. 2010, Springer: New York. p. 29-37.

457. Møller, A.R. and S. Shore, Interaction between somatosensory and auditory systems, in Textbook of Tinnitus, A.R. Møller, et al., Editors. 2010, Springer: New York. p. 69-76.

458. Møller, A.R., Hearing: Anatomy, Physiology, and Disorders of the Auditory System, 3rd Ed. 2012, San Diego: Plural Publishing.

459. Møller, A.R., Hearing, Anatomy, Physiology, and Disorders of the Auditory System, 3rd Ed. 2013, San Diego: Plural Publishing Inc.

460. Møller, A.R., Sensory Systems: Anatomy and Physiology. 2014, Aage R. Møller Publishing: Dallas.

461. Møller, A.R., Pain: Its Anatomy, Physiology and Treatment. 2014, Dallas: Aage R. Møller Publishing. 406.

462. Møller, A.R., Microvascular Decompression Surgery for Disabling Positional Vertigo and Tinnitus, in Microvascular Decompression Surgery, S.-T. Li, et al., Editors. 2016, Springer.

463. Møller, M.B., et al., Diagnosis and surgical treatment of disabling positional vertigo. J. Neurosurg., 1986. 64: p. 21-28.

464. Møller, M.B., Disabling positional vertigo, in Advances in Otolaryngology -- Head and Neck Surgery,, E.N. Myers, et al., Editors. 1990, Mosby Year Book, Inc.: Chicago, Illinois,. p. 81-106.

465. Møller, M.B. and A.R. Møller, Vascular compression syndrome of the eighth nerve: Clinical correlations and surgical findings., in Neurologic Clinics: Diagnostic Neurotology and Otoneurology, I.K. Arenberg and D.B. Smith, Editors. 1990, WB Saunders Publishing Co: Philadelphia. p. 421-439.

466. Møller, M.B., et al., Vascular decompression surgery for severe tinnitus: Selection criteria and results. Laryngoscope, 1993. 103: p. 421-427.

467. Møller, M.B., et al., Microvascular decompression of the eighth nerve in patients with disabling positional vertigo: Selection criteria and operative results in 207 patients. Acta Neurochir. (Wien), 1993. 125: p. 75-82.

468. Møller, M.B., Audiological evaluation. J. Clin. Neurophysiol., 1994. 11: p. 309-318.

469. Montoya, J., et al., Cytokine signature associated with disease severity in chronic fatigue syndrome patients. Proc Nat Acad Sci USA, 2017.

470. Morest, D.K., M.D. Ard, and D. Yurgelun-Todd, Degeneration in the central auditory pathways after acoustic deprivation or over-stimulation in the cat. Anat. Rec., 1979. 193: p. 750.

471. Morest, D.K. and B.A. Bohne, Noise-induced degeneration in the brain and representation of inner and outer hair cells. Hear. Res., 1983. 9: p. 145-152.

472. Morgan, D.H., Temporomandbular joint surgery. Correction of pain, tinnitus, and vertigo. Dental Radiography and Photography, 1973. 46(2): p. 27-46.

473. Morgan, D.H., Tinnitus of TMJ origin. J. Craniomandibular practice, 1992. 10(2): p. 124-129.

474. Morgan, M.M. and P. Carrive, Activation of periaqueductal gray reduces locomotion but not mean arterial blood pressure in awake, freely moving rats. Neuroscience, 2001. 102: p. 905-10.

475. Moseley, G. and H. Flor, Phantom limb pain and bodily awareness: current concepts and future directions. Neurorehabil Neural Repair, 2012. 26(6): p. 646-52.

476. Mountcastle, V.B., Neural mechanisms in somesthesia, in Medical Physiology, V.B. Mountcastle, Editor. 1974, Mosby: St Louis.

477. Mufson, E.J., et al., Human cholinergic basal forebrain: chemoanatomy and neurologic dysfunction. J Chem Neuroanat., 2003. 26(4): p. 233-42.

478. Mühlnickel, W., et al., Reorganization of auditory cortex in tinnitus. Proc. Nat. Acad. Sci. USA, 1998. 95(17): p. 10340-3.

479. Multon, S. and J. Schoenen, Pain control by vagus nerve stimulation: from animal to man and back. Acta Neurol Belg. , 2005. 105(2): p. 62-7.

480. Munhall, K.G., et al., Dynamic visual speech perception in a patient with visual form agnosia. NeuroReport, 2002. 13(14): p. 1793-6.

481. Murray, C.D., et al., The treatment of phantom limb pain using immersive virtual reality: three case studies. Disabil Rehabil., 2007. 29(18): p. 1465-9.

482. Nabavi, S., et al., Engineering a memory with LTD and LTP. NATURE REVIEWS | IMMUNOLOGY, 2014. 511: p. 348-352.

483. Nair, V., Young, BM, La, C, Reiter, P, Nadkarni, TN, Song, J, Vergun, S, Addepally, NS, Mylavarapu, K, Swartz, JL, Jensen, MB, Chacon, MR, Sattin, JA, Prabhakaran, V., Functional connectivity changes in the language network during stroke recovery. Ann Clin Transl Neuro, 2015. 2(2): p. 185-95.

484. Naito, A., Y.J. Sun, and Y. Yanagidaira, Electromyographic (EMG) study of cold shivering in the chronic spinal dog. Jap. J. Physiol., 1997. 47(1): p. 81-6.

485. Nakai, O., S. Itagaki, and S. Saito, Electromyographic analysis of spasmodic torticollis. Tenth Meeting of the World Society for Stereotactic and Functional Neurosurgery. Abstract, 1989.

486. Nakashima, K., et al., An exteroceptive reflex in the sternocleidomastoid muscle produced by electrical stimulation of the supraorbital nerve in normal subjects and patients with spasmodic torticollis. Neurology, 1989. 39: p. 1354-1358.

487. Napadow, V. and R. Harris, What has functional connectivity and chemical neuroimaging in fibromyalgia taught us about the mechanisms and management of 'centralized' pain? Arthritis Res Ther. , 2014. 16(4): p. 425.

488. Narins, C.R., et al., Clinical implications of silent versus symptomatic exercise-induced myocardial ischemia in patients with stable coronary disease. J. Am. Col. Cardiol., 1997. 29(4): p. 756-63.

489. Nemeroff, C.B., et al., VNS therapy in treatment-resistant depression: clinical evidence and putative neurobiological mechanisms. Neuropsychopharmacology, 2006. 31(7): p. 1345-55.

490. Newham, D.J. and K.R. Mills, Muscles, tendons and ligaments, in Handbook of Pain, P.D. Wall and R. Melzack, Editors. 1999, Churchill Livingstone: Edinburgh. p. 517-538.

491. Nguyen, J.P., et al., Treatment of deafferentation pain by chronic stimulation of the motor cortex. Report of a series of 20 cases. Acta Neurochiur. Suppl (Wien), 1997. 8(54-60).

492. Nichols, J.A., et al., Vagus nerve stimulation modulates cortical synchrony and excitability through the activation of muscarinic receptors. Neuroscience., 2011. 189: p. 207-14.

493. Nicoll, R.A. and R.C. Malenka, Expression mechanisms underlying NMDA receptor-dependent long-term potentiation. Ann. N.Y. Acad. Sci., 1999. 868: p. 515-25.

494. Nielsen, V.K., Pathophysiological aspects of hemifacial spasm. Part I. Evidence of ectopic excitation and ephaptic transmission. Neurology, 1984. 34: p. 418-426.

495. Nielsen, V.K., Pathophysiology of hemifacial spasm: II. Lateral spread of the supraorbital nerve reflex. Neurology, 1984. 34: p. 427-31.

496. Nijs, J., et al., Brain-derived neurotrophic factor as a driving force behind neuroplasticity in neuropathic and central sensitization pain: a new therapeutic target? Expert Opin Ther Targets., 2015. 19(4): p. 565-76.

497. Nikolopoulos, T.P., I. Johnson, and G.M. O'Donoghue, Quality of life after acoustic neuroma surgery. Laryngoscope, 1998. 108(9): p. 1382-1385.

498. Nucci, C., et al., Apoptosis in the mechanisms of neuronal plasticity in the developing visual system. Eur. J. Ophthalmol., 2003. 13(Suppl. 3): p. 36-43.

499. Ochoa, J.L., The newly recognized painful ABC syndrome: Thermographic aspects. Thermology, 1986. 2: p. 65-107.

500. Okado, N. and R. Oppenheim, Cell death of motoneurons in the chick embryo spinal cord: XI. Acetylcholine receptors and synaptogenesis in skeletal muscle following the reduction of motoneuron death by neuromuscular blockade. J. Neurosci., 1984. 4(6): p. 1639-1652.

501. Ollat, H., Pharmacology of hemifacial spasm, in Hemifacial Spasm: A Multidisciplinary Approach, M. Sindou, Y. Keravel, and A. Møller, Editors. 1997, Springer-Verlag: Wien.

502. Olson, E.J., B.F. Boeve, and M.H. Silber, Rapid eye movement sleep behaviour disorder: demographic, clinical and laboratory findings in 93 cases. Brain, 2000. 123(2): p. 231-239.

503. Oppenheimer, S.M., et al., Distribution of cardiovascular related cells within the human thalamus. Clinical Autonomic Research., 1998. 8(3): p. 173-9.

504. Ottesen, O., How hardwired is the brain? Technological advances provide new insights into the brain malleability and neurotransmission. Nutr. rev, 2010. Suppl 2: p. S60-4.

505. Page, N.G., J.P. Bolger, and M.D. Sanders, Auditory evoked phosphenes in optic nerve disease. J. Neurol. Neurosurg. Psych., 1982. 45(1): p. 7-12.

506. Pagni, C.A., M. Lanotte, and S. Canavero, How frequent is anesthesia dolorosa following spinal posterior rhizotomy? A retrospective analysis of fifteen patients. Pain, 1993. 54(3): p. 323-7.

507. Paolino, M. and V. Ghulyan-Bedikian, Ménière's disease and tinnitus, in Textbook of Tinnitus, A.R. Møller, et al., Editors. 2010, Springer: New York. p. 477-486.

508. Park, T., Youngchai, Ko, Soo Joo, Lee, Kyung Bok, Lee, Jun, Lee, Moon-Ku, Han, Jong-Moo Park, Yong-Jin Cho, Keun-Sik Hong, Dae-Hyun Kim,g Jae-Kwan Cha, et al, Identifying Target Risk Factors Using Population Attributable Risks of Ischemic Stroke by Age and Sex. J Stroke., 2015. 17(3): p. 302–311.

509. Parnes, L.S. and R.G. Price-Jones, Particle repositioning maneuver for benign paroxysmal positional vertigo. Ann. Otol. Rhinol. Laryngol., 1993. 102: p. 325-331.

510. Passe, E.G., Sympathectomy in relation to Ménière's disease, nerve deafness and tinnitus. A report of 110 cases. Proc. Roy. Soc. Med., 1951. 44: p. 760-772.

511. Paula-Lima, A.C., J. Brito-Moreira, and S.T. Ferreira, Deregulation of excitatory neurotransmission underlying synapse failure in Alzheimer's disease. J Neurochem, 2013. 126(2): p. 191-202.

512. Peacock, W.J., L.J. Arens, and B. Berman, Cerebral palsy spasticity: Selective posterior rhizotomy. Pediatr. Neurosci., 1987. 13: p. 61-66.

513. Penfield, W. and E. Boldrey, Somatic motor and sensory representation in the cerebral cortex of man as studied by electrical stimulation. Brain, 1937. 60: p. 389-443.

514. Pensak, M.L., et al., Sudden hearing loss and cerebellopontine angle tumors. Laryngoscope, 1985. 95(10): p. 1188-93.

515. Perkin, G.D. and R.D. Illingworth, The association of hemifacial spasm and facial pain. J. Neurol. Neurosurg. Psychiatry, 1989. 52: p. 663-665.

516. Petzoldt, A., J. Lützkendorf, and S. Sigrist, Mechanisms controlling assembly and plasticity of presynaptic active zone scaffolds. Curr Opin Neurobiol., 2016. 39: p. 69-76.

517. Phillips, M.L., C. Ladouceur, and W. Drevets, A neural model of voluntary and automatic emotion regulation: implications for understanding the pathophysiology and neurodevelopment of bipolar disorder. Mol Psychiatry, 2008. 13(9): p. 833-57.

518. Pichler, M., et al., Block of P/Q-type calcium channels by therapeutic concentrations of aminoglycoside antibiotics. Biochemistry, 1996. 35: p. 14659-14664.

519. Pierrot-Deseilligny, E., Propriospinal transmission of part of the corticospinal excitation in humans. Muscle & Nerve., 2002. 26(2): p. 155-72.

520. Pillay, P.K. and S.J. Hassenbusch, Bilateral MRI-guided stereotactic cingulotomy for intractable pain. Stereotact. Funct. Neurosurg., 1992. 59(1-4): p. 33-8.

521. Plautz, E.J., et al., Post-infarct cortical plasticity and behavioral recovery using concurrent cortical stimulation and rehabilitative training: A feasibility study in primates. Neurol. Res., 2003. 25: p. 801-810.

522. Plewnia, C., M. Bartels, and C. Gerlof, Transient suppression of tinnitus by transcranial magnetic stimulation. Ann. Neurol., 2003. 53(2): p. 263-266.

523. Podda, G. and C. Constantinescu, Nabiximols in the treatment of spasticity, pain and urinary symptoms due to multiple sclerosis. Expert Opin Biol Ther, 2012. 12(11): p. 1517-31.

524. Podivinsky, F., Torticollis, in Handbook of Clinical Neurology, Diseases of the Basal Ganglia, P.J. Vinken and G.W. Bruyn, Editors. 1968, North Holland Publishing Co: New York. p. 567-603.

525. Porter, R. and R. Lemon, Cortical function and voluntary movement. 1993, Oxford: Clarendon Press.

526. Portmann, G., The saccus endolymphaticus and an operation for draining the same for the relief of vertigo. J. Laryng. Otol., 1927. 42: p. 809.

527. Portmann, M., R. Dauman, and J.M. Aran, Audiometric and electrophysiological correlations in sudden deafness. Acta Otolaryngol, 1985. 99(3-4): p. 363-8.

528. Price, D.D., S. Long, and C. Huitt, Sensory testing of pathophysiological mechanisms of pain in patients with reflex sympathetic dystrophy. Pain, 1992. 49: p. 163-173.

529. Price, D.D., Psychological and neural mechanisms of the affective dimension of pain. Science, 2000. 288: p. 1769-1772.

530. Priuska, E.M. and J. Schacht, Formation of free radical by gentamycin and iron and evidence for an iron/gentamycin complex. Biochem. Pharmacol., 1995. 50: p. 1749-52.

531. Procacci, P., M. Zoppi, and M. Maresca, Heart, vascular and haemopathic pain, in Textbook of Pain, P.D. Wall and R. Melzack, Editors. 1999, Churchill Livingstone: Edinburgh. p. 621-639.

532. Pruitt, D., Schmid, AN, Kim, LJ, Abe, CM, Trieu, JL, Choua, C, Hays, SA, Kilgard, MP, Rennaker, RL., Vagus Nerve Stimulation Delivered with Motor Training Enhances Recovery of Function after Traumatic Brain Injury. J.Neurotrauma, 2016. 33(9): p. 871-9.

533. Pulec, J.L., Early decompression of the facial nerve in Bell's palsy. Ann. Otol. Rhinol.Laryngol., 1981. 90(6): p. 570-7.

534. Pulec, J.L., Total facial nerve decompression: technique to avoid complications. Ear, Nose, & Throat Journal, 1996. 75(7): p. 410-415.

535. Punte, A.K., O. Meeus, and P. Van de Heyning, Cochlear Implants and tinnitus, in Textbook of Tinnitus, A.R. Møller, et al., Editors. 2010, Springer: New York. p. 619-624.

536. Puretic, M.B. and V. Demarin, Neuroplasticity mechanisms in pathophysiology of chronic pain. Acta Clin Croat, 2012. 51(3): p. 425-9.

537. Qian, Y., H. Forssberg, and R. Diaz Heijtz, Motor Skill Learning Is Associated with Phase- Dependent Modifications in the Striatal cAMP/PKA/DARPP-32 Signaling Pathway in Rodents. PLoS One,, 2015.

538. Quasthoff, S. and C. Sommer, Peripheral mechanisms, in Pain in Peripheral Nerve diseases. Pain Headache, C. Sommer, Editor. 2001, Karger: Basel. p. 110-148.

539. Quattrocki, E. and K. Friston, Autism, oxytocin and interoception. Neurosci Biobehav Rev., 2014. 47: p. 410–430.

540. Rahko, T. and V. Kotti, Tinnitus treatment by transcutaneous nerve stimulation (TNS). Acta Otolaryngol. (Stockh), 1997. Suppl 529: p. 88-89.

541. Ralston, D.D. and H.J. Ralston, The termination of the corticospinal tract axons in the macaque monkey. J. Comp. Neurol., 1985. 242: p. 325-337.

542. Ramachandran, V.S., D. Rogers-Ramachandran, and M. Stewart, Perceptual correlates of massive cortical reorganization. [letter; comment]. Science, 1992. 258: p. 1159-60.

543. Ramachandran, V.S., Plasticity and functional recovery in neurology. Clin Med., 2005. 5(4): p. 368-73.

544. Ramachandran, V.S. and E.L. Altschuler, The use of visual feedback, in particular mirror visual feedback, in restoring brain function. Brain, 2009. 132(7)): p. 1693-710.

545. Rand, R.W. and T.L. Kurze, Facial nerve preservation by posterior fossa transmeatal microdissection in total removal of acoustic tumours. J. Neurol. Neurosurg. Psychiat., 1965(28): p. 311-316.

546. Rapkin, A.J., Chronic pelvic pain, in Textbook of pain, P.D. Wall and R. Melzack, Editors. 1999, Churchill Livingstone: Edinburgh. p. 641-659.

547. Rasminsky, M., Ephaptic transmission between single nerve fibers in the spinal nerve roots of dystrophic mice. J. Physiol. (Lond.), 1980. 305: p. 151-169.

548. Rauschecker, J.P., Auditory cortical plasticity: a comparison with other sensory systems. Trends Neurosci., 1999. 22: p. 74-80.

549. Rauschecker, J.P. and S.K. Scott, Maps and streams in the auditory cortex: nonhuman primates illuminate human speech processing. Nat Neurosci., 2009. 12(6): p. 718-24.

550. Reed, G.F., An audiometric study of 200 cases of subjective tinnitus. Arch. Otolaryngol., 1960. 71: p. 94-104.

551. Reisfield, G., M., Medical cannabis and chronic opioid therapy. J Pain Palliat Care Pharmacother. , 2010. 24(4): p. 356-61.

552. Rexed, B.A., Cytoarchitectonic atlas of the spinal cord. J. Comp. Neurol., 1954. 100: p. 297-379.

553. Rey-Dios, R. and A. Cohen-Gadol, Current neurosurgical management of glossopharyngeal neuralgia and technical nuances for microvascular decompression surgery. Neurosurg Focus, 2013. 34(3): p. E8.

554. Rice, A., Cannabinoids and pain. Curr Opin Investig Drugs., 2001. 2(3): p. 399-414.

555. Rice, D. and S.J. Barone, Critical periods of vulnerability for the developing nervous system: evidence from humans and animal models. Environ Health Perspect., 2000. 108 Suppl 3: p. 511-33.

556. Rioult-Pedotti, M.S., et al., Dopamine Promotes Motor Cortex Plasticity and Motor Skill Learning via PLC Activation. PLoS One,, 2015. 10: p. e0124986.

557. Rizzi, M.D. and K. Hirose, Aminoglycoside ototoxicity. Curr Opin Otolaryngol Head Neck Surg., 2007. 15(5): p. 352-7.

558. Roberts, L.E. and D.J. Bosnyak, Auditory Training in Tinnitus, in Textbook of Tinnitus, A.R. Møller, et al., Editors. 2010, Springer: New York. p. 563-574.

559. Robertson, D. and D.R. Irvine, Plasticity of frequency organization in auditory cortex of guinea pigs with partial unilateral deafness. J. Comp. Neurol., 1989. 282(3): p. 456-471.

560. Robertson, D., B.M. Johnstone, and T. McGill, Effects of loud tones on the inner ear: A combined electrophysiological and ultrastructural study. Hear. Res., 1990. 2: p. 39-53.

561. Robillard, R.B., R.L. Hilsinger Jr, and K.K. Adour, Ramsay Hunt facial paralysis: clinical analyses of 185 patients. Otolaryngol Head Neck Surg, 1986. 95(3): p. 292-7.

562. Rocco, A.G., Radiofrequency lumbar sympatholysis. Regional Anesthesia, 1995. 20: p. 3-12.

563. Romanski, L.M., et al., Dual streams of auditory afferents target multiple domains in the primate prefrontal cortex. Nature Neurosci., 1999. 2(12): p. 1131-1136.

564. Rondanelli, M., et al., Update on the role of melatonin in the prevention of cancer tumorigenesis and in the management of cancer correlates, such as sleep-wake and mood disturbances: review and remarks. Aging Clin Exp Res., 2013. 25(5): p. 499–510.

565. Rosas-Ballina, M. and K.J. Tracey, Cholinergic control of inflammation. J Intern Med., 2009. 256(6): p. 663-79.

566. Rosen, J.B., et al., A direct projection from the central nucleus of the amygdala to the acoustic startle pathway: Anterograde and retrograde tracing studies. Behav. Neurosci., 1991. 105: p. 817-25.

567. Rosenkranz, K., A. Kacar, and J.C. Rothwell, Differential modulation of motor cortical plasticity and excitability in early and late phases of human motor learning. J Neurosci, 2007. 27: p. 12058-12066.

568. Rosenow, J.M., et al., Deep brain stimulation for movement disorders. Neurol. Res., 2004. 26: p. 9-20.

569. Rösler, K.M., Transcranial magnetic brain stimulation: a tool to investigate central motor pathways. News Physiol. Sci., 2001. 16: p. 297-302.

570. Ross, B., J. Nedzelski, and A. McLean, Efficacy of feedback training in long-standing facila nerve paresis. Laryngoscope, 2009. 101(7): p. 744-50.

571. Rubel, E. and B. Fritzsch, Auditory system development: primary auditory neurons and their targets. Ann. Rev. Neurosci, 2002. 25: p. 51-101.

572. Rubinstein, J.T., et al., Electrical suppression of tinnitus with high-rate pulse trains. Otology & Neurotology, 2003. 24: p. 478-485.

573. Rudomin, P., Presynaptic control of synaptic effectiveness of muscle spindle and tendon organ afferents in the mammalian spinal cord, in The segmental motor system, M.D. Binder and L.M. Mendell, Editors. 1990, Oxford University Press: Oxford. p. 349-380.

574. Rushworth, G., Some aspects of the pathophysiology of spasticity and rigidity. Clin. Pharmacol. Therapeutics, 1964. 6: p. 828-36.

575. Saito, S. and A.R. Møller, Chronic electrical stimulation of the facial nerve causes signs of facial nucleus hyperactivity. Neurol Res., 1993. 15(4): p. 225-31.

576. Saito, S., et al., Abnormal response from the sternocleidomastoid muscle in patients with spasmodic torticollis: Observations during microvascular decompression operations. Acta Neurochir (Wien), 1993. 124: p. 92-98.

577. Salt, A.N., Regulation of endolymphatic fluid volume. Ann N Y Acad Sci., 2001. 942: p. 306-12.

578. Sandyk, R. and M.A. Gillman, Baclofen in hemifacial spasm. Int. J. Neurosci., 1987. 33: p. 261-4.

579. Sanes, D.H. and E.J. Walsh, Development of central auditory processing, in Development of the auditory system, E.W. Rubel, A.N. Popper, and R.R. Fay, Editors. 1998, Springer: New York. p. 271-314.

580. Sanes, J.N., S. Suner, and J.P. Donoghue, Dynamic organization of primary motor cortex output to target muscles in adult rat. I. Long term patterns of reorganization following motor or mixed peripheral nerve lesions. Exp. Brain Res., 1990. 79: p. 479-491.

581. Sarvey, J.M., E.C. Burgard, and G. Decker, Long-term potentiation: studies in the hippocampal slice. J. Neurosci. Methods, 1989. 28(1-2): p. 109-24.

582. Sathe, S., Migraine and neurogenetic disorders. Curr Pain Headache Rep., 2013. 17(9): p. 360.

583. Scadding, J.W., et al., Clinical trial of propranolol in post-traumatic neuralgia. Pain, 1982: p. 283-92.

584. Scadding, J.W., Peripheral neuropathies, in Textbook of pain, P.D. Wall and R. Melzack, Editors. 1999, Churchill Livingstone: Edinburgh. p. 815-834.

585. Scadding, J.W., Complex regional pain syndrome, in Textbook of pain, P.D. Wall and R. Melzack, Editors. 1999, Churchill Livingstone: Edinburgh. p. 835-849.

586. Schaefer, N., et al., The malleable brain: plasticity of neural circuits and behavior - A review from students to students. J Neurochem. , 2017.

587. Schäfers, M. and C. Sommer, Polyneuropathies, in Pain in Peripheral Nerve diseases. Pain Headache, C. Sommer, Editor. 2001, Karger: Basel. p. 53-108.

588. Schenck, C.H., et al., Prominent eye movements during NREM sleep and REM sleep behavior disorder associated with fuoxetine treatment of depression and obsessive -compulsive disorder. Sleep, 1992. 15(3): p. 226-35.

589. Schenck, C.H., J.L. Boyd, and M.W. Mahowald, A parasomnia overlap disorder involving sleepwalking, sleep terrors, and REM sleep behavior disorder in 33 polysomnographically confirmed cases. Sleep, 1997. 20(11): p. 972-81.

590. Schieppati, M., The Hoffman reflex: a means of assessing spinal reflex excitability and its descending control in man. Prog. Neurobiol., 1987. 28: p. 345-376.

591. Schinder, A.F. and M. Poo, The neurotrophin hypothesis of synaptic plasticity. Trends Neurosci., 2000. 23(12): p. 639-45.

592. Schlee, W., et al., Using auditory steady state responses to outline the functional connectivity in the tinnitus brain. PLoS One, 2008. 3(11).

593. Schlee, W., et al., Mapping cortical hubs in tinnitus. BMC Biol., 2009. 7: p. 80.

594. Schlee, W., et al., A Global Brain Model of Tinnitus, in Textbook of Tinnitus, A.R. Møller, et al., Editors. 2010, Springer: New York. p. 161-170.

595. Schlee, W., et al., Does tinnitus distress depend on age of onset? PLoS One, 2011. 6(11): p. e27379.

596. Schlee, W., et al., Age-related changes in neural functional connectivity and its behavioral relevance. BMC Neurosci., 2012. 13(1).

597. Schlee, W., et al., Development of large-scale functional networks over the lifespan. Neurobiol Aging, 2012. 33(10): p. 2411-21.

598. Schleuning, A.J., Management of the patient with tinnitus. Med. Clin. N. Am., 1991. 75: p. 1225-1237.

599. Schreiner, C.E. and J.A. Winer, Auditory cortex mapmaking: principles, projections, and plasticity. Neuron., 2007. 56(2): p. 356-65.

600. Schwaber, M.K., Neuroplasticity of the adult primate auditory cortex following cochlear hearing loss. Am. J. Otol., 1993. 14(3): p. 252-258.

601. Searchfield, G.D., et al., Counseling and Psycho-education for Tinnitus Management, in Textbook of Tinnitus, A.R. Møller, et al., Editors. 2010, Springer: New York. p. 535-556.

602. Sehgal, N. and J.R. McGuire, Beyond Ashworth: Electrophysiologic quantification of spasticity. Physical Medicine and Rehabilitation Clinics of North America, 1998. 9(4): p. 949-979.

603. Sekhar, L.N. and A.R. Møller, Operative management of tumors involving the cavernous sinus. J. Neurosurg., 1986(64): p. 879-889.

604. Sekiya, T., et al., Vestibular nerve injury as a complication of microvascular decompression. Neurosurgery, 1991(29): p. 773-775.

605. Selemon, L.D., A role of synaptic plasticity in the adolescent development of execute function. Transl. Psychiatry, 2013. 3: p. 238.

606. Seligmann, H., et al., Drug-induced tinnitus and other hearing disorders. Drug Safety, 1996. 14(3): p. 198-212.

607. Seltzer, Z. and M. Devor, Ephaptic transmission in chronically damaged peripheral nerves. Neurology, 1979. 29: p. 1061-1064.

608. Sen, C.N. and A.R. Møller, Signs of hemifacial spasm created by chronic periodic stimulation of the facial nerve in the rat. Exp. Neurol., 1987. 98: p. 336-349.

609. Serhan, C.N., et al., Novel anti-inflammatory--pro-resolving mediators and their receptors. Curr Top Med Chem, 2011. 11(6): p. 629-47.

610. Sessle, B.J., Recent development in pain research: Central mechanism of orofacial pain and its control. J. Endodon., 1986. 12: p. 435-444.

611. Seth, A., Interoceptive inference, emotion, and the embodied sel. Trends Cogn Sci., 2013. 17(11): p. 565-73.

612. Shambaugh, G.E., Surgery of the endolymphatic sac. Arch. Otol., 1966. 83: p. 302.

613. Sharma, A., M.F. Dorman, and A.J. Spahr, Rapid development of cortical auditory evoked potentials after early cochlear implantation. Neuroreport, 2002. 13(10): p. 1365-8.

614. Sharma, A., M.F. Dorman, and A.J. Spahr, A sensitive period for the development of the central auditory system in children with cochlear implants: implications for age of implantation. Ear Hear., 2002. 23(6): p. 532-9.

615. Sharma, A., M.F. Dorman, and A. Kral, The influence of a sensitive period on central auditory development in children with unilateral and bilateral cochlear implants. Hear Res., 2005. 203: p. 134-43.

616. Sharma, A. and M.F. Dorman, Central Auditory Development in Children with Cochlear Implants: Clinical Implications, in Cochlear and Brainstem Implants, A.R. Møller, Editor. 2006, Karger: Basel. p. 66-88.

617. Sharma, A., et al., Deprivation-induced cortical reorganization in children with cochlear implants. Int J Audiol., 2007. 46(9): p. 494-9.

618. Sherriff, F.E. and Z. Henderson, The paragigantocellular nucleus of the ventral medulla: a secondary source of cholinergic innervation of rat brainstem nuclei. Brain Res., 1994. 636: p. 119-25.

619. Shore, S., J. Zhou, and S. Koehler, Neural mechanisms underlying somatic tinnitus, in Tinnitus: Pathophysiology and Treatment, Progress in Brain Research, B. Langguth, et al., Editors. 2007, Elsevier: Amsterdam. p. 107-123.

620. Shore, S.E., et al., Connections between the cochlear nuclei in guinea pig. Hear. Res., 1992. 62(1): p. 16-26.

621. Shore, S.E., et al., Trigeminal ganglion innervates the auditory brainstem. J Comp. Neurol., 2000. 419(3): p. 271-285.

622. Shulman, A., J. Tonndorf, and B. Goldstein, Electrical tinnitus control. Acta Otolaryngol., 1985. 99(3-4): p. 318-25.

623. Sie, K.C.Y. and E.W. Rubel, Rapid Changes in Protein Synthesis and Cell Size in the Cochlear Nucleus following Eighth Nerve Activity Blockade and Cochlea Ablation. J. Comp. Neurol., 1992. 320: p. 501-508.

624. Silberstein, S. and R. Lipton, Epidemiology of Migraine. Neuroepidemiology, 1993. 12: p. 179–194.

625. Silverstein, H., et al., Conservative management of acoustic neuroma in the elderly patients. Laryngoscope, 1985. 95: p. 766-70.

626. Silverstein, H., et al., The unrecognized rotation of the vestibular and cochlear nerves from the labyrinth to the brain stem: Its implications to surgery of the eighth cranial nerve. Otolaryngol. Head Neck Surg., 1986. 95: p. 543-549.

627. Silverstein, H., et al., Direct round window membrane application of gentamicin in the treatment of Ménière's disease. Otolaryngol. Head & Neck Surg., 1999. 120(5): p. 649-55.

628. Simone, D.A., et al., Neurogenic hyperalgesia: central neural correlates in responses of spinothalamic tract neurons. J. Neurophys., 1991. 66: p. 228-246.

629. Simons, D.G. and S. Mense, Understanding and measurement of muscle tone as related to clinical muscle pain. Pain, 1998. 75(1): p. 1-17.

630. Simopoulos, A., Omega-3 fatty acids in health and disease and in growth and development. Am J Clin Nutr, 1991. 54(3): p. 438-63.

631. Simpson, J.J. and E. Davies, Recent advances in the pharmacological treatment of tinnitus. Trends Pharmacol. Sci., 1999. 20: p. 12-18.

632. Sindou, M. and D. Jeanmonod, Microsurgical-DREZ-otomy for treatment of spasticity and pain in the lower limbs. Neurosurgery, 1989. 24: p. 655-670.

633. Sindou, M. and P. Mertens, Microvascular decompression (MVD) in trigeminal and glosso-vago-pharyngeal neuralgias. A twenty year experience. Acta Neurochir. (Wien), 1993. 58: p. 168-170.

634. Sindou, M. and P. Mertens, Selective spinal cord procedures for spasticity and pain, in Neurophysiology in Neurosurgery, V. Deletis and J.L. Shils, Editors. 2002, Academic Press: Amsterdam. p. 93-117.

635. Sindrup, S.H. and T.S. Jensen, Efficacy of pharmacological treatments of neuropathic pain: an update and effect related to mechanism of drug action. Pain, 1999. 83: p. 389-400.

636. Sipski, M.L., C.J. Alexander, and R.R. Rosen, Sexual arousal and orgasm in women: Effects of spinal cord injury. Ann. Neurol., 2001. 49(1): p. 35-44.

637. Sloan, T., Anesthesia and motor evoked potential monitoring, in Neurophysiology in Neurosurgery, V. Deletis and J.L. Shils, Editors. 2002, Elsevier Science: Amsterdam. p. 451-474.

638. Smith, P.F., The Endocannabinoid System In The Cochlear Nucleus And Its Implications For Tinnitus Treatment, in Textbook of Tinnitus, A.R. Møller, et al., Editors. 2010, Springer: New York. p. 639-648.

639. Sola, A.E., Upper extremity pain, in Handbook of Pain, P.D. Wall and R. Melzack, Editors. 1999, Churchill Livingstone: Edinburgh. p. 559-578.

640. Sommer, C. and F. Birklein, Resolvins and inflammatory pain. F1000 Med Rep. , 2011. 3: p. 19.

641. Song, B.B., S.H. Sha, and J. Schacht, Iron chelators protect from aminoglycoside-induced cochleo- and vestibulotoxitity in guinea pig. Free Rad. Biol. Med., 1998. 25: p. 189-195.

642. Song, J., et al., Distressed aging: the differences in brain activity between early- and late-onset tinnitus. Neurobiol Aging, 2013. 34(7): p. 1853-63.

643. Sorensen, J., et al., Fibromyalgia - are there different mechanisms in the processing of pain? A double blind crossover comparison of analgesic drugs. J. Rheumatololgy, 1997. 24: p. 1615-1621.

644. Soros, P., et al., Phantom eye syndrome: Its prevalence, phenomenology, and putative mechanisms. Neurology, 2003. 60(9): p. 1542-3.

645. Spencer, R.F., et al., Changes in calcium-binding protein expression in the auditory brainstem nuclei of the jaundiced Gunn rat. Hear. Res., 2002. 171: p. 129-141.

646. Spoendlin, H., Structural basis of peripheral frequency analysis, in Frequency analysis and periodicity detection in Hearing, R. Plomp and G.F. Smoorenburg, Editors. 1970, A. W. Sijthoff: Leiden. p. 2-36.

647. Spoendlin, H., Anatomical changes following noise exposure, in Effects of Noise on Hearing, D. Henderson, et al., Editors. 1976, Raven Press: New York.

648. Spoendlin, H. and A. Schrott, Analysis of the human auditory nerve. Hear. Res., 1989. 43: p. 25-38.

649. Spoor, A., Presbycusis values in relation to noise induced hearing loss. Int. Audiol., 1967. 6: p. 48-57.

650. Stein, R., Letter to the Editor. Paraplegia, 1991. 29: p. 495-497.

651. Sterr, A., et al., Perceptual correlates of changes in cortical representation of fingers in blind multifinger Braille readers. J. Neurosci., 1998. 18(11): p. 4417-23.

652. Sugimoto, T., G.J. Bennett, and K.C. Kajander, Transsynaptic degeneration in the superficial dorsal horn after sciatic nerve injury: effects of chronic constriction injury, transection, and strychnine. 42, 1990: p. 205-213.

653. Sun, F., et al., Functional connectivity of cortical networks involved in bimanual motor sequence learning. Cereb Cortex, 2007. 17: p. 1227-1234.

654. Sunderland, S., Microvascular relations and anomalies at the base of the brain. J. Neurol. Neurosurg. Psychiatry, 1948. 11: p. 243-257.

655. Sunderland, S., A classification of peripheral nerve injuries producing loss of function. Brain, 1951. 74: p. 491-516.

656. Sunderland, S., Cranial nerve injury. Structural and pathophysiological considerations and a classification of nerve injury, in The Cranial Nerves, M. Samii and P.J. Jannetta, Editors. 1981, Springer-Verlag;: Heidelberg, Germany. p. 16-26.

657. Surén, P., et al., Association Between Maternal Use of Folic Acid Supplements and Risk of Autism Spectrum Disorders in Children. JAMA, 2013. 309(6): p. 570-577.

658. Sutton, M.A. and E.M. Schuman, Dendritic protein synthesis, synaptic plasticity, and memory. Cell, 2006. 127: p. 49-58.

659. Sweet, W.H., Deafferentation pain after posterior rhizotomy, trauma to a limb, and herpes zoster. Neurosurgery, 1984. 15(6): p. 928-32.

660. Sweet, W.H., Percutaneous methods for the treatment of trigeminal neuralgia and other faciocephalic pain: Comparison with microvascular decompression. Semin. Neurol., 1988. 8: p. 272-279.

661. Syka, J., N. Rybalko, and J. Popelar, Enhancement of the Auditory Cortex Evoked Responses in Awake Guinea Pigs After Noise Exposure. Hear. Res., 1994. 78: p. 158-168.

662. Syka, J., J. Popelar, and E. Kvasnak, Response properties of neurons in the central nucleus and external and dorsal cortices of the inferior colliculus in guinea pig. Exp. Brain Res., 2000. 133: p. 254-266.

663. Syka, J., Plastic changes in the central auditory system after hearing loss, restoration of function, and during learning. Physiol Rev, 2002. 82(3): p. 601-36.

664. Szczepaniak, W.S. and A.R. Møller, Interaction between auditory and somatosensory systems: A study of evoked potentials in the inferior colliculus. Electroencephologr. Clin. Neurophysiol., 1993. 88: p. 508-515.

665. Szczepaniak, W.S. and A.R. Møller, Effects of (-)-baclofen, clonazepam, and diazepam on tone exposure-induced hyperexcitability of the inferior colliculus in the rat: possible therapeutic implications for pharmacological management of tinnitus and hyperacusis. Hear. Res., 1996. 97: p. 46-53.

666. Szczepaniak, W.S. and A.R. Møller, Evidence of neuronal plasticity within the inferior colliculus after noise exposure: A study of evoked potentials in the rat. Electroenceph. Clin. Neurophysiol., 1996. 100: p. 158-164.

667. Tabbaa, M., Paedae, B, Liu, Y, Wang, Z, Neuropeptide Regulation of Social Attachment: The Prairie Vole Model. Compr Physiol. , 2016: p. 81-104.

668. Tanimoto, T., M. Takeda, and S.S. Matsumoto, Suppressive effect of vagal afferents on cervical dorsal horn neurons responding to tooth pulp electrical stimulation in the rat. Experimental Brain Research, 2002. 145(4): p. 468-79.

669. Tasker, R.R., Reflex sympathetic dystrophy - neurosurgical approaches, in Reflex sympathetic dystrophy, M. Stanton-Hicks, W. Jänig, and R.A. Roas, Editors. 1990, Kluwer Academic: MA. p. 125-34.

670. Taub, E., G. Uswatte, and T. Elbert, New treatments in neurorehabilitation founded on basic research. Nature Rev. Neurosci., 2002. 3(3): p. 228-36.

671. Tetzlaff, W., M.B. Graeber, and G.W. Kreutzberg, Reaction on motoneurons and their microenvironment to axotomy. Exp Brain Res, 1986. 3(Suppl,13): p. 3-8.

672. Thayer, J.F. and E.M. Sternber, Neural aspects of immunomodulation: Focus on the vagus nerve. Brain Behav Immun., 2010. 24(8): p. 1223–1228.

673. Thompson, S.W.N., A.E. King, and C.J. Woolf, Activity-Dependent Changes in Rat Ventral Horn Neurons in vitro; Summation of Prolonged Afferent Evoked Postsynaptic Depolarizations Produce a d-2-Amino-5-Phosphonovaleric Acid Sensitive Windup. Eur. J. Neurosci., 1990. 2: p. 638-649.

674. Tolosa, E.S. and J. Pena, Involuntary vocalizations in movement disorders. Adv. Neurol., 1988. 49: p. 343-363.

675. Tomimatsu, Y., et al., Proteases involved in long-term potentiation. Life Sci., 2002. 72(4-5): p. 355-61.

676. Topka, H., et al., Reorganization of corticospinal pathways following spinal cord injury. Neurology, 1991. 41(8): p. 1276-1283.

677. Towle, V.L., et al., ECoG Gamma Activity: Differentiating expressive and receptive speech areas. Brain, 2008. 131: p. 2013-27.

678. Tracey, K., Physiology and immunology of the cholinergic antiinflammatory pathway. Journal of Clinical Investigation, 2007. 117(2): p. 289–96.

679. Travell, J. and D.G. Simons, Myofascial pain and dysfunction, the trigger point manual. 1983, New York: Williams and Wilkins.

680. Tsubokawa, T., et al., Chronic motor cortex stimulation for the treatment of central pain. Acta Neurochir Suppl (Wien), 1991. 52: p. 137-9.

681. Turner, J.G. and J.F. Willott, Exposure to an augmented acoustic environment alters auditory function in hearing-impaired DBA/2J mice. Hear. Res., 1998. 118: p. 101-113.

682. Ulloa, L., The vagus nerve and the nicotinic anti-inflammatory pathway. Nat Rev Drug Discov, 2005. 4(8): p. 673-84.

683. Ungerleider, L.G. and J.V. Haxby, "What" and "Where" in the human brain. Curr. Opin. Neurobiol., 1994. 4: p. 157-165.

684. Vandenheede, M. and J. Schoenen, Central mechanisms in tension-type headaches. Curr. Pain Headache Rep., 2002. 6(5): p. 392 400.

685. VanSwearingen, J. and J. Brach, Changes in facial movement and synkinesis with facial neuromuscular reeducation. Plast Reconstr Surg, 2003. 111(7): p. 2370-5.

686. Vasama, J.P., M.B. Møller, and A.R. Møller, Microvascular decompression of the cochlear nerve in patients with severe tinnitus. Preoperative findings and operative outcome in 22 patients. Neurol. Res., 1998. 20: p. 242-248.

687. Vernon, J., The loudness of tinnitus. Hear Speech Action, 1976. 44: p. 17-19.

688. Vernon, J.A. and M.B. Meikle, Masking devices and alprazolam treatment for tinnitus. Otolaryngol Clin North Am., 2003. 36(2): p. 307-20.

689. Vitek, J.L., et al., Microelectrode-guided pallidotomy: Technical approach and application for treatment of medically intractable Parkinson's disease. J. Neurosurg., 1998. 88: p. 1027-43.

690. Vitek, J.L., et al., Neuronal activity in the basal ganglia in patients with generalized dystonia and hemiballismus. Ann. Neurol., 1999. 46(1): p. 22-35.

691. Vitureira, N. and Y. Goda, Cell biology in neuroscience: the interplay between Hebbian and homeostatic synaptic plasticity. J Cell Biol., 2013. 203(2): p. 175-86.

692. Voscopoulos, C. and M. Lema, When does acute pain become chronic? Br J Anaesth, 2010. Suppl 1: p. 69-85.

693. Wada, J.A., Kindling 2. 1981, New York: Raven Press.

694. Wahlig, J.B., et al., Intraoperative loss of auditory function relieved by microvascular decompression of the cochlear nerve. Can J Neurol Sci., 1999. 26(1): p. 44-7.

695. Wall, J.T., et al., Functional reorganization in somatosensory cortical areas 3b and 1 of adult monkeys after median nerve repair: possible relationships to sensory recovery in humans. J. Neurosci., 1986. 6(1): p. 218-233.

696. Wall, J.T., J. Xu, and X. Wang, Human brain plasticity: an emerging view of the multiple substrates and mechanisms that cause cortical changes and related sensory dysfunctions after injuries of sensory inputs from the body. Brain Res. Rev., 2002. 39(2-3): p. 181-215.

697. Wall, P.D., The presence of ineffective synapses and circumstances which unmask them. Phil. Trans. Royal Soc. (Lond.), 1977. 278: p. 361-372.

698. Wall, P.D. and M. Devor, Sensory afferent impulses originate from dorsal root ganglia as well as from periphery in normal and nerve injured rats. Pain, 1983. 17: p. 321-339.

699. Walsh, E.G., Muscles, Masses and Motion: The Physiology of Normality, Hypotonicity, Spasticity and Rigidity. 1992, Oxford: Blackwell.

700. Walton, K.D. and R.R. Llinás, Central Pain as a Thalamocortical Dysrhythmia. A Thalamic Efference Disconnection?, in Translational Pain Research: From Mouse to Man, L. Kruger and A.R. Light, Editors. 2010, CRC Press: Boca Raton, FL.

701. Wang, J., et al., Gamma-aminobutyric acid circuits shape response properties of audiory cortex neurons. Brain Res., 2002. 944(219-31).

702. Warr, W.B., Organization of olivocochlear systems in mammals, in The mammalian auditory pathway: Neuroanatomy, D.B. Webster, A.N. Popper, and R.R. Fay, Editors. 1992, Springer-Verlag: New York.

703. Warren, E.H. and M.C. Liberman, Effects of contralateral sound on auditory-nerve responses. I. Contributions of cochlear efferents. Hear. Res., 1989. 37: p. 89-104.

704. Warrick, J.W., Stellate ganglion block in the treatment of Ménière's disease and in the symptomatic relief of tinnitus. Br. J. Otol., 1969. 41: p. 699-702.

705. Weber, H., The natural history of disc herniation and the influence of intervention. Spine, 1994. 19: p. 2234-2238.

706. Weinberg, R.J. and A. Rustioni, A cuneocochlear pathway in the rat. Neuroscience, 1987. 20: p. 209-219.

707. Weiss, T., et al., Rapid functional plasticity of the somatosensory cortex after finger amputation. Exp. Brain Res., 2000. 134(2): p. 199-203.

708. Weisz, N., et al., Tinnitus perception and distress is related to abnormal spontaneous brain activity as measured by magnetoencephalography. PLoS Med, 2005. 2(6): p. e153.

709. Whipple, B. and B.R. Komisaruk, Brain (PET) responses to vaginal-cervical self-stimulation in women with complete spinal cord injury: preliminary findings. J. Sex & Marital Therapy, 2002. 28(1): p. 79-86.

710. Whitaker, S., Idiopathic sudden hearing loss. Am. J. Otol., 1980. 1: p. 180-3.

711. White, J.C. and W.H. Sweet, Facial and cephalic neuralgias: Trigeminal neuralgia, in Pain. 1955, Charles C. Thomas. p. 433-493.

712. White, S.R. and R.S. Neuman, Facilitation of spinal motoneuron by 5-hydroxytryptamine and noradrenaline. Brain Res., 1980. 185: p. 1-9.

713. Whurr, R., et al., The use of botulinum toxin in the treatment of adductor dysphonia. J. Neurol. Neurosurg. Psych., 1993. 56: p. 526-530.

714. Wiesel, T.N. and D.H. Hubel, Effects of visual deprivation on morphology and physiology of cells in the cats lateral geniculate body. J. Neurophysiol., 1963. 26: p. 973-93.

715. Wiesel, T.N. and D.H. Hubel, Extent of recovery from the effects of visual deprivation in kittens. J. Neurophysiol., 1965. 28: p. 1060-1072.

716. Wiesel, T.N. and D.H. Hubel, Comparison of the effects of unilateral and bilateral eye closure on cortical unit responses in kittens. J. Neurophysiol., 1965. 28(6): p. 1029-40.

717. Wiesendanger, M., The pyramidal tract. its structure and function., in Handbook of behavioral neurobiology, A.L. Towe and E.S. Luschei, Editors. 1981, Plenum: New York. p. 401-490.

718. Willer, J., Relieving effect of TENS on painful muscle contraction produced by an impairment of reciprocal innervation: an electrophysiological analysis. Pain, 1988. 32(3): p. 271-4.

719. Willott, J.F. and S.M. Lu, Noise induced hearing loss can alter neural coding and increase excitability in the central nervous system. Science, 1981. 16: p. 1331-1332.

720. Willott, J.F., Neurogerontology. 1999, New York: Springer Publishing Company.

721. Willott, J.F., J.G. Turner, and V.S. Sundin, Effects of exposure to an augmented acoustic environment on auditory function in mice: roles of hearing loss and age during treatment. Hear. Res., 2000. 142: p. 79–88.

722. Willott, J.F., T.H. Chisolm, and J.J. Lister, Modulation of presbycusis: current status and future directions. Audiol. Neurotol., 2001. 6: p. 231-249.

723. Wilsey, B., et al., Low-dose vaporized cannabis significantly improves neuropathic pain. J Pain., 2012. 14(2): p. 136-48.

724. Winer, J.A., et al., Auditory cortical projections to the cat inferior colliculus. J. Comp. Neurol., 1998. 400(2): p. 147-74.

725. Wise, L.Z. and D.R.F. Irvine, Auditory response properties of neurons in deep layers of cat superior colliculus. J. Neurophysiol., 1983. 49: p. 674-685.

726. Wladislavorsky-Wasserman, P., et al., Ménière's Disease: A 30 year epidemiologic and clinical study in Rochester, MN, 1951-1980. Laryngoscope, 1984. 94: p. 1098-1102.

727. Wolpaw, J.R. and J.A. O'Keefe, Adaptive plasticity in the primate spinal stretch reflex: Evidence of a two-phase process. J. Neuro. Sci., 1984. 4: p. 2718-24.

728. Wolpaw, J.R., Acquisition and maintenance of the simplest motor skill: investigation of CNS mechanisms. Med. Sci. Sports Exerc., 1994. 26(12): p. 1475-9.

729. Woolf, C.J. and S.W.N. Thompson, The induction and maintenance of central sensitization is dependent on N-methyl-D-aspartic acid receptor activation: Implications for the treatment of post-injury pain hypersensitivity states. Pain, 1991. 44: p. 293-299.

730. Woolf, C.J., P. Shortland, and R.E. Cogershall, Peripheral nerve injury triggers central sprouting of myelinated afferents. Nature, 1992. 355: p. 75-78.

731. Woolf, C.J. and M.W. Salter, Neural plasticity: Increasing the gain in pain. Science, 2000. 288: p. 1765-1768.

732. Wu, W.J., et al., Aminoglycoside ototoxicity in adult CBA, C57BL and BALB mice and the Sprague-Dawley rat. Hear. Res., 2001. 158: p. 165-178.

733. Wu, W.J., S.H. Sha, and J. Schacht, Recent advances in understanding aminoglycoside ototoxicity and its prevention. Audiol. Neurootol., 2002. 7(171-4).

734. Xenellis, J.E. and F.H. Linthicum, On the myth of the glial/schwann junction (Obersteiner-Redlich zone): Origin of vestibular nerve schwannomas. Otol. Neurotol., 2003. 24(1): p. 1.

735. Yakhnitsa, V., B. Linderoth, and B.A. Meyerson, Spinal cord stimulation attenuates dorsal horn hyperexcitability in a rat model of mononeuropathy. Pain, 1999. 79: p. 223-233.

736. Yaksh, T.L., Preclinical models of nociception, in Anesthesia: biological functions, T.L. Yaksh, et al., Editors. 1997, Lippincott-Raven Publishers: Philadelphia.

737. Yaksh, T.L., Central pharmacology of nociceptive transmission, in Textbook of pain, P.D. Wall and R. Melzack, Editors. 1999, Churchill Livingstone: Edinburgh. p. 253-308.

738. Yan, J., et al., Sensitization of dural afferents underlies migraine-related behavior following meningeal application of interleukin-6 (IL-6). Mol Pain., 2012. 8(6).

739. Yang, Y.a.C., N. (2013) Presynaptic long-term plasticity. Front Synaptic Neurosci, 5, 8., Presynaptic long-term plasticity. Front Synaptic Neurosci,, 2013. 5: p. 8.

740. Yeh, H.S.H. and J.M. Tew, Tic convulsif, the combination of geniculate neuralgia and hemifacial spasm relieved by vascular decompression. Neurology, 1984. 34: p. 682-683.

741. Yger, P. and M. Gilson, Models of Metaplasticity: A Review of Concepts. Front Comput Neurosci., 2015. 10(9): p. 138.

742. Yoshida, M., A. Rabin, and A. Anderson, Monosynaptic inhibition of pallidal neurons by axon collaterals of caudatonigral fibers. Exp. Brain Res, 1972. 15: p. 33-347.

743. Yoshida, N. and M.C. Liberman, Sound conditioning reduces noise-induced permanent threshold shift in mice. Hear. Res., 2000. 148: p. 213-219.

744. Young, R.F., et al., Technique of stereotactic medical thalamotomy with the Leksell gamma knife for treatment of chronic pain. Neurol. Res., 1995. 17(1): p. 59-65.

745. Youngs, R., H. Ludman, and S. Smith, Transtympanic surgery for hemifacial spasm. Clin Otolaryngol, 1988(13): p. 331-333.

746. Yrjänheikki, J., et al., A tetracycline derivative, minocycline, reduces inflammation and protects against focal cerebral ischemia with a wide therapeutic window. Proc Natl Acad Sci U S A., 1999. 96(23): p. 13496-500.

747. Yu, H. and J. Neimat, The treatment of movement disorders by deep brain stimulation. Neurotherapeutics, 2008. 5(1): p. 26-36.

748. Zakrzewska, J., et al., Safety and efficacy of a Nav1.7 selective sodium channel blocker in trigeminal neuralgia: a double-blind, placebo-controlled, randomised withdrawal phase 2a trial. . The Lancet Neurology, 2017.

749. Zhou, J. and S. Shore, Projections from the trigeminal nuclear complex to the cochlear nuclei: a retrograde and anterograde tracing study in the guinea pig. J. Neurosci. Res., 2004. 78(6): p. 901-907.

750. Zhou, J. and S. Shore, Convergence of spinal trigeminal and cochlear nucleus projections in the inferior colliculus of the guinea pig. J Comp Neurol., 2006. 495(1): p. 100-12.

751. Zittermann, A., The estimated benefits of vitamin D for Germany. Mol Nutr Food Res., 2010. 54(8): p. 1164-71.

752. Zochodne, D.W., Epineurial peptides: a role in neuropathic pain? Canadian. J. Neurol Sci., 1993. 20(1): p. 69-72.

www.ingramcontent.com/pod-product-compliance
Lightning Source LLC
Chambersburg PA
CBHW081719220526
45468CB00008B/1900